THE CLINICIAN'S GUIDE TO
Acid/Peptic Disorders and Motility Disorders of the Gastrointestinal Tract

The Clinician's Guide to
Acid/Peptic Disorders and Motility Disorders of the Gastrointestinal Tract

Henry P. Parkman, MD
Gastroenterology Section
Department of Medicine
Temple University Hospital
Philadelphia, Pa

Robert S. Fisher, MD
Chief, Gastroenterology Section
Department of Medicine
Temple University Hospital
Philadelphia, Pa

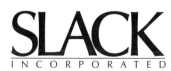

SLACK
INCORPORATED

Delivering the best in health care information and education worldwide

www.slackbooks.com

ISBN-10: 1-55642-716-6
ISBN-13: 978-1-55642-716-9

SLACK Incorporated uses a review process to evaluate submitted material. Prior to publication, educators or clinicians provide important feedback on the content that we publish. We welcome feedback on this work.

Published by: SLACK Incorporated
                     6900 Grove Road
                     Thorofare, NJ 08086 USA
                     Telephone: 856-848-1000
                     Fax: 856-853-5991
                     www.slackbooks.com

Contact SLACK Incorporated for more information about other books in this field or about the availability of our books from distributors outside the United States.

Library of Congress Cataloging-in-Publication Data
The clinician's guide to acid/peptic disorders and motility disorders of
  the gastrointestinal tract / edited by Henry Parkman and Robert S.
  Fisher.
    p. ; cm.
  Includes bibliographical references and index.
  ISBN-13: 978-1-55642-716-9 (alk. paper)
  ISBN-10: 1-55642-716-6 (alk. paper)
  1. Gastrointestinal system--Diseases. 2. Gastrointestinal system
--Motility. 3. Gastroesophageal reflux.   I. Parkman, Henry.
II. Fisher, Robert S. (Robert Stephen)
  [DNLM: 1. Gastrointestinal Diseases. 2. Gastroesophageal Reflux.
WI 140 C6409 2006]
RC817.C65 2006
616.3'3--dc22

WI
140
C6409
2006

                              2006007041

Printed in the United States of America.
Last digit is print number: 10   9   8   7   6   5   4   3   2   1

Contents

Acknowledgments

The editors wish to thank the authors, who took time away from their busy schedules to contribute concise, contemporary, and well-written chapters for this book. We also wish to acknowledge our colleagues, fellows, nurses, and clerical and administrative staffs at the Temple University Gastroenterology Section and Digestive Disease Center for their commitment to excellence in clinical care, medical education, and research.

About the Authors

Henry P. Parkman is Professor of Medicine in the Gastroenterology Section of the Department of Medicine at Temple University School of Medicine, Philadelphia, Pa. Dr. Parkman's gastroenterology training began with a gastrointestinal (GI) fellowship at the University of Pennsylvania. His research investigated the inhibitory neural circuitry of the lower esophageal sphincter (LES), the barrier preventing gastroesophageal reflux. At the University of Pennsylvania, he also compared the clinical outcomes and costs of pneumatic dilation and surgical esophagomyotomy for treatment of patients with achalasia, a disorder involving abnormal LES neural control. Dr. Parkman extended his research training with an NIH research training fellowship in the Department of Physiology at Mayo Clinic where he studied the neural reflexes governed by the inferior mesenteric ganglion.

Since joining the faculty of Temple University School of Medicine in 1990, Dr. Parkman has been actively involved in studying GI motility at both the basic science and clinical levels. His basic research has focused on gaining greater insights into excitation-contraction mechanisms for gastric and gallbladder muscle.

Dr. Parkman is Director of the Clinical GI Motility Laboratory at Temple University Hospital. He has developed expertise in a comprehensive array of GI motility tests for clinical evaluation of patients, including specialized tests of gastric motility. His clinical research studies have focused primarily on esophageal and gastric motility in normal individuals and on clinical motility disorders of the esophagus and stomach, primarily achalasia and gastroparesis. He is funded with an NIH K24 Midcareer Investigator Award in Patient-Oriented Research Award entitled "Novel Evaluation & Treatment of Gastric Dysmotility." This grant allows him the time to perform research and mentor others.

Dr. Parkman holds several positions for Temple University, the School of Medicine, and the Department of Medicine, including Director of the Clinical Research Center, Medical Director of the Office of Clinical Research, Vice Chair of the Research Committee for the Department of Medicine, and Chair of the IRB Adverse Events Committee.

Dr. Parkman has been on the Council of the American Motility Society (AMS) for the last 6 years and has been President of the AMS for the last 2 years. The AMS is the national GI motility organization that seeks to foster excellence in research and medical practice in neurogastroenterology and GI motility. Dr. Parkman has been co-director of the highly successful biennial AMS Clinical Motility Courses.

Robert S. Fisher is Professor of Medicine and Chief of the Gastroenterology Section and Digestive Disease Center at Temple University School of Medicine. Dr. Fisher obtained an undergraduate degree in Engineering from Princeton University. He attended medical school at the University of Pennsylvania School of Medicine following which he completed a straight medical internship at the Chicago Wesley Memorial Hospital of Northwestern University Medical School.

Dr. Fisher spent a year studying medical applications of LASER energy at the United States Army Medical Research Laboratories in Fort Knox, Ken before serving 1 year in South Vietnam where he was awarded a Vietnamese Honor Medal by the South Vietnamese government and a Bronze Star by the U.S. Army. Dr. Fisher then completed a medical residency and chief residency at Temple University Hospital under the tutelage of Dr. Sol Sherry. He obtained training in gastroenterology at the Hospital of the University of Pennsylvania before returning to the Temple University School of Medicine in 1972. Dr. Fisher has been Chief of the Gastroenterology Section at Temple for 21 years.

Dr. Fisher's research has spanned the GI tract. Early in his career, he published a series of studies defining the physiology of the pyloric sphincter and its abnormality in patients with gastric ulcer disease. This was followed by the development of a number of scintigraphic techniques to quantitate aboral and retrograde movement of luminal contents through the gastrointestinal tract. The techniques included esophageal transit, gastroesophageal reflux, gastric emptying, enterogastric reflux, small bowel transit, and colonic transit, as well as whole gut scintigraphy. Dr. Fisher was the first investigator to demonstrate decreased gallbladder emptying as a pathogenetic factor in the pathogenesis of cholesterol gallstones. This observation was followed by a series of studies on the physiology of gallbladder motility.

In more recent years, Dr. Fisher has focused on the distribution of acid in the upper gastrointestinal tract as it relates to gastroesophageal reflux disease and Barrett's esophagus. Years ago, he opened the first multidisciplinary Functional Gastrointestinal Disease Center in the country. During his tenure, Dr. Fisher's research has been funded by the NIH as well as a host of pharmaceutical companies.

Dr. Fisher has published more than 130 peer-reviewed articles, 130 invited chapters or reviews, and more than 150 abstracts.

Contributing Authors

Paul J. Bandini Jr, MD
Assistant Professor of Medicine
Gastroenterology Section
Temple University School of Medicine
Philadelphia, Pa

Dilip Bearelly, MD
Internal Medicine Resident
Temple University Hospital
Philadelphia, Pa

Donald O. Castell, MD
Division of Gastroenterology and
Hepatology
Medical University of South Carolina
Charleston, SC

Daniel T. Dempsey, MD, FACS
Professor and Chairman
Department of Surgery
Temple University School of Medicine
Philadelphia, Pa

Nikhil Deshpande, MD
Fellow in Gastroenterology
Temple University Hospital
Philadelphia, Pa

Ram Dickman, MD
The Neuro-Enteric Clinical Research
Group
Research Fellow
Southern Arizona VA Health Care
System
University of Arizona Health Sciences
Center
Tucson, Ariz

Ronnie Fass, MD, FACP, FACG
Head, the Neuro-Enteric Clinical
Research Group
Professor of Medicine
University of Arizona
Director, GI Motility Laboratory at
Southern Arizona VA Health Care
System
Tucson, Ariz

Frank K. Friedenberg, MD
Associate Professor of Medicine
Gastroenterology Section
Temple University School of Medicine
Philadelphia, Pa

William L. Hasler, MD
Gastroenterology Section
University of Michigan Medical Center
Ann Arbor, Mich

Brenda J. Horwitz, MD
Assistant Professor of Medicine
Section of Gastroenterology
Temple University School of Medicine
Philadelphia, Pa

David A. Katzka, MD
Hospital of the University of
Pennsylvania
Gastroenterology Section
Philadelphia, Pa

Annapurna Korimilli, MD
Fellow in Gastroenterology
Temple University Hospital
Philadelphia, Pa

Benjamin Krevsky, MD, MPH
Professor of Medicine
Gastroenterology Section
Temple University School of Medicine
Philadelphia, Pa

Alex S. Kuryan, MD
West Chester Gastrointestinal Associates
West Chester, Pa

Mark Lee, BS
Consultant in GI Research
Temple University School of Medicine
Philadelphia, Pa

John G. Lieb II, MD
Fellow in Gastroenterology
University of Florida
Gainesville, Fla

Harvey Licht, MD
Associate Professor of Medicine
Gastroenterology Section
Temple University School of Medicine
Philadelphia, Pa

Henry C. Lin, MD
Division of Gastrointestinal and Liver
Diseases
Department of Medicine
Keck School of Medicine
University of Southern California
Los Angeles, Calif

Robert C. Lowe, MD
Assistant Professor of Medicine
Director of Education
Boston University School of Medicine
and Boston Medical Center
Boston, Mass

Kathleen Lukaszewski, DO
Gastroenterology Fellow
Temple University Hospital
Philadelphia, Pa

Larry S. Miller, MD
Professor of Medicine
Gastroenterology Section
Temple University School of Medicine
Philadelphia, Pa

Ann Ouyang, MB, BS
Professor of Medicine
Milton S. Hershey Medical Center
College of Medicine
Pennsylvania State University
Hershey, Pa

Kashyap V. Panganamamula, MD
Clinical Instructor of Medicine
Gastroenterology Section
Temple University School of Medicine
Philadelphia, Pa

Marianne T. Ritchie, MD
Assistant Professor of Medicine
Gastroenterology Section
Temple University School of Medicine
Philadelphia, Pa

Joel E. Richter, MD
Professor and Chairman
Department of Medicine
Temple University School of Medicine
Philadelphia, Pa

Ian Roy Schreibman, MD
Milton S. Hershey Medical Center
College of Medicine
Pennsylvania State University
Hershey, Pa

Rupa N. Shah, MD
Gastroenterology Fellow
Temple University Hospital
Philadelphia, Pa
Private Practice
Tuscon, Ariz

Jonathan T. Simon, MD
Section of Gastroenterology
Boston University School of Medicine
Boston Medical Center
Boston, Mass

Kevin S. Skole, MD
Gastroenterology Fellow
Temple University Hospital
Philadelphia, Pa

Stuart J. Spechler, MD
Professor of Medicine
University of Texas Southwestern School
of Medicine
Dallas Veterans Affairs Medical Center
Division of Gastroenterology
Dallas, Tex

Radu Tutuian, MD
Division of Gastroenterology and Hepatology
Medical University of South Carolina
Charleston, SC

Gregg W. Van Citters, PhD
Research Fellow
Department of Gene Regulation &
Drug Discovery
City of Hope National Medical Center/
Beckman Research Institute
Duarte, Calif

Arnold Wald, MD
Section of Gastroenterology and
Hepatology
University of Wisconsin School of
Medicine and Public Health
Madison, Wis

M. Michael Wolfe, MD
Professor of Medicine
Research Professor of Physiology and
Biophysics
Boston University School of Medicine
Chief, Section of Gastroenterology
Boston Medical Center
Boston, Mass

Preface

This handbook on acid/peptic and motility disorders of the gastrointestinal tract is the third in the series for the *Clinician's Guide to Gastroenterology*. It provides an up-to-date guide of the current status of important topics in gastroesophageal reflux disease, GI motility disorders, and functional bowel disorders. The handbook is intended to be a user-friendly manual with a primary focus for clinicians—whether a gastroenterologist, internist, primary care physician, GI fellow, or medical resident. The chapters highlight clinical advances and progress made in the care of patients in clinically important areas. Each chapter stresses the symptoms, causes, evaluation, and treatment of major GI disorders.

GI motility disorders, functional bowel disorders, and gastroesophageal reflux disease are important areas for the health of the United States. GI motility and functional bowel disorders, such as achalasia, gastroesophageal reflux, gastroparesis, functional dyspepsia, irritable bowel syndrome, colonic inertia, pelvic floor dyssynergia, and fecal incontinence, affect up to 30% of the US population. These disorders comprise about 40% of GI problems for which patients seek health care. GI motility disorders affect patients, not only by causing symptoms and posing a heavy burden of illness, but also by decreasing quality of life leading to decreased work productivity and increased absenteeism. Unfortunately, these disorders are often ignored or sidelined because the underlying mechanisms are not understood and appropriate therapy is not available. Motility disorders can be complex and difficult to treat. Understanding the GI motility dysfunction underpins the appropriate management. This handbook serves as a guide to help clinicians care for these patients.

Gastrointestinal dysmotility also impacts on the quality of life of patients with other disorders. For example, a significant percentage of patients with diabetes have gastrointestinal dysmotility. Gastrointestinal complications of diabetes can affect one or more parts of the gut and produce nausea, vomiting, abdominal pain, constipation, diarrhea, dysphagia, and heartburn. Abnormal gastric emptying, or gastroparesis, may lead to poor glucose control and complications of diabetes. Likewise, esophageal and GI motor dysfunction is often present in Parkinson's disease and may lead to trouble swallowing or evacuating the bowels.

The role of GI motility in nutrition, obesity, and drug delivery is not always appreciated. Nutrition depends on the controlled delivery of food for digestion and optimal assimilation from the gastrointestinal tract. Signaling of satiety is dependent on proper control of GI motility and release of GI hormones; obesity can result when satiety and GI motility are altered. Bioavailability of orally administered drugs is controlled in large part by GI motility.

We trust that this book will be useful for doctors to help care for patients affected by gastroesophageal reflux, peptic ulcer disease, GI motility disorders, and/or functional bowel disorders.

Henry P. Parkman, MD
Robert S. Fisher, MD

Section I

Acid/Peptic Disorders

Presentations and Evaluations of Gastroesophageal Reflux Disease

Joel E. Richter, MD

Gastroesophageal reflux disease (GERD) is the failure of the normal antireflux barrier to protect against frequent and abnormal amounts of gastroesophageal reflux (GER) (ie, gastric contents moving retrograde effortlessly from the stomach to the esophagus). GER itself is not a disease but rather a normal physiological process. It occurs multiple times each day especially after large meals, without producing symptoms or mucosal damage. In contrast, GERD is a spectrum of disease usually producing symptoms of heartburn and acid regurgitation. Most patients have no visible mucosal damage at the time of endoscopy (non-erosive GERD), while others have esophagitis; peptic strictures; Barrett's esophagus; or evidence of extraesophageal manifestations such as chest pain, pulmonary, or ear, nose and throat symptoms. GERD is a multifactorial process, one of the most common diseases of mankind, and impacts greatly on health care, contributing to the expenditure in the United States of nearly $6 billion per year for acid-suppressing medications.

Clinical Manifestations

CLASSIC REFLUX SYMPTOMS

Heartburn is the classic symptom of GERD (Table 1-1) with patients generally reporting a burning feeling that rises from the stomach or lower chest and radiates toward the neck, throat, and occasionally the back.[1] It occurs postprandially, particularly after large meals or after eating spicy foods, citrus products, fats, chocolates, and alcohol. The supine position and bending over may exacerbate heartburn. Nighttime heartburn may cause sleeping difficulties and impair next-day function.[2] When heartburn dominates the patient's complaints, it has high specificity (89%), but low sensitivity (38%) for GERD as diagnosed by 24-hour esophageal pH testing.[3] GERD is usually diagnosed symptomatically by the occurrence of heartburn 2 or more days a week, although less frequent symptoms do not preclude the disease.[4] Although

Table 1-1

SYMPTOMS AND SIGNS SUGGESTING THE DIAGNOSIS OF GASTROESOPHAGEAL REFLUX DISEASE

Classic Symptoms	Extraesophageal Manifestations
Heartburn	Angina-like chest pain
Acid regurgitation	Asthma with wheezing
Dysphagia	Aspiration pneumonia
Odynophagia	Chronic bronchitis
Water brash	Bronchiectasis
Burping	Interstitial pulmonary fibrosis
Hiccups	Throat clearing
Nausea	Hoarseness
Vomiting	Globus
	Dysphonia
	Recurrent sore throat
	Posterior laryngitis
	Vocal cord ulcers/granulomas
	Leukoplakia
	Dental erosion

heartburn is an aid to diagnosis, its frequency and severity do not predict the degree of esophageal damage.[5]

Other common symptoms of GERD are acid regurgitation and dysphagia. The effortless regurgitation of acidic fluid, especially after meals and worsened by stooping or the supine position, is highly suggestive of GERD.[3] Among patients with daily regurgitation, lower esophageal sphincter (LES) pressure is usually low and associated gastroparesis and esophagitis are common, making this symptom more difficult to treat medically than classic heartburn. Dysphagia is reported by more than 30% of individuals with GERD.[6] It usually occurs in the setting of long-standing heartburn with slowly progressive dysphagia for solids. Weight loss is uncommon as patients have good appetites. The most common causes are a peptic stricture or Schatzki's ring, but other etiologies include severe esophageal inflammation alone, peristaltic dysfunction, and esophageal cancer arising from Barrett's esophagus.

Less common symptoms associated with GERD include water brash, odynophagia, burping, hiccups, nausea, and vomiting.[7] Water brash is the sudden appearance of a slightly sour or salty fluid in the mouth. It is not regurgitated fluid, but rather secretions from the salivary glands in response to acid reflux.[8] Odynophagia (ie, pain on swallowing) may be seen with severe ulcerative esophagitis. However, its presence should raise the suspicion of an alternative cause of esophagitis, especially infections or pills.

Some patients with GERD are asymptomatic. This is particularly true in the elderly patient because of decreased acidity of the reflux material or decreased pain perception. Many elderly patients present first with complications of GERD because of long-standing disease with minimal symptoms. For example, up to one third of patients with Barrett's esophagus are insensitive to acid at the time of presentation.[9]

EXTRAESOPHAGEAL MANIFESTATIONS

GER may be the cause of a wide spectrum of conditions, including noncardiac chest pain, asthma, posterior laryngitis, chronic cough, recurrent pneumonitis, and even dental erosion.[9] Some of these patients have classic reflux symptoms, but many are "silent refluxers" contributing to problems in making the diagnosis. Furthermore, it may be difficult to establish a causal relationship even if GER can be documented by testing (eg, pH studies) because individuals may simply have 2 common diseases without a cause-and-effect relationship.

Chest Pain

GER-related chest pain may mimic angina pectoris, having a squeezing or burning quality, being substernal in location, and radiating to the back, neck, jaw, or arms. It frequently is worse after meals, can awaken the patient from sleep, and may worsen during emotional stress. Heavy exercise, even treadmill testing, may provoke GER.[10] Reflux-related chest pain may last for minutes to hours, often resolves spontaneously, and may be eased with antacids. The majority of patients with GERD-induced chest pain have heartburn symptoms.[11]

Multiple studies over the past 15 years identify GER, rather than spastic motility disorders, as the most common esophageal cause of noncardiac chest pain. Overall, these reports found that 41% of patients had abnormal 24-hour pH test results, whereas 32% had chest pain that was clearly associated with acid reflux.[12] The mechanism for GERD-related chest pain is poorly understood and probably is multifactorial related to H+ ion concentration, volume and duration of acid reflux, secondary esophageal spasm, and prolonged contractions of the longitudinal muscles.[13]

Asthma and Other Pulmonary Diseases

The prevalence of GERD in asthmatics is estimated between 34% and 89%, depending on the group of patients studied and how GER is defined (eg, symptoms or 24-hour pH monitoring).[14] Symptomatic GERD is an important comorbid condition in asthma patients and is associated with greater asthma severity.[15] GERD should be considered in asthmatics who present in adulthood, those without an intrinsic component, and those not responding to bronchodilators or steroids.[16] Up to 30% of patients with GERD-related asthma have no other esophageal complaints. Other pulmonary diseases possibly associated with GERD include aspiration pneumonia, interstitial pulmonary fibrosis, chronic bronchitis, bronchiectasis, and possibly cystic fibrosis, neonatal bronchopulmonary dysplasia, and sudden infant death syndrome.

Proposed mechanisms of reflux-induced asthma include aspiration of gastric contents into the lungs with secondary bronchospasm or activation of a vagal reflex from the esophagus to the lungs, causing bronchoconstriction. Animal[17] and human[18] studies report bronchoconstriction after esophageal acidification, but the response is mild and inconsistent. On the other hand, intratracheal infusion of even small amounts of acid induces profound and reproducible bronchospasm in cats.[17] The reflux of acid into the trachea as compared to the esophagus alone predictably caused marked changes in peak expiratory flow rates in asthmatic patients.[19] Although both mechanisms may trigger reflux-induced asthma, patients with severe asthma probably suffer from intermittent microaspiration.

Ear, Nose, and Throat Diseases

GERD may be associated with a variety of laryngeal symptoms and signs, of which "reflux laryngitis" is the most common.[20,21] These patients present with hoarseness, globus sensation, frequent throat clearing, recurrent sore throat, and prolonged voice warm-up. Ear, nose, and throat (ENT) signs attributed to GERD include posterior laryngitis with edema and redness, vocal cord ulcers and granulomas, leukoplakia, and even carcinoma. These changes are usually limited to the posterior third of the vocal cords and interarytenoid areas, both in close proximity to the upper esophageal sphincter (UES). GERD is the third leading cause of chronic cough (after sinus problems and asthma), accounting for 20% of cases.[22] Dental erosion (ie, the loss of tooth structure by nonbacterial chemical processes) can be caused by GER in healthy subjects and patients with bulimia.[23] Microaspiration of gastric contents is the most likely etiology of these complaints. Animal studies find that the combination of acid, pepsin, and conjugated bile acids is very injurious to the larynx.[24] Human studies report that proximal esophageal acid exposure, especially while sleeping, is significantly increased in patients with laryngeal symptoms and signs.[25]

Pathophysiology

The pathophysiology of GERD is complex, resulting from an imbalance between defensive factors protecting the esophagus (antireflux barriers, esophageal acid clearance, tissue resistance) and aggressive factors from the stomach (gastric acidity, volume, and duodenal contents) (Figure 1-1).

The key to both physiologic and pathologic GER is the LES and the presence and reducibility of the hiatal hernia. In the healthy state, the distal smooth muscle of the esophagus contributes to basal LES pressure. The crural diaphragm provides extrinsic squeeze to this intrinsic LES, contributing to resting pressure during inspiration and augmenting LES pressure during periods of increased abdominal pressure, such as coughing, sneezing, or bending.[26]

Importantly, basal LES pressure, as measured by esophageal manometry, does not correlate with the severity of GERD. Rather, the transient relaxation of an otherwise normal LES, precipitated by gastric distention and not triggered by swallowing, is the primary mechanism for nearly all physiologic reflux and in some series, the majority of pathologic reflux.[27] In the latter group of patients, especially those with esophagitis or Barrett's esophagus, a hypotensive LES is present in 25% to 40% of reflux episodes.[27] The presence of a hiatal hernia results in displacement of the LES from the crural diaphragm into the chest, thereby reducing LES basal pressure and shortening the length of the high pressure zone by eliminating the intra-abdominal LES segment. Hiatus hernia eliminates the increased LES pressure that occurs during straining, impairs esophageal acid clearance due to the "pinch-cock" effect of the crural diaphragm, and reduces compliance at the EG junction, thereby increasing liquid flow 6-fold across the barrier.[28,29] Statistical modeling has revealed a significant interaction between

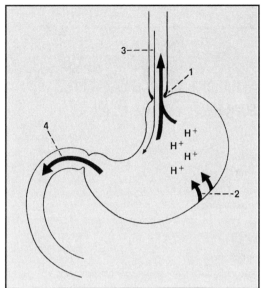

Figure 1-1. Pathophysiology of GERD. Multifactorial process including 1) impairment of antireflux barrier, 2) gastric acidity and volume, 3) esophageal acid clearance, and 4) delayed gastric emptying.

hiatus hernia and LES pressure, such that the likelihood of GER is increased as basal LES pressure decreases, an effect substantially amplified by the presence and as the hernia size increases.[30]

Esophageal peristalsis clears acid volume in both the upright and supine positions. However, small residual amounts of acid remain and are neutralized by swallowed saliva with a pH of 6.4 to 7.8.[31] Peristaltic dysfunction and weak esophageal motor activity increase in frequency with the severity of esophagitis, further impairing acid clearance. Cigarette smoking and head and neck radiation decrease saliva production and may aggravate acid clearance.

Gastric factors (volume and ingredients in the gastric refluxate) are critical in the production of reflux esophagitis. Acid combined with activated pepsin at pH <4 is the key ingredient of the gastric contents causing mucosal damage.[32] Conjugated bile acids from duodenal reflux into the stomach may augment this damage, but there is minimal evidence that "alkaline" bile reflux alone in the human causes esophagitis.[33] Gastric acid secretion is normal in GERD patients. However, recent studies find that *H. pylori* infection, especially with the cagA+ virulent strain, is a "biological antisecretory agent" that lowers gastric acidity thereby protecting the esophagus from the development of severe esophagitis and Barrett's esophagus.[34] Acid output is decreased by 2 mechanisms: 1) the associated severe corpus gastritis, which over time progresses to multifocal atrophic gastritis, and 2) the production of ammonia by the bacteria itself. Finally, delayed gastric emptying increases gastric volume and episodes of transient LES relaxation, which may aggravate GER.

Table 1-2

COMMONLY USED TESTS FOR ASSESSING THE PRESENCE, MECHANISM, AND CONSEQUENCES OF GASTROESOPHAGEAL REFLUX DISEASE*

Tests for Reflux
- Intraesophageal pH monitoring
- Ambulatory bilirubin monitoring
- Intraesophageal pH and impedance monitoring
- Radionuclide 99mTc scintiscanning
- Barium esophagogram

Tests to Assess Symptoms
- Empiric trial of acid suppression
- Intraesophageal pH monitoring with symptoms correlation
- Acid perfusion (Bernstein) test

Tests to Assess Esophageal Damage
- Endoscopy
- Esophageal biopsy
- Barium esophagogram

Tests to Assess Pathogenesis of GERD
- Esophageal manometry with impedance
- Gastric analysis
- Radionuclide 99mTc scintiscanning

* Order of presentation represents the order of diagnostic usefulness.

Diagnostic Tests

A range of tests are available to the physician pursuing the diagnosis of GERD. Many times, these studies are unnecessary because the patient's history is sufficiently revealing to identify the presence of troubling reflux disease.[3] However, this may not be the case, and the clinician must decide which tests to use to arrive at a diagnosis in a reliable, timely, and cost-effective manner (Table 1-2). Furthermore, the various esophageal tests need to be selected carefully depending upon the information desired. For example, identifying the presence of GERD is different than proving that the patient's symptoms are due to reflux episodes. Additionally, defining that acid reflux exists may not be enough. To tailor appropriate medical or surgery therapy requires knowing whether complications of GERD are present as well as possible mechanisms by which abnormal GER occurs.

EMPIRIC TRIAL OF ACID SUPPRESSION

The simplest and most definitive method for diagnosing GERD and assessing its relationship to symptoms (either classical or atypical) is the empiric trial of acid suppression. Unlike other tests that only suggest an association (eg, esophagitis at endoscopy or positive symptom index on pH testing), the response to antireflux therapy assures a cause-and-effect relationship between GERD and symptoms. Therefore, it has become the "first" test used in patients with classical or atypical reflux symptoms without alarm complaints. The popularity of this approach was aided by the introduction of the proton pump inhibitors (PPIs), which, unlike the histamine 2 receptor antagonists (H2RAs), could drastically reduce the amount of acid reflux into the esophagus. Symptoms usually responded to a PPI trial in 7 to 14 days. If symptoms disappear with therapy and then return when the medication is stopped, GERD may be assumed.

In the reported empiric trials with heartburn, the initial dose of PPI was high (eg, omeprazole 40 to 80 mg/day) and given for not less than 14 days. A positive response is defined as at least 50% improvement in heartburn. Using this approach, the PPI empiric trial had a sensitivity of 68% to 83% for determining the presence of GERD.[35,36] In noncardiac chest pain, Fass et al[37] found that a 7-day trial of omeprazole 40 mg AM and 20 mg PM had a sensitivity of 78% and specificity of 86% for predicting GERD when compared to traditional tests. Likewise, Ours et al[38] found omeprazole 40 mg twice a day (BID) for 2 weeks a very reliable method for identifying acid-related cough. Empiric trials using a 2- to 4-month regimen of BID PPIs also are commonly used in patients with suspected asthma and ENT-related GERD complaints.

An empiric trial of PPIs for diagnosing GERD has many advantages. The test is office based, easily performed, relatively inexpensive, available to all physicians, and avoids many needless procedures. For example, Fass et al[37] showed a savings of greater than $570 per average patient due to a 59% reduction in the number of diagnostic tests performed for noncardiac chest pain. Disadvantages are few, including a placebo response and uncertain symptomatic endpoint, if symptoms don't totally resolve with extended treatment.

ENDOSCOPY

Upper endoscopy is the "gold standard" for documenting the type and extent of mucosal injury to the esophagus. It identifies the presence of esophagitis and excludes other etiologies for the patient's complaints. However, only 40% to 60% of patients with abnormal esophageal reflux by pH testing have endoscopic evidence of esophagitis. Thus, the sensitivity of endoscopy for GERD is 60% at best, but it has excellent specificity at 90% to 95%.[39]

The earliest endoscopic signs of acid reflux include edema and erythema. Neither finding is specific for GERD, and both are very dependent upon the quality of endoscopic visual images.[39] More reliable are the findings of friability, granularity, and red streaks. Friability (ie, easy bleeding) occurring with gentle pressure on the mucosa results from the development of enlarged capillaries near the mucosal surface in response to acid. Red streaks may extend upward from the EG junction along the ridges of the esophageal folds. In studies evaluating these stigmata, nearly all patients had GERD.[40] With progressive acid injury, erosions develop (Figure 1-2). These are

Figure   1-2.   Endoscopic esophagitis with linear erosions. This would be classified as grade II esophagitis by the Savary-Miller and Hetzel system and as grade B by the Los Angeles scale.

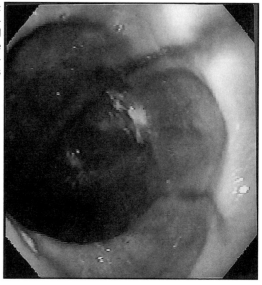

characterized by shallow thinning of the mucosa associated with a white or yellow exudate surrounded by erythema. Commonly located just above the EG junction, erosions may be either single lesions or coalesced regions. Typically, they occur along the tops of mucosal folds, areas most prone to acid exposure. Erosions may also be caused by nonsteroidal anti-inflammatory drug (NSAID) use, heavy smoking, and infectious esophagitis.[40] Ulcers reflect more severe esophageal damage. They have depth into the mucosa, tend to have either a white or yellow discolored base, and may be seen either isolated along a fold or surrounding the EG junction.

Beyond these mucosal findings, other complications of acid reflux disease often are noted at endoscopy, including rings, strictures, or Barrett's mucosa. The Schatzki's ring is a thin, pearly white tissue structure located at the squamocolumnar junction. Its etiology is controversial but recent debate suggests it as a complication of GERD for several reasons: 1) the mucosa above the ring resembles the mucosa of chronic reflux, devoid of submucosal vessels; 2) the ring may be associated with other evidence of endoscopic esophagitis; and 3) some rings progress to strictures.[41] Peptic strictures cause narrowing of the distal esophagus because of chronic acid-induced inflammation, which eventually stimulates collagen formation and the creation of a shortened, thick, noncompliant region of scarring. Like rings, peptic strictures tend to occur distally at the EG junction. They are typically short and less than 1 cm in length. If they are longer, other etiologies such as Zollinger-Ellison syndrome, pill esophagitis, or mechanical trauma from a long-term indwelling nasogastric (NG) tube should be sought.[41] Further evidence of esophagitis is often seen proximal to the stricture. Barrett's esophagus, which appears as a salmon or pink colored mucosa in the tubular esophagus, is another complication of GERD (Figure 1-3). Although the diagnosis can be suggested at endoscopy, mucosal biopsies are always necessary to confirm the presence of specialized intestinal metaplasia.[42]

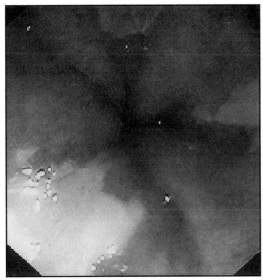

Figure 1-3. Barrett's esophagus with reddish pink columnar mucosa with tongue like projections 4 to 5 cm into the tubular esophagus.

Endoscopic grading of GERD depends upon the endoscopist's interpretation of these visual images. Unfortunately, there exists no standard classification scheme for endoscopic findings. Instead, several grading systems are available but none is completely satisfactory (Table 1-3). In Europe, the most popular scheme is the Savary-Miller classification,[43] which is based on degree of mucosal erosions. In the United States, the Hetzel and Los Angeles systems are most popular. The Hetzel system grades severity not by the number of erosions but instead by the area of mucosal injury.[44] In the Los Angeles system, the number, length, and location of mucosal breaks determine the degree of esophagitis.[45] These different classification systems diverge the most when defining the subtlest degree of injury. When erythema, edema, and indistinct Z-line are included, the sensitivity of diagnosing GERD rises at the expense of specificity.

Most patients with reflux disease are treated initially without endoscopy. The important exception is the patient experiencing "alarm" symptoms: dysphagia, odynophagia, weight loss, and gastrointestinal (GI) bleeding. With such symptoms, endoscopy should be performed early to rule out other entities such as infections, ulcers, cancer, or varices. The role of endoscopy in GERD patients without alarm symptoms is more controversial and evolving in the era of PPI therapy. Initially, endoscopy was used to characterize patients into 2 groups, nonerosive or mild erosive disease and severe erosive disease, and better direct their management. However, this practice is now unnecessary with the widespread use of PPIs as first-line therapy for GERD. Because these drugs treat both groups equally well, early endoscopy has less impact on the choice of therapy. Currently, guidelines suggest the major role of endoscopy is to define Barrett's esophagus and to diagnose and treat GERD complications, especially peptic strictures.[46] Using this rationale, the majority of patients with chronic GERD need only one endoscopy while on therapy.

Table 1-3

ENDOSCOPIC GRADING SYSTEMS FOR ESOPHAGITIS

	Savary-Miller Classification	*Hetzel Classification*
Grade 0	Not applicable	Normal appearing mucosa
Grade I	Single, erosive, or exudative lesion on one longitudinal fold	Mucosal edema, hyperemia, friability of mucosa
Grade II	Multiple erosions on more than one longitudinal fold	Superficial erosions involving <10% of mucosal surface of last 5 cm of distal esophagus
Grade III	Circumferential erosions	Superficial erosion involving 10% to 50% of distal esophagus
Grade IV	Ulcer, stricture, or short esophagus isolated or associated with grade I to III lesion	Deep ulceration or confluent erosions >50% of distal esophagus
Grade V	Barrett's + grade I to III lesion	Not applicable

Los Angeles Classification

Grade A	One or more mucosal breaks confined to folds, no longer than 5 mm
Grade B	One or more mucosal breaks >5 mm confined to folds but not continuous between tops of mucosal folds
Grade C	Mucosal breaks continuous between tops of 2 or more mucosal folds but not circumferential
Grade D	Circumferential mucosal break

ESOPHAGEAL BIOPSY

The ability to obtain tissue during endoscopy is very important. Biopsies of the esophagus help to identify reflux injury, exclude other esophageal diseases, and confirm the presence of complications, especially Barrett's esophagus. Microscopic changes indicative of reflux may occur even when the mucosa appears normal endoscopically.[47]

The most sensitive histological markers of GERD are reactive epithelial changes characterized by an increase in the basal cell layer greater than 15% of the epithelium thickness or papilla elongation into the upper third of the epithelium (Figure 1-4). These changes represent increased epithelial turnover of the squamous mucosa. Papillae, or rete peg, height increases due to loss of surface cells from acid injury, while basal cell hyperplasia is indicative of mucosal repair. Unfortunately, these changes are also noted in up to 50% of normal individuals when biopsies are taken from the distal

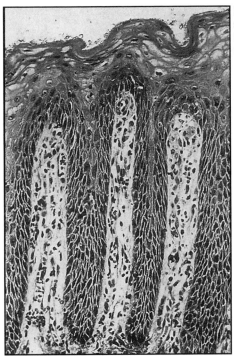

Figure 1-4. Reparative changes secondary to acid reflux characterized by basal cell hyperplasia and marked elongation of the rete pegs.

2 to 3 cm of the esophagus.[48] Hence, these changes are sensitive markers for GERD but have poor specificity.

Acute inflammation characterized by the presence of neutrophils and eosinophils is very specific for esophagitis.[48] Acid reflux injury to the vascular bed of the esophagus releases vasoactive substances that promote edema and migration of neutrophils and eosinophils into the area. Neutrophils are specific for acute esophagitis but are an insensitive marker, being present in only 15% to 40% of GERD patients.[49] Eosinophils are found more often on biopsy (19% to 63% of subjects) but are less specific, being present in up to 33% of healthy adults.[50] Interestingly, the sensitivity and specificity of eosinophils in children is much stronger, reflecting the lack of eosinophils in the juvenile inflammatory response.[48,51]

Further evaluation of microscopic changes associated with reflux disease can be assessed with electron microscopy. Studies with transmission electron microscopy performed on human esophageal biopsies demonstrate the presence of dilated intercellular spaces in patients with both erosive and nonerosive reflux disease.[52] This finding precedes the onset of gross morphological damage thus representing one of the earliest alterations in GERD.

Barrett's esophagus is suspected at endoscopy and confirmed by biopsy and histological examination. The characteristic histologic finding in Barrett's esophagus is the distinctive specialized intestinal epithelium. This is a glandular epithelium with mucin-type cells and the distinguishing presence of goblet cells (Figure 1-5). These

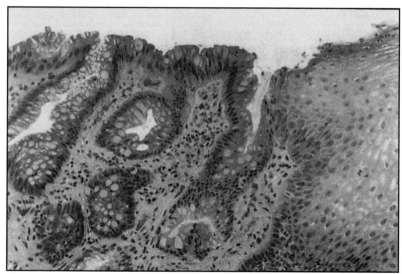

Figure 1-5. Barrett's esophagus with histology characterized by specialized intestinal metaplasia with glandular epithelium and classic goblet cells (white cells intermittently seen in mucosa) on the left side of the picture. Normal squamous mucosa of the esophagus is to the right.

are easily seen on hematoxylin and eosin-stain sections and can be demonstrated more prominently in sections stained with Alcian blue. It occupies most or all of the columnar lined area and is the type of epithelium in which adenocarcinoma arises.[53] Other types of epithelium seen with Barrett's esophagus include gastric, fundic, and cardia type epithelia, but these alone do not satisfy modern criteria for the diagnosis of Barrett's esophagus, nor are they associated with adenocarcinoma.

Like endoscopy, the role of esophageal biopsies in evaluating GERD has evolved over the years. Recent studies show there is little value for histological examination of normal-appearing squamous mucosa to either confirm or exclude pathological reflux.[54] In patients with classic esophagitis, biopsies are usually not taken unless needed to exclude cancer, infection, pill injury, or bullous skin disease. Therefore, the current primary indication for esophageal biopsies is to determine the presence of Barrett's epithelium. When the diagnosis is suspected, biopsies are mandatory and best done when esophagitis is healed.

ESOPHAGEAL pH MONITORING

Ambulatory intraesophageal pH monitoring is now the standard for establishing pathologic reflux.[55,56] The test is performed with a pH probe passed nasally and positioned 5 cm above the manometrically determined LES. The probe is connected to a battery-powered data logger capable of collecting pH values every 4 to 6 seconds. An event marker is activated by the subject in response to symptoms, meals, and body position changes. Patients are encouraged to eat normally and have regular

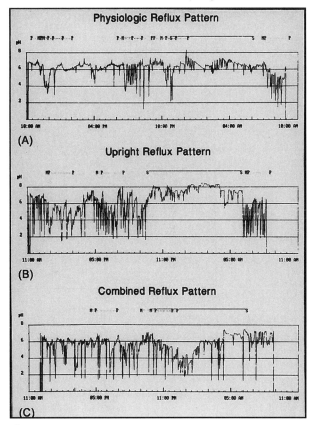

Figure 1-6. Common patterns of 24-hour esophageal reflux by pH monitoring (A). The physiological pattern of GER in healthy subjects. Reflux is noted after meals (m) but not while asleep (s). A reflux episode is defined as a pH drop to less than 4 (B). Upright reflux pattern with extensive daytime GER, but none at night. These patients have frequent symptoms, but esophagitis is uncommon. Combined pattern with daytime and nocturnal GER (C). Most of these patients have esophagitis.

daily activities. Monitoring is carried out usually for 18 to 24 hours. Reflux episodes are detected by a drop in pH to below 4. Commonly measured parameters include percent total time pH <4, percent time upright and supine pH <4, total number of reflux episodes, duration of longest reflux episode, and number of episodes greater than 5 minutes.[55] The total percent time pH <4 is the most reproducible measurement for GERD with reported upper limits of normal values ranging from 4% to 5.5%.[56] Ambulatory pH testing can discern positional variations in GER, meals, and sleep-related episodes and help relate symptoms to reflux events (Figure 1-6). As the result

Figure 1-7. New tubeless Bravo pH device attached to the esophageal mucosa 6 cm above the normal z-line.

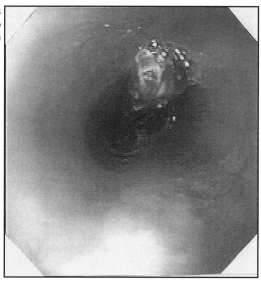

of its reliability for measuring GER across normal activities, ambulatory pH testing has replaced other older studies, such as the standard acid reflux (Tuttle) test and radionuclide scintigraphy.

One important problem with esophageal pH monitoring is the absence of an absolute threshold value that reliably identifies pathologic GER. Validation studies comparing the presence of esophagitis with abnormal pH tests report sensitivities ranging from 77% to 100% with specificities from 85% to 100%.[56] However, these patients rarely need pH testing; rather the patients with a normal endoscopy and suspected reflux symptoms should benefit most from ambulatory pH monitoring. Unfortunately, the data are much less conclusive in this group with considerable overlap between controls and nonerosive refluxers.[56] Other drawbacks of pH testing include possible equipment failure, the pH probe missing a reflux event because it is buried in a mucosal fold, and false-negative studies due to dietary or activity limitations from poor tolerability of the nasal probe.

A new tubeless device (Bravo pH probe, Medtronics, Minneapolis, Minn) has been recently developed to overcome many of the disadvantages of traditional pH monitoring.[57] The size of a vitamin pill, it is attached endoscopically to the mucosa about 6 cm above the normal z-line (Figure 1-7). The capsule is painless, does not interfere with normal activities or sleep, and gathers pH data for 2 days. Over 10 to 14 days, the capsule detaches from the mucosa and passes harmlessly in the stool. Early studies suggest 100% sensitivity in discriminating esophagitis patients and 60% sensitivity and 85% specificity in identifying patients with nonerosive reflux disease.[57]

An important advantage of ambulatory esophageal pH monitoring is its ability to record and correlate symptoms with reflux episodes over extended periods of time. For this indication, it has essentially replaced the shorter acid perfusion (Bernstein) test. Because only about 10% to 20% of reflux episodes are associated with reported symptoms, different statistical analyses have evolved attempting to define a significant association between these 2 variables, including the symptom index, symptom sensitivity index, and symptom association probability.[58] Unfortunately, no studies to date have defined the accuracy of any of these symptom scores in predicting response to therapy. Therefore, pH testing and symptom correlation can define an association between complaints and GER, but only treatment trials address the true definition of a causal relationship.

Definite clinical indications for ambulatory pH monitoring have been established.[56] Prior to fundoplication, pH testing should be performed in patients with normal endoscopy to identify the presence of pathological reflux. If esophagitis is present, pH testing is not necessary because the disease has been established. After antireflux surgery, persistent or recurrent symptoms warrant repeat pH testing. In these situations, pH monitoring is performed with the patient off all antireflux medications (PPIs for 1 week, H2RAs for 2 days). Esophageal pH testing is particularly helpful in the evaluation of patients with reflux symptoms resistant to treatment with normal or equivocal endoscopic findings. For this indication, pH testing is usually done on therapy to define 2 populations: those with and those without continued abnormal esophageal acid exposure times. The group with persistent GER needs intensification of the medical regimen, while those patients with symptoms and good acid control have another etiology for their complaints. Finally, ambulatory pH testing may help in defining patients with extraesophageal manifestations of GERD. In this situation, pH testing is usually done with additional pH probes placed in the proximal esophagus or pharynx.[59] Initially, most of these studies were done off antireflux medications to confirm the coexistence of GERD; however, this does not guarantee symptom causality. Therefore, the current approach is to treat aggressively with PPIs first, reserving pH testing only for those patients not responding after 4 to 12 weeks of therapy.[60]

BARIUM ESOPHAGOGRAM

The barium esophagogram is an inexpensive, readily available, and noninvasive esophageal test. Techniques vary according to the question being asked and the suspected underlying pathology, yet all phases of testing involve the patient ingesting a quantity of barium contrast followed by radiographic monitoring. The double-contrast method displays the esophagus by having the upright patient swallow high density barium as well as a gas-forming agent. Initially, double-contrast views of the esophagus are obtained that detail the esophageal mucosa, attempting to highlight mucosal lesions. Next, double-contrast views of the gastric cardia are gathered to check for possible causes of dysphagia. The patient is then placed in the prone position and esophageal motility assessed fluoroscopically by observing multiple swallows of barium separated by 20 seconds to allow for esophageal recovery. In the same position, single contrast views of the esophagus can be obtained while the patient quickly ingests a thin barium solution. This acts maximally to delineate the esophagus and esophagogastric junction, revealing subtle strictures, rings, and hiatal hernias. Finally, various maneuvers are performed to provoke reflux, including coughing, rolling side-to-side, leg lifting, and the water siphon test.[61]

The barium esophagogram is most useful in demonstrating structural narrowing of the esophagus and assessing the presence and reducibility of a hiatal hernia. Subtle findings such as Schatzki's rings, webs, or minimally narrowed peptic strictures are

Figure 1-8. (Left) Barium esophagogram suggests a subtle stricture. (Right) Same patient with ring well defined with hiatal hernia after Valsalva's maneuver.

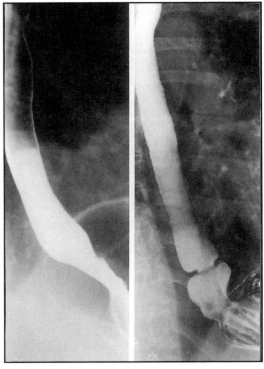

often seen only with an esophagogram, being missed by endoscopy, which may not adequately distend the esophagus (Figure 1-8). Swallowing a 13-mm radiopaque pill or marshmallow along with the barium liquid is the most sensitive test for detecting esophageal narrowing with sensitivity values reported between 95% and 100%.[62] By giving the patient swallows of barium in the prone oblique position, the barium esophagogram also allows good assessment of peristalsis and is helpful preoperatively in identifying a weak esophageal pump.[62]

The ability of the barium esophagogram to detect esophagitis varies considerably. While sensitivities of 79% to 100% have been reported with moderate to severe esophagitis, mild esophagitis is usually missed.[62] Barium testing also falls short when addressing the presence of a Barrett's esophagus. Barium studies can identify GER when contrast moves in a retrograde fashion from the stomach into the esophagus. If this occurs spontaneously, repeatedly, or to a significant degree into the mid or proximal esophagus, the test is positive but it only has a sensitivity of about 40% for defining GERD.[63] Provocative maneuvers such as leg lifting, coughing, Valsalva's, or water siphon test can be used to elicit stress reflux. Although these tests can improve the sensitivity of the barium esophagogram, some argue that they also decrease its specificity.[64]

The barium esophagogram is primarily used in evaluating the GERD patient with new-onset dysphagia because it can define subtle strictures and rings as well as assess motility. On the other hand, endoscopy is preferred in the patient with recurrent dysphagia known to have a stricture or for the assessment of esophagitis or Barrett's esophagus.

ESOPHAGEAL MANOMETRY

Esophageal manometry provides information on the functional ability of the esophageal muscles by quantifying the contractile activities of the esophageal sphincters and body during swallowing. The equipment necessary to perform manometric testing includes a catheter, pressure transducers, and a recorder. Testing is performed by first passing the catheter apparatus into the stomach and pulling it back across the LES into the esophagus. The assembly is capable of recording multiple pressure readings simultaneously from within the esophagus. The number of readings is dependent upon the number of sensors, typically spaced 3 to 5 cm apart along the catheter. Anywhere from 3 to 8 sensors are connected to transducers that convert the physical changes of pressure to electrical signals. These signals are transmitted to a recorder that transforms the information to a visual display by way of a polygraph. Either a water-perfused catheter system or one based on solid-state circuitry is typically employed. The solid-state systems are more expensive and fragile; however, they are better able to accurately record pressures in both the proximal esophagus and pharynx, and testing can be performed with solid and semi-solid boluses in addition to water. With this technology, resting pressures of the lower and upper esophageal sphincters as well as the timing and completeness of the relaxation are recorded. In the esophageal body, peristalsis is evaluated by assessing the presence, propagation velocity, amplitude, and duration of contraction waves in response to wet swallows.[65]

The measurement of LES pressures logically should be associated with the severity of GERD because of its importance as a major barrier to reflux. However, esophageal manometry is generally not indicated in the evaluation of the uncomplicated GERD patient because the vast majority of these individuals have a normal resting LES pressure, with transient LES relaxation being the primary mechanism by which their reflux occurs. It is an integral component of traditional catheter pH testing to accurately define LES location, a task poorly performed by endoscopy, fluoroscopy, or the pH pull-through technique.

Esophageal manometry to document adequate esophageal peristalsis is traditionally recommended before antireflux surgery.[66] If ineffective peristalsis (low amplitude or frequent failed peristalsis) is identified,[67] then a complete fundoplication may be contraindicated. However, this assumption has recently been challenged by several studies finding that reflux control was better and dysphagia no more common in patients with weak peristalsis after a complete as opposed to a partial fundoplication.[68] An improvement of traditional manometry (ie, combining it with multichannel intraluminal impedance testing) is helping to clarify this controversy. Impedance measurement is a new technique that measures the electrical impedance of the esophagus, the opposite of conductivity, using a catheter system similar to standard manometry.[69] Used as an esophageal function test, it can correlate the amplitude of peristaltic contractions and the frequency of peristalsis with the transport of a bolus along the esophagus.[70] This may help to better define the presence of a weak esophageal pump. Using this technique, a recent study found that less than 50% of patients with ineffective peristalsis had a significant delay in esophageal bolus transit measured by impedance.[71] Therefore, potentially only these patients with a significant physiological defect in motility will require a modified fundoplication.

MISCELLANEOUS TESTS

Radiolabelled 99 Technetium-sulfur colloid scintiscanning is useful as a semiquantitative test for detecting GER.[72] After instilling 300 mL of radioisotope in saline via a NG tube into the stomach, gamma counts over the esophagus are obtained in the supine position before and after provocation with abdominal compression. Although test specificity approaches 90%, the sensitivity is quite variable from 14% to 90%.[73]

The acid perfusion (Bernstein) test is useful for detecting the relationship of symptoms to esophageal acidification.[74] The study is done upright with a NG tube positioned in the midesophagus. Initially, normal saline is infused at 120 drops per minute for 5 to 15 minutes, followed by an infusion of 0.1 N HCl. If symptoms develop with acid infusion, saline is reinfused to assess symptom relief. Symptoms during acid infusion but not saline infusion constitute a positive test. The sensitivity of the Bernstein's test for GERD ranges from 32% to 100% and its specificity from 40% to 100%.[75] In clinical practice, 24-hour esophageal pH testing has generally replaced both of these tests.

Bile reflux can be measured using ambulatory esophageal bilirubin monitoring (Bilitec [Medtronics, Minneapolis, Minn]),[76] which utilizes the spectrophotometric property of bilirubin, the most common pigment in bile. Similar to pH testing, a fiberoptic light source is introduced into the esophagus with a data collection system worn on a waist belt. A spectrophotometer measures the wavelength absorption at 450 nm (bilirubin) and at 565 nm (reference) every 8 seconds. An integrated microcomputer calculates the difference of the absorbances, which is directly proportional to the bilirubin concentration in the sample.[76,77] This allows a pH-independent assessment of duodenogastroesophageal reflux, which is preferable to the older method employing an esophageal pH >7.[78]

Combining impedance with pH monitoring using an ambulatory system allows the measurement of both acid and nonacid reflux.[79,80] However, unlike the Bilitec device, it does not identify the origin of the nonacid reflux (ie, duodenal contents versus neutralized gastric contents after a meal). This new technology may be particularly helpful in patients with persistent symptoms despite an adequate medical trial and allows more efficient monitoring of reflux in patients on PPI therapy. It has been especially useful in defining nonacid reflux in patients with troubling regurgitation symptoms despite BID PPIs.

References

1. Carlsson R, Dent J, Bolling-Sternevold E, et al. The usefulness of a structured questionnaire in the assessment of symptomatic gastroesophageal reflux disease. *Scand J Gastroenterol*. 1998;33:1023.

2. Shaker R, Castell DO, Schoenfeld PS, Spechler SJ. Nighttime heartburn is an underappreciated clinical problem that impacts sleep and daytime function: the results of a Gallup survey conducted on behalf of the American Gastroenterological Association. *Am J Gastroenterol*. 2003;98:1487-1493.

3. Klauser AG, Schindlebeck NE, Muller-Lissner SA. Symptoms of gastroesophageal reflux disease. *Lancet*. 1990;335:205.

4. Dent J, Brun J, Fendrick AM, et al. An evidence-based appraisal of reflux disease management—the Genval report. *Gut*. 1999;44(Suppl 2):S1.

5. Johnson DA, Fennerty MB. Heartburn severity underestimates erosive esophagitis severity in elderly patients with GERD. *Gastroenterology*. 2004;126:660-664.

6. Jacob P, Kahrilas PJ, Vanagunos A. Peristaltic dysfunction associated with nonobstructive dysphagia in reflux disease. *Dig Dis Sci*. 1990;35:939.

7. Brzana RJ, Koch KL. Gastroesophageal reflux disease presenting with intractable nausea. *Ann Intern Med*. 1997;126:704.

8. Helms JF, Dodds WJ, Hogan WJ, et al. Acid neutralizing capacity of human saliva. *Gastroenterology*. 1987;83:69-74.

9. Extraesophageal presentations of gastroesophageal reflux disease. *Am J Gastroenterol*. 2000;25(Supplement):51-544.

10. Schofied PM, Bennettt DH, Whorwell PJ, et al. Exertional gastroesophageal reflux: a mechanism for symptoms in patients with angina pectoris and normal coronary angiograms. *BMJ*. 1987;294:1459-1461.

11. Hewson EG, Sinclair JW, Dalton CB, et al. Twenty-four hour esophageal pH monitoring. The most useful test for evaluating non-cardiac chest pain. *Am J Med*. 1991;90:576.

12. Richter JE. Approach to the patient with non-cardiac chest pain. In: Yamada T, ed. *Textbook of Gastroenterology*. 2nd ed. Philadelphia: JB Lippincott; 1995:648.

13. Balaban D, Yamamoto Y, Liu J, et al. Sustained esophageal contraction: a marker of esophageal chest pain identified by intraluminal ultrasonography. *Gastroenterology*. 1999;116:29-37.

14. Harding SM, Sontag SJ. Asthma and gastroesophageal reflux. *Am J Gastroenterol*. 2000;95:S23.

15. Liou A, Grubb JR, Schechtman KB, Hamilos DC. Causative and contributive factors to asthma severity and patterns of medication use in patients seeking specialized asthma care. *Chest*. 2003;124:1781-1788.

16. Irwin RS, Curley FJ, French CL. Difficult-to-control asthma: contributing factors and outcome of a systematic protocol. *Chest*. 1993;103:1662.

17. Tuchman DN, Boyle JT, Pack AI, et al. Comparison of airway responses following tracheal or esophageal acidification in the cat. *Gastroenterology*. 1984;87:872.

18. Schan CA, Harding SM, Haile JM, et al. Gastroesophageal reflux-induced bronchoconstriction: an intraesophageal acid infusion study using state-of-the-art technology. *Chest*. 1994;105:731.

19. Jack CIA, Calverley PMA, Donnelly RJ, et al. Simultaneous tracheal and esophageal pH measurements in asthmatics patients with gastro-esophageal reflux. *Thorax*. 1995;50:201.

20. Koufman JA. The otolaryngologic manifestations of gastroesophageal reflux disease. A clinical investigation of 225 patients using ambulatory 24-hour pH monitoring and an experimental investigation of the role of acid and pepsin in the development of laryngeal injury. *Laryngoscope*. 1978;88:339.

21. Wong RKH, Hanson DG, Waring PJ, Shaw G. ENT manifestations of gastroesophageal reflux. *Am J Gastroenterol*. 2000;95:S15.

22. Irwin RS, Richter JE. Gastroesophageal reflux and cough. *Am J Gastroenterol*. 2000;95:S39.

23. Lazarchik DA, Filler SJ. Dental erosion: predominant oral lesion in gastroesophageal reflux disease. *Am J Gastroenterol*. 2000;95:S33.

24. Adhami T, Goldblum JR, Richter JE, Vaezi MF. The role of gastric and duodenal agents in laryngeal injury: an experimental canine model. *Am J Gastroenterol*. 2004;99(11)2095-2106.

25. Jacob P, Kahrilas PH, Herzon G. Proximal esophageal pH—manometry in patients with "reflux laryngitis. *Gastroenterology.* 1991;100:305.
26. Mittal RK, Balaban DH. The esophagogastric junction. *N Engl J Med.* 1997;336:924.
27. Dent J, Holloway RH, Toouli J, Dodds WJ. Mechanisms of lower esophageal sphincter incompetence in patients with symptomatic gastroesophageal reflux. *Gut.* 1988;29:1020.
28. Kahrilas PJ, Lin S, Chen J, Manka M. The effect of hiatus hernia on gastro-esophageal junction pressure. *Gut.* 1999;44:476.
29. Mittal RK, Lange RC, McCallum RW. Identification and mechanism of delayed esophageal acid clearance in subjects with hiatus hernia. *Gastroenterology.* 1987;92:130.
30. Sloan S, Rademaker AW, Kahrilas PJ. Determinants of gastroesophageal junction incompetence: hiatal hernia, lower esophageal sphincter, or both? *Ann Intern Med.* 1992;117:977.
31. Helm JF, Dodds WJ, Pek LR, et al. Effect of esophageal emptying and saliva on clearance of acid from the esophagus. *N Engl J Med.* 1984;310:284.
32. Orlando RC, Bryson JC, Powell DW. Mechanisms of H+ injury in rabbit esophageal epithelium. *Am J Physiol.* 1984;246:G718.
33. Champion G, Richter JE, Vaezi MF, et al. Duodenogastroesophageal reflux: relationship to pH and importance in Barrett's esophagus. *Gastroenterology.* 1994;107:747.
34. Labenz J, Malfertheiner P. *H. pylori* in gastro-esophageal reflux disease: causal agent, independent or protective factor. *Gut.* 1997;41:277.
35. Schindlebeck NE, Klauser AG, Voderholzer WA, Mueller-Lissner S. Empiric therapy for gastroesophageal reflux disease. *Arch Intern Med.* 1995;155:1808-1812.
36. Fass R, Ofman JJ, Granelk I, et al. Clinical and economic assessment of the omeprazole test in patients with symptomatic suggestive of gastroesophageal reflux disease. *Arch Intern Med.* 1999;159:2161-2167.
37. Fass R, Fennerty MB, Ofman JJ. The clinical and economic value of a short course of omeprazole in patients with non-cardiac chest pain. *Gastroenterology.* 1998;115:42-49.
38. Ours TM, Kavuru MS, Schilz R, Richter JE. A prospective evaluation of esophageal testing and a double-blind, randomized study of omeprazole in a diagnostic and therapeutic algorithm for chronic cough. *Am J Gastroenterol.* 1999;94:3131-3138.
39. Richter JE. Severe reflux esophagitis. *Gastrointest Endosc Clin North Am.* 1994;4:677-697.
40. Johnson LF, DeMeester T, Haggitt RC. Endoscopic signs of gastroesophageal reflux objectively evaluated. *Gastrointest Endosc.* 1976;22:151-155.
41. Richter JE. Peptic strictures of the esophagus. *Gastroenterol Clin North Am.* 1999;28:875-891.
42. Falk GF. Barrett's esophagus. *Gastroenterology.* 2002;122:1569-1591.
43. Ollyo JB, Lang F, Fontolliet C, Monnier P. Savary-Miller's new endoscopic grading of reflux-esophagitis: a simple, reproducible, logical, complete and useful classification. *Gastroenterology.* 1990;98:A100.
44. Hetzel DJ, Dent J, Reed WD, et al. Healing and relapse of severe peptic esophagitis after treatment with omeprazole. *Gastroenterology.* 1988;95:903-912.
45. Armstrong D, Bennett JR, Blum AL, et al. The endoscopic assessment of esophagitis: a progress report of observer agreement. *Gastroenterology.* 1996;111:85-92.
46. DeVault KR, Castell DO. Updates guidelines for the diagnosis and treatment of gastroesophageal reflux disease. *Am J Gastroenterol.* 2004;100(1):190-200.

47. Funch-Jensen P, Kock K, Christensen LA, et al. Microscopic appearance of the esophageal mucosa in a consecutive series of patients submitted to endoscopy. Correlation with gastroesophageal reflux symptoms and microscopic findings. *Scand J Gastroenterol.* 1986;21:65-69.

48. Riddell RH. The biopsy diagnosis of gastroesophageal reflux disease, "carditis," and Barrett's esophagus. *Am J Surg Pathol.* 1996;20:31-50.

49. Seefeld U, Krejs GJ, Siebenmann RE, Blum AL. Esophageal histology in gastroesophageal reflux. Morphometric findings in suction biopsies. *Dig Dis Sci.* 1977;22:956-964.

50. Tunmmala V, Barwick KW, Sontag S, et al. The significance of intraepithelial eosinophils in the histological diagnosis of gastroesophageal reflux disease. *Am J Clin Pathol.* 1987;87:43-48.

51. Winters HS, Madara JL, Stafford RJ, et al. Intraepithelial eosinophils: a new diagnostic criterion for reflux esophagitis. *Gastroenterology.* 1982;83:818-823.

52. Tobey NA, Carson JL, Alkiek RA, Orlando RC. Dilated intercellular spaces: a morphological feature of acid reflux-damaged human esophageal epithelium. *Gastroenterology.* 1996;111:1200-1205.

53. Paull A, Trier JS, Dalton MD, et al. The histologic spectrum of Barrett's esophagus. *N Engl J Med.* 1976;295:476-482.

54. Schindlbeck NE, Wiebecke B, Klause AG, et al. Diagnostic value of histology in nonerosive gastroesophageal reflux disease. *Gut.* 1996;39:151-154.

55. DeMeester TR, Johnson LF, Joseph GJ, et al. Pattern of gastroesophageal reflux in health and disease. *Ann Surg.* 1976;184:459-470.

56. Kahrilas PJ, Quigley EMM. Clinical esophageal pH recording: a technical review for practice guidelines development. *Gastroenterology.* 1996;110:1982-1996.

57. Pandolfino JE, Richter JE, Ours TM, et al. Ambulatory esophageal pH monitoring using a wireless system. *Am J Gastroenterol.* 2003;98(4):740-749.

58. Weusten BLAM, Snout AJPM. Symptom analysis in 24-hour esophageal pH monitoring. In: Richter JE, ed. *Ambulatory Esophageal pH Monitoring. Practical Approach and Clinical Application.* 2nd ed. Baltimore, Md: Williams and Wilkins; 1997:97-105.

59. Shaker R, Milbrath M, Ren J, et al. Esophagopharyngeal distribution of refluxed gastric acid in patients with reflux laryngitis. *Gastroenterology.* 1995;109:1575-1582.

60. Richter JE. Extraesophageal presentations of gastroesophageal reflux disease: the case for aggressive diagnosis and treatment. *Cleveland Clinic Journal Medicine.* 1997;64:37-42.

61. Ott DJ. Gastroesophageal reflux disease. *Radiol Clin North Am.* 1994;32:1147-1166.

62. Ott DJ, Kelley TF, Chen MYM, et al. Use of a marshmallow bolus for evaluating lower esophageal mucosal rings. *Am J Gastroenterol.* 1991;86:817-820.

63. Thompson JK, Koehler RE, Richter JE. Detection of gastroesophageal reflux: value of the barium studies compared with 24-hour pH monitoring. *Am J Roentgerol.* 1994;162:621-626.

64. Johnston BT, Troshinsky MB, Castell JA, Castell DO. Comparison of barium radiology with esophageal pH monitoring in the diagnosis of gastroesophageal reflux disease. *Am J Gastroenterol.* 1996;91:1181-1185.

65. Ergun GA, Kahrilas PJ. Clinical application of esophageal manometry and pH monitoring. *Am J Gastroenterol.* 1996;91:1077-1089.

66. Waring JP, Hunter JG, Oddsdottir M. The preoperative evaluation of patients considered for laparoscopic antireflux surgery. *Am J Gastroenterol.* 1995;90:35-38.

67. Leite LP, Johnston BT, Barrett J, et al. Ineffective esophageal motility. The primary finding in patients with non-specific esophageal motility disorder. *Dig Dis Sci.* 1997;42:1859-1865.

68. Oleynikov D, Eubanks TR, Oelschlager BK, Pelligrini CA. Total fundoplication is the operation of choice for patients with gastroesophageal reflux and defective peristalsis. *Surg Endosc.* 2002;16:909-913.

69. Silny J. Intraluminal multiple electric impedance procedures for measurement of gastrointestinal motility. *J Gastrointest Motil.* 1991;3:151-162.

70. Srinivasan R, Vela MF, Katz PO, et al. Esophageal function testing using multichannel intraluminal impedance. *Am J Physiol Gastrointest Liver Physiol.* 2001;280:G457-G462.

71. Tutuian R, Castell DO. Clarification of the esophageal function defect in patients with manometric ineffective esophageal motility: studies using combined impedance-manometry. *Gastroenterology.* 2004;2:230-236.

72. Fisher RS, Malmud LS, Robert GS, et al. Gastroesophageal scintiscanning to detect and quantitate GE reflux. *Gastroenterology.* 1976;70:301-308.

73. Jenkins AF, Cowan RJ, Richter JE. Gastroesophageal scintigraphy: is it a sensitive screening test for gastroesophageal reflux disease? *J Clin Gastroenterol.* 1985;7:127-131.

74. Bernstein LM, Baker LA. A clinical test for esophagitis. *Gastroenterology.* 1958;34:760-781.

75. Richter JE. Disorders of esophageal function. In: Mc Callum RW, Phillips SF, Reynolds JC, eds. *Gastrointestinal Motility Disorders for the Clinician: Practical Guidelines for Patient Care.* New York: Academy Professional Information Services; 1998:5.1-5.28.

76. Bechi P, Pucciani F, Baldini F, et al. Long-term ambulatory enterogastric reflux monitoring in the validation of a new fiberoptic technique. *Dig Dis Sci.* 1993;38:1297-1302.

77. Vaezi MF, Richter JE. Role of acid and duodenogastroesophageal reflux in gastroesophageal reflux disease. *Gastroenterology.* 1996;111:1192-1199.

78. Pellegrini CA, DeMeester TR, Wernly JA, et al. Alkaline gastroesophageal reflux. *Am J Surg.* 1978;75:177-182.

79. Vela MF, Comacho-Lobato L, Srinivasan R, et al. Intraesophageal impedance and pH measurements of acid and nonacid reflux: effect of omeprazole. *Gastroenterology.* 2001;120:1599-1606.

80. Shay S, Bomeli S, Richter JE. Multichannel intraluminal impedance accurately detects fasting, recumbent reflux events and their clearing. *Am J Physiol Gastrointest Liver Physiol.* 2002;283:G376-G383.

Medical Treatment of Gastroesophageal Reflux Disease

Kevin S. Skole, MD and Robert S. Fisher, MD

The goal of treatment for gastroesophageal reflux disease (GERD) has evolved over the past 30 years from short-term symptom relief to long-term symptom control. The treatment philosophies vary. A stepped approach involves initiating simple, cost-efficient treatment modalities, and then progressing to more advanced medical therapies and possibly endoscopic or surgical interventions. Generally, this progresses as follows: phase 1: lifestyle modifications and the use of over-the-counter (OTC) treatments; phase 2: initiating prescription medications for acid suppression; phase 3: increasing the dose and combining acid suppression medications and/or adding promotility agents; and phase 4: consideration of endoscopic or surgical interventions. The authors recognize that alternative theories are to start treatment with proton pump inhibitors (PPI), eventually "stepping-down" to an effective and less costly treatment,[1,2] or to start PPI therapy with the intent to use maintenance therapy only when symptoms recur (step-in approach).[3]

Stepped Approach to Treating Gastroesophageal Reflux Disease

PHASE 1: LIFESTYLE CHANGE AND OVER-THE-COUNTER ANTACIDS, H2 RECEPTOR ANTAGONISTS OR PROTON PUMP INHIBITORS

The first step in treating GERD is to institute some simple lifestyle (behavioral) modifications (Table 2-1). These measures include alterations in eating habits such as dietary restrictions and weight loss, postural changes during sleep, changes in medications if possible, and refraining from smoking. While lifestyle changes are frequently recommended, the evidence demonstrating their clinical efficacy is weak. They are generally considered of limited value and are employed as an adjunct to standard medical therapy.[1,4]

Table 2-1

LIFESTYLE (BEHAVIORAL) MODIFICATIONS IN GASTROESOPHAGEAL REFLUX DISEASE

- Alter eating habits
  * Eat small meals
  * Do not lie down after eating
  * Avoid bedtime snacks
- Change diet
  * Avoid fatty foods
  * Limit intake of chocolate, peppermint, and alcohol
  * Reduce intake of citrus fruit, coffee, and tomato-based products
- Reduce weight
- Wear loose fitting clothing
- Change posture during sleep (ie, elevate head of bed; sleep on left side)
- Adjust current medications
- Refrain from cigarette smoking

Gastric distention has been implicated as an aggravating factor in GERD.[5] Therefore, large meals should be avoided and small, frequent meals encouraged. Patients do not have to follow a bland diet but should avoid foods that cause heartburn (Table 2-2). Foods containing a high fat content, chocolate (rich in fat and xanthines), and carminatives (such as peppermint) may aggravate heartburn by decreasing the resting LES pressure.[6-9] Other foods such as citrus fruits, tomato-based products, onions, and coffee may increase heartburn by a direct irritating effect on sensitive esophageal mucosa.[7,10,11] Alcohol and carbonated beverages have also been associated with exacerbations of reflux symptoms.[12]

Maintaining an upright position for 2 to 3 hours following meals, as well as avoiding complete recumbency during sleep may be important both to decrease the number of reflux episodes and to improve esophageal clearance when reflux has occurred.[4,13,14] Therefore, lying down after eating, as well as snacking at night, should be discouraged. The trunk of the body is best elevated during sleep by placing blocks (bricks, cinder blocks, or customized wooden blocks) under the head of the bed frame, by using a wedge-shaped bolster, or by using a mechanical hospital bed and placing the patient in a reversed Trendelenburg's position. Sleeping on the left side has also been proposed as being beneficial.[15] Although elevating the head of the bed has been shown to decrease esophageal acid exposure and improve esophageal clearance, improved symptoms and accelerated healing of esophagitis have not been demonstrated.

Wearing loose-fitting clothing has been advocated, as tight clothes may increase intragastric pressure and thus change the pressure gradient across the LES.[16] The impact of obesity on LES pressures has also led to advocacy of weight loss to control

Table 2-2

MECHANISM BY WHICH FOODS AND MEDICATIONS PREDISPOSE TO REFLUX SYMPTOMS

Mechanism	Decrease in LES Pressure	Direct Esophageal Irritant
Foods	Fatty foods	Citrus fruit
	Chocolate	Tomato-based products
	Peppermint	Coffee
	Alcohol	Onions
	Carbonated beverages	
Medications	Anticholinergics	Aspirin/NSAIDS
	Benzodiazepines	Ascorbic acid
	B-agonists	Iron and potassium prepara-
	Calcium channel blockers	tions
	Opioids	Bisphosphonates
	Progesterone-containing	Quinidine
	medications	Tetracycline
	Xanthines	

GERD symptoms, although study results have been mixed.[17] Some have suggested that the beneficial effects of weight loss may be due to dietary change rather than weight loss itself. Smoking has been associated with decreased LES pressure and increased esophageal acid exposure, which should provide patients who smoke with further incentive to pursue smoking cessation.[18]

Certain medications may aggravate heartburn by presumably reducing LES pressure (see Table 2-2).[6] This group includes xanthines such as theophylline; anticholinergic agents, including propantheline (Pro-Banthine), dicyclomine, and tricyclic antidepressants; narcotic analgesics; calcium channel blockers such as nifedipine, verapamil, and diltiazem; benzodiazepines; B-adrenergic agonists; and progesterone-containing oral contraceptives. Other medications, including tetracycline and its derivatives, quinidine preparations, aspirin and other NSAIDs, alendronate sodium, both iron and potassium preparations, and ascorbic acid may injure the esophageal mucosa directly and produce "pill esophagitis."[6,19] Most patients with pill esophagitis will complain of odynophagia (ie, painful swallowing) as well as heartburn, chest pain, and dysphagia. If at all possible, use of medications that aggravate GERD whether by increasing reflux of gastric contents or by irritating the esophageal mucosa directly should be reduced in patients with symptomatic GERD.

For many years antacids were the mainstay of therapy for patients with symptomatic GERD. Antacids remain a popular choice when patients self-medicate for heartburn because antacids provide rapid relief, presumably by neutralizing gastric and esophageal acidity. Some investigators have suggested, however, that heartburn is relieved not by acid neutralization but by the primary esophageal peristaltic wave stimulated by swallowing antacids, which rapidly clears the esophagus of refluxate. Studies have not been convincing that antacids are superior to placebo in controlling acid reflux-related esophagitis symptoms.[20,21] Alginic acid has been added to antacids in an attempt to improve efficacy. Antacid/alginic acid combinations (eg, Gaviscon [GlaxoSmithKline, Brentford, Middlesex, UK]) produce a hydrophobic viscous "raft" that floats on the liquid meniscus on top of the stomach.[22] Whether this viscous layer selectively delivers antacid into the esophagus during reflux episodes, acts as a mechanical barrier to diminish reflux quantitatively, or both has not been clearly determined. Antacid/alginic acid combinations are available in liquid and tablet form.

Because of their proven safety and efficacy, subprescription-dose H2 receptor antagonists have been available OTC for several years.[23] Controlled studies have demonstrated that OTC H2 receptor antagonists relieve heartburn and can even, when taken prophylactically, prevent its occurrence.[24-26] Interestingly, there is very little controlled evidence that OTC H2 receptor antagonists improve symptoms or reduce antacid use when compared to antacid alone.[27] Of interest, even before OTC H2 receptor antagonists were available, approximately 70% of patients with heartburn did not seek medical care from their doctors. With the recent approval of OTC omeprazole, this percentage may increase further. These observations suggest that phase 1 treatment, primarily with lifestyle change, OTC antacids, and OTC acid suppressants, may be effective in relieving symptoms in the majority of people with heartburn.

Phase 2: Use of Prescription-Dose H2 Receptor Antagonists or Proton Pump Inhibitors

The majority of patients who seek physician care for symptomatic GERD have already implemented and failed to respond to many of the lifestyle changes, as well as available OTC pharmacologic agents. From the late 1970s through the 1980s, H2 receptor antagonists in prescription doses were the cornerstones of medical treatment for GERD. Since the late 1980s, however, the use of PPIs has become so prevalent that they are considered by many to be first-line treatment for GERD.[28] This section will address the evidence supporting the use of prescription-dose H2 receptor antagonists and/or once daily PPI (Table 2-3).

By decreasing the acid output and the volume of parietal cell secretions, H2 receptor antagonists raise the pH of the gastric contents, thus raising the pH of the refluxate to the esophagus. Four H2 receptor antagonists are currently available in North America: cimetidine (Tagamet [GlaxoSmithKline, Brentford, Middlesex, UK]),[29] ranitidine (Zantac [GlaxoSmithKline, Brentford, Middlesex, UK]),[30] famotidine (Pepcid [Johnson and Johnson-Merck Pharmaceuticals, Whitehouse Station, NJ]),[31] and nizatidine (Axid [Reliant Pharmaceuticals, Liberty Corner, NJ]).[32] Although numerous studies have demonstrated the safety and efficacy of H2 receptor antagonists in diminishing the symptoms of GERD,[33] about 25% to 40% of patients may not experience symptomatic relief.[34,35] Moreover, 40% to 60% of GERD patients with erosive reflux esophagitis will not experience full mucosal healing of erosions with standard doses of H2 receptor antagonists.[36,37] Symptomatic relief of GERD seems to require greater suppression of acid secretion than is the case in patients with duodenal or gastric ulcer.[38] This, coupled with the fact that H2 receptor antagonists have a

Table 2-3

DOSING OF H2 RECEPTOR ANTAGONISTS AND PROTON PUMP INHIBITORS IN GASTROESOPHAGEAL REFLUX DISEASE PATIENTS

H2 Receptor Antagonists	Dose	PPI	Dose
Cimetidine (Tagamet)	300 to 400 mg BID	Omeprazole (Prilosec)	20 to 40 mg QD
Ranitidine (Zantac)	150 to 300 mg BID	Lansoprazole (Prevacid)	15 to 30 mg QD
Famotidine (Pepcid)	20 to 40 mg BID	Rabeprazole (Aciphex)	20 mg QD
Nizatidine (Axid)	150 mg BID	Pantoprazole (Protonix)	40 mg QD
		Esomeprazole (Nexium)	20 to 40 mg QD
		Omeprazole NaHCO$_3$ (Zegerid)	40 mg PO

QD = daily; BID = twice daily

relatively short duration of action (4 to 8 hours), means that twice-daily dosing with H2 receptor antagonists is recommended for treatment of GERD.[39] To achieve consistent healing of reflux esophagitis (>70% at 12 weeks), even greater acid suppression is often necessary, and yet higher doses of H2 receptor antagonists may be required.[40] Moreover, as will be discussed later, tachyphylaxis is often associated with H2 receptor antagonists, which may limit their efficacy in long-term use.

As a group, H2 receptor antagonists are among the safest drugs currently in use to treat any disorder. Nevertheless, a few side effects have been reported. Cimetidine, by virtue of its imidazole ring, may affect the hepatic cytochrome P-450 mixed-function oxidase system and alter the metabolism of some coadministered pharmaceutical agents. In addition, cimetidine in high doses has been reported to cause gynecomastia, impotence, decreased sperm counts, and mental confusion. High doses of ranitidine have been associated with mild, transient elevation in hepatic transaminase levels. Famotidine has been reported to have a deleterious effect on cardiac output. Nizatidine has been used relatively infrequently in comparison to the other H2 receptor antagonists; therefore, little has been written about its side effects. All of the H2 receptor antagonists have been reported to suppress bone marrow in selected cases.

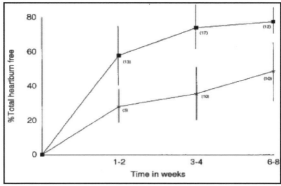

Figure 2-1. Comparison of H2RA and PPI for acute symptom relief. Symptom relief-time curve expressed as the mean total heartburn relief for each drug class corrected for patients free of heartburn at baseline at 1-2, 3-4, and 6-8 weeks. By week 2, more patients treated with PPIs are asymptomatic compared with H2RA, even after a much longer duration of treatment (8 weeks), implying a substantial therapeutic gain despite the fact that both drug classes achieve greater symptom relief with longer durations of treatment. The number of studies is shown in parentheses. •, PPI; *, H2RA. (Reprinted with permission from Chiba N, De Gara CJ, Wilkinson JM, Hunt RH. Speed of healing and symptom relief in grade II to IV gastroesophageal reflux disease: a meta-analysis. *Gastroenterology.* 1997;112:1798-1810.)

PPIs are substituted benzimidazoles that inhibit the proton pump (hydrogen/ potassium adenosine triphosphatase enzyme) within the parietal cells of the stomach by noncompetitive, generally irreversible antagonism.[41] Controlled trials assessing various PPIs have consistently shown earlier improvement in reflux symptoms and greater endoscopic healing of reflux esophagitis than when conventional, BID doses of H2 receptor antagonists are used.[37,42-44] The enhanced clinical efficacy of PPIs over H2 receptor antagonists is directly related to a greater degree of acid suppression.[45] It should be noted that there are numerous classifications of esophagitis that have been used to gauge responses to treatment.

Currently, there are 6 commercially available PPIs in the United States: omeprazole (Prilosec [Proctor and Gamble, USA]), lansoprazole (Prevacid [TAP Pharmaceuticals, Lake Forest, Ill]), rabeprazole (Aciphex [Eisai Co Ltd, Tokyo, Japan]), pantoprazole (Protonix [Wyeth Pharmaceuticals, Madison, NJ]), esomeprazole (Nexium [AstraZeneca, Coral Gables, Fla]), and a combination of omeprazole with sodium bicarbonate (Zegerid [Santarus Inc, San Diego, Calif]). They are available in enteric-coated tablets, gelatin capsules containing enteric-coated microspheres, sublingual lozenges, intravenous forms, and uncoated granules. For phase 2 therapy, all PPIs are taken daily; symptom relief can be expected in 62% to 94% of cases; esophageal healing occurs in 71% to 96%.[46,47] According to a 1997 meta-analysis, when compared to H2 receptor antagonists, symptomatic relief occurred in 78% of cases versus 48%, and esophagitis healed in 84% versus 52% (Figures 2-1 and 2-2).[36]

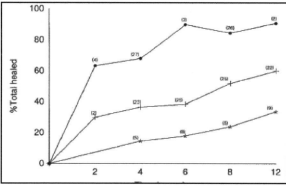

Figure 2-2. Comparison of H2RA and PPI for acute healing of esophagitis. Healing time curve expressed as the mean total healing for each drug class per evaluation time in weeks. By week 4, PPIs heal more patients than any other drug class, even after a much longer duration of treatment (12 weeks), implying a substantial therapeutic gain despite the fact that all drug classes achieve higher healing with longer durations of therapy. The number of studies shown in parentheses. •, PPI; *, H2RA. (Reprinted with permission from Chiba N, De Gara CJ, Wilkinson JM, Hunt RH. Speed of healing and symptom relief in grade II to IV gastroesophageal reflux disease: a meta-analysis. *Gastroenterology.* 1997;112:1798-1810.)

The issue of superiority of one PPI over the others has generated some controversy. Much of the published literature has been sponsored by interested pharmaceutical companies; studies favoring each PPI are easily found. Independent one-on-one comparisons have consistently shown the first-generation PPIs (ie, omeprazole, lansoprazole, pantoprazole, and rabeprazole) to be essentially equivalent in healing rates (80%) and intragastric pH profiles; however, there are several reports suggesting that rabeprazole has a faster onset of action (ie, day 1 effect) than the others.[48-51] A comparison of all 5 available PPIs in controlling 24-hour intragastric pH showed a statistically significant advantage for esomeprazole, on day 5 of therapy.[52] While clinical endpoints were not considered in this study, the ability to maintain gastric pH >4 has been associated with esophageal healing.[53] A meta-analysis done in 2003 also found esomeprazole to be superior to omeprazole, but otherwise noted no significant differences among PPIs in the short-term treatment of GERD.[54] Two recent studies have also favored esomeprazole over omeprazole and lansoprazole, respectively, in terms of healing and symptom control.[55,56] The subtle differences in pharmacodynamics, individual variability, and insurance coverage tend to dictate which PPI is chosen for phase 2 therapy. Switching from one PPI to another is a reasonable approach to patients who fail to respond to initial daily PPI therapy.[57]

Short-term side effects of PPIs occur in 1% to 3% of patients and include headache, diarrhea, constipation, nausea, rash, and pruritis. Rare serious side effects include hepatitis, interstitial nephritis, and visual disturbances. Hypergastrinemia is a common finding in patients on chronic PPI therapy, but concerns for subsequent increased risks of atrophic gastritis, gastric intestinal metaplasia, and gastric and/or colonic neoplasm have not been borne out in long-term follow-up studies to date.

PHASE 3: MEDICAL TREATMENT OF REFRACTORY GASTROESOPHAGEAL REFLUX DISEASE

When reflux symptoms fail to resolve or when esophagitis does not heal in response to phase 2 treatment with BID H2 receptor antagonist or once daily PPI, 3 options are available prior to consideration of endoluminal or surgical intervention: (1) use of a PPI BID, (2) induction of robust acid suppression using BID PPI along with an evening double dose of H2 receptor antagonist, or (3) combining a PPI with a prokinetic agent.

Proton Pump Inhibitor Twice Daily

As noted, PPIs have been demonstrated to offer the maximum acid suppression, esophageal healing, and symptom control when compared to other forms of GERD medical therapy. Most studies evaluating the efficacy of PPIs have emphasized once daily dosing. Nonresponders, however, are often defined as those with persistent symptoms despite BID dosing.[58] In the United States, increasing a PPI to BID is fairly common,[59] in part because some patients appear to be PPI resistant, especially during nighttime hours.[60] Studies have shown that BID PPI, taken 30 minutes before breakfast and dinner, offers better gastric acid control and suppression of nocturnal acid breakthrough.[61] The timing is very important, as PPIs are most effective when taken in the fasting state and when they arrive at the parietal cells when large numbers of active proton pumps are present.[62] As with daily dosing, switching from one PPI to another can offer more symptom control, as individual responses to PPIs vary, even at BID dosing.[63] As will be addressed shortly, there are concerns about costs of using PPIs; in addressing this, one study has shown that those on BID PPI can often be weaned to once daily dosing.[64]

Proton Pump Inhibitor Twice Daily Plus Evening Histamine Antagonist

Even with vigorous acid suppression via BID PPI, nocturnal acid breakthrough, defined as intragastric pH of <4 for more than 1 hour overnight, can occur in up to 73% of GERD patients and healthy volunteers.[65] Because excess esophageal exposure to gastric acid, or hypersensitivity to gastric acid, is believed to be the main component to GERD symptoms, Peghini et al proposed that bedtime ranitidine might help control GERD symptoms in patients on PPI therapy by further suppressing nocturnal gastric acid.[66] This was supported by a study showing a correlation between increased nocturnal gastric acid levels and supine esophageal acid exposure.[67] In addition, Katz et al found that nocturnal esophageal acid exposure was seen in 33% of GER patients, 50% of Barrett's esophagus patients, and 8% of normal controls on BID PPI therapy.[68] Adachi et al also found higher nocturnal esophageal acid exposure in patients with significant esophagitis.[69] In a study of 25 healthy volunteers and patients with GERD symptoms, however, Ours et al failed to find significant improvement in gastric pH, nocturnal acid breakthrough, esophageal acid exposure, or symptom control when PPI with hour of sleep (HS) ranitidine was compared to other acid suppression treatment regimens.[70] Orr et al also showed that 150 mg of ranitidine at bedtime did not significantly alter the occurrence of sleep-related GER.[71] Moreover, any benefit from the addition of an evening dose of H2 receptor antagonists may be transient, as tachyphylaxis to the H2 receptor antagonists can set in as early as 1 week after continuous use.[72] The significance of H2RA use at bedtime to control nocturnal acid breakthrough is an area that remains unsettled.[73]

Promotility and Additional Agents

A promotility drug that reduces GER and decreases the contact time between the potentially toxic gastric refluxate and the esophageal mucosa may be an attractive alternative in many cases. Ideally, this agent would increase resting LES pressure, decrease the frequency of transient LES relaxations, and stimulate distal esophageal contractions to improve esophageal clearance while avoiding gastric distention by stimulating gastric emptying. A prokinetic drug might be especially useful when heartburn is accompanied by no or mild to moderate esophagitis or by symptoms suggestive of a diffuse motility disturbance, such as regurgitation, excessive nocturnal choking, coughing, wheezing, nausea, or abdominal bloating with distention. However, prokinetics are limited by their availability and side effects.

Metoclopramide and bethanechol are the currently available promotility agents that have been used for the treatment of GERD.[74] Metoclopramide blocks dopamine type 2 receptors not just at the LES, in the stomach, and in the proximal portion of the small intestine but also in the chemoreceptor trigger zone of the medulla oblongata and in the vomiting center within the blood-brain barrier.[75] It augments the effect of acetylcholine at cholinergic receptors within the enteric nervous system. Therefore, it increases LES pressure, improves esophageal clearance, decreases GER, and accelerates stomach emptying.[76] At a dose of 10 mg 30 minutes before meals and at bedtime, metoclopramide has been reported to improve reflux symptoms better than placebo and as well as H2 receptor antagonists.[77] Healing of esophagitis has not been convincingly demonstrated with metoclopramide alone, but when used in conjunction with an H2 receptor antagonist such as cimetidine, accelerated healing rates have been observed.[78] The use of metoclopramide has been limited by its safety profile. Because of effects at the nigrostriatal region of the brain, about 20% to 40% of patients experience lethargy, stupor, somnolence, agitation, akathisia, extrapyramidal reactions sometimes simulating Parkinson's disease, or tardive dyskinesia.[79] These side effects are dose related and almost always reversible, although irreversible tardive dyskinesia has been reported, especially in elderly patients on prolonged high-dose regimens.[80]

Bethanechol, a cholinomimetic agent, increases the amplitudes of resting LES pressure and esophageal contraction.[81] Another potentially salutary effect is increased secretion of saliva, which contains bicarbonate. Studies in children and adults have demonstrated improvement in GERD symptoms and healing of esophagitis in patients treated with bethanechol alone or in conjunction with an H2 receptor antagonist.[82,83] The recommended dosage of bethanechol for adults is 25 mg 30 minutes before meals and at bedtime and has been associated with bladder spasm, urinary frequency, abdominal cramps, blurred vision, and wheezing.

Both metoclopramide and bethanechol are available in generic form; therefore, they are affordable. Because of the limitations noted above, however, these medications are generally used only when the other phase 3 treatments have been unsuccessful.

Prior to being removed from the US market in 2001, cisapride had been approved for nighttime control of GERD symptoms. Studies had shown that cisapride alone could provide symptom relief,[84] and cisapride in combination with PPI or H2 receptor antagonists had been shown to have superior treatment and maintenance control over either PPI or H2 receptor antagonists alone.[85-87] However, recent European studies have questioned the efficacy of combining cisapride with a PPI. Smythe et al found that the addition of cisapride to PPI did not improve esophageal motility or reduce esophageal reflux in patients with Barrett's esophagus.[88] Van Rensburg et al found no difference in esophageal healing or symptom control when cisapride was added to pantoprazole.[89] Hatlebakk et al found that cisapride was an ineffective maintenance medication after symptom relief had been achieved with PPI or H2 receptor antagonists.[90] Poe et al, however, did find cisapride a useful adjunct to PPI in diagnosing GERD-related cough.[91] Given these conflicting studies, should cisapride again become available in the United States, its addition to PPI therapy as an evening adjunct is worth attempting, provided no contraindications are noted.

Domperidone, a peripheral dopamine antagonist, stimulates the upper GI tract in a pattern similar to metoclopramide. Trials evaluating the clinical efficacy of domperidone in GERD have produced inconsistent results.[92-94] Domperidone does not readily cross the blood-brain barrier and thus has few central side effects. As with metoclopramide, domperidone is associated with hyperprolactinemia and results in breast engorgement, nipple tenderness, galactorrhea, and amenorrhea in some women. Domperidone has long been used in Canada and Europe, but remains unavailable in the United States.

Tegaserod (Zelnorm [Novartis, Basel, Switzerland]), a partial 5HT4 receptor agonist, is used to treat women with constipation-predominant irritable bowel syndrome and both men and women with chronic constipation.[95] In a crossover study of 19 patients with mild-moderate GERD, tegaserod 1 mg/day caused a more than 50% decrease in acid exposure in the postprandial period in patients with abnormal acid exposure.[96] Its role in the treatment of GERD, either as sole therapy or in combination with a PPI, remains unclear.[97]

As noted earlier, characteristics of the ideal prokinetic would include reducing contact time between gastric acid and the esophagus by reducing transient lower esophageal relaxations (TLESR). Research has shown that GERD symptoms, especially in those with nonerosive reflux disease or minimal esophagitis, may be attributable to TLESR, which have been associated with 55% to 80% of reflux episodes in GERD patients.[98,99] Several agents, including cholecystokinin A antagonists, anticholinergic agents, nitric oxide synthase inhibitors, morphine, and gamma-aminobutyric acid B (GABAB) agonists, are noted to reduce TLESRs. The only agent available for oral therapy is baclofen, a GABA agonist. Several studies have shown that 10 to 20 mg of baclofen 3 to 4 times daily reduces 24-hour esophageal pH, reflux event, and symptoms in GERD patients, although this has not been a uniform finding.[100-103] Studies of baclofen have been of short duration only (up to 4 weeks); studies involving longer follow-up are necessary prior to widespread use of baclofen to treat GERD. Moreover, the benefits of baclofen are limited by central nervous system (CNS) side effects, leading to support for the development of additional GABA agonists and other medications to address TLESR.[104]

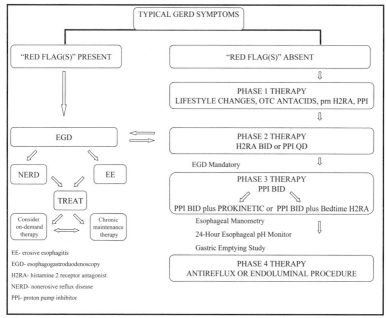

Figure 2-3. Algorithm for diagnosis and treatment of GERD.

Empirical Treatment of Gastroesophageal Reflux Disease (by Physicians) and the Role of *Helicobacter pylori*

Empirical treatment by physicians without extensive testing is appropriate and cost-effective for many patients with classic reflux symptoms (Figure 2-3). "Extensive testing" usually refers to endoscopy, which is used to determine if there is esophageal mucosal damage, including erosions, ulceration, stricture, Barrett's esophagus, or cancer. The majority of GERD patients will have no such findings; therefore, the standard of care supports empiric treatment in the absence of "alarm" (red flag) symptoms.[105-107] In some cases, however, prolonged esophageal pH monitoring and esophageal motility studies may be helpful. Empirical treatment usually consists of lifestyle modifications, OTC antacids or OTC H2 receptor antagonists (phase 1), or a 2- to 4-week trial of prescription-dose H2 receptor antagonists in a twice-daily regimen or a PPI trial in a once-daily regimen (phase 2). Alarm (red flag) symptoms or signs such as anorexia, weight loss, dysphagia, odynophagia, severe vomiting or hematemesis, blood in the stool, jaundice, anemia, or pulmonary symptoms indicate that empirical treatment should not be used. Additionally, institution of treatment without diagnostic testing is unwarranted when reflux symptoms are very severe, when symptoms are refractory after 2 to 4 weeks of empirical treatment, when symptoms recur after discontinuation of empirical treatment, when maintenance therapy is anticipated, and in patients older than 55 years. An evaluation is also reasonable in persons with an increased risk of esophageal or gastric cancer, including those of Asian descent and those with a family history of esophageal and/or gastric cancer. High-risk patients with severe coincident disease in whom a complication of GERD might be devastating are also not candidates for empirical treatment. Some gastroenterologists believe that all patients with heartburn, especially those with severe symptoms, deserve a once-in-a-lifetime endoscopy before any treatment is initiated and do not advocate empiric therapy for any GERD patients.[108]

Whether being *H. pylori*-positive is beneficial to patients with GERD is a question that has generated great controversy. Epidemiologic studies have shown that *H. pylori* may have a protective effect when addressing esophageal acid exposure; nocturnal acid exposure has been better controlled in *H. pylori*-positive patients on BID PPI.[109-111] Further studies have associated this phenomenon with strains of *H. pylori* with the cytotoxin-associated gene A (cagA).[112] Most randomized controlled studies, however, have not shown that *H. pylori* eradication worsens GERD symptoms,[113-115] although this is not uniform.[116] Recently, a systematic review of the literature seemed to verify that GERD is not worsened by *H. pylori* eradication.[117] In addition, one recent, double-blind study that used symptom scores, urea breath tests, endoscopy, and 24-hour pH monitoring demonstrated that there are no clinically significant differences in clinical or laboratory-related GERD manifestations between *H. pylori*-infected and noninfected GERD patients.[118] Nonetheless, there are studies that support the presence of *H. pylori* as protective from erosive esophagitis, and there are current recommendations that support eradication of *H. pylori* in GERD patients requiring long-term PPI therapy.[119,120] This is an unsettled area.

Endoluminal/Surgical Therapies

Endoluminal or surgical treatment of GERD is generally reserved for patients who have not responded acceptably to the conventional medical therapies described above or for those who cannot or do not desire to be on chronic medical therapy.[121] These include younger patients who have few or no other medical comorbidities and patients with significant drug allergies or interactions with other medications. Surgical therapy refers to Toupet (270 degree wrap around the distal esophagus) and Nissen (360 degree wrap around the distal esophagus) fundoplication. Long-term data have shown surgery to be effective in improving symptoms and reducing medication needs while maintaining an acceptable risk profile. For those who meet the surgical criteria but cannot or are unwilling to undergo surgery, recent developments in endoluminal therapy offer alternatives. These include injection of an inert polymer circumferentially around the region of the LES, administration of radiofrequency current to the distal esophagus, LES and gastric cardia, and endoscopic suturing devices. Plication of the gastric cardia with titanium pledgets has also been described. Endoluminal methods hold promise, but long-term data are still forthcoming.

Nonerosive Reflux Disease

Because fewer than half of patients with typical reflux symptoms have evidence of mucosal injury on endoscopy, the term nonerosive reflux disease (NERD) has come into widespread use in the past 5 years.[122,123] Technically, NERD patients have typical GERD symptoms, such as heartburn, acid reflux, regurgitation, etc; a nega-

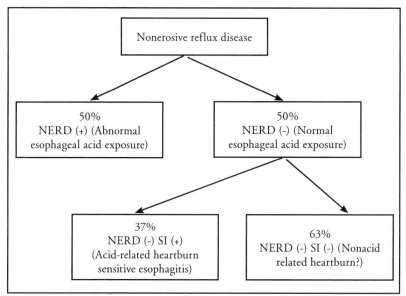

Figure 2-4. 24-hour acid and symptom patterns in nonerosive reflux disease (NERD). (Reprinted with permission from Martinez SD, Malagon IB, Garewal HS, Cui H, Fass R. Non-erosive reflux disease (NERD)—acid reflux and symptom patterns. *Aliment Pharmacol Ther.* 2003;17:537–545.)

tive endoscopy; and confirmation of abnormal esophageal acid exposure or a positive symptom index (SI) by 24-hour esophageal pH testing. Those with normal esophageal pH monitoring are considered to have a functional disorder, which is sometimes called functional heartburn (Figure 2-4).[124] A recent study found that 50% of NERD patients have normal acid exposure.[125] Thirty-seven percent of these, however, showed a close correlation between their symptoms and acid reflux events (ie, a positive SI).

The treatment for NERD patients is similar to that for patients with erosive esophagitis, with the understanding that several studies have shown that NERD patients are 10% to 30% less likely to respond to PPI therapy than patients with mucosal injury.[126-128] Moreover, while PPIs have been shown to be better than prokinetics, a recent meta-analysis did not show clear superiority of PPI over H2 receptor antagonists in patients with NERD.[129] Nonetheless, PPI therapy is commonly prescribed for NERD, and a recent publication demonstrated it to be effective in this group when compared to placebo.[130] This systematic review of 3 published studies and 4 Food and Drug Administration (FDA) reports concluded that PPI provided a 30% to 35% therapeutic gain over placebo for "sufficient" heartburn control and 25% to 30% for complete heartburn control.

These same authors also evaluated the literature to compare the symptomatic response rates of patients with NERD to response rates in patients with erosive esophagitis (Table 2-4). In 2 randomized controlled trials, symptomatic responses at 4 weeks were 56% for erosive esophagitis patients, compared to 37% for NERD patients.[131,132] Because there are no endoscopic findings to evaluate in NERD, and

Table 2-4

COMPARISON OF NONEROSIVE REFLUX DISEASE AND EROSIVE ESOPHAGITIS

Finding	NERD	EE
Abnormal endoscopy	No	Yes
Abnormal esophageal acid exposure	50%	75%
Complete heartburn resolution at 4 weeks	37%	56%
Well-controlled by on-demand therapy	Yes	No

Adapted from Dean BB, Gano AD Jr, Knight K, Ofman JJ, Fass R. Effectiveness of proton pump inhibitors in nonerosive reflux disease. *Clin Gastroenterol Hepatol.* 2004;2(8):656-664.

as response rates are clearly lower than for those with esophagitis, the actual goals of therapy for NERD patients are controversial. Most physicians aim for substantial but not absolute symptom relief.[133] Current recommendations for NERD treatment are an initial 2- to 8-week period of daily PPI, followed by an assessment of long-term needs (ie, continuous versus noncontinuous maintenance therapy).[134] An evaluation of noncontinuous therapy will be presented later in this chapter.

Long-Term Therapy

MAINTENANCE THERAPY WITH ACID SUPPRESSION

Most agree that GERD is a chronic, relapsing disorder. Recurrent reflux symptoms and mild esophagitis can be controlled in the majority of patients by phase 1 or phase 2 treatment. Many patients with erosive esophagitis, however, will experience rapid clinical or endoscopic relapse when a successful antireflux treatment is discontinued. In 1988 Hetzel and colleagues[135] demonstrated 60% and 82% relapse rates of endoscopically confirmed esophagitis within 4 and 6 months, respectively, after discontinuation of treatment in patients originally healed with omeprazole. Multiple subsequent studies have shown relapse rates to range from 23% to 96% at 12 months when acute treatment is discontinued.[86,136,137] This explains why more than 50% of patients with recurrent symptoms remain on maintenance therapy for at least 3 years.[138,139]

There is some evidence to suggest that the relapse rates may be higher in those initially healed with a PPI than in those who took an H2 receptor antagonists or a prokinetic agent for initial healing (Figure 2-5). This will be addressed in more detail shortly, as will the copious data pertaining to maintenance with PPIs. Unfortunately, data on placebo-controlled maintenance studies with an H2 receptor antagonist or prokinetic agent are limited. One study did show that ranitidine 150 mg at bedtime

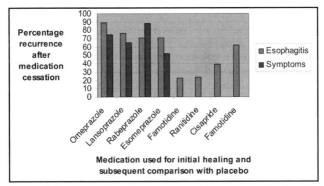

Figure 2-5. Comparison of recurrence with those on placebo after initial healing—6- to 12-month follow up. References in order: 1) *Scand J Gastroenterol Suppl.* 1994;201:69-73. 2) *Ann Int Med.* 1996;15:859-867. 3) *Eur J Gastroenterol Hepatol.* 2000;12:889-897. 4) *Am J Gastroenterol.* 2001;96;27-34. 5) *Gastroenterology.* 1989;96:A39. 6) *Gastroenterology.* 1986;91:1198-1205. 7) *Gut.* 1991;32:1280-1285.

was no better than placebo as maintenance therapy,[140] and another that cisapride monotherapy was no more effective that placebo in maintenance therapy in patients whose symptoms were initially controlled by PPI.[141] PPIs are clearly better maintenance therapy than H2 receptor antagonists or prokinetics, but in patients with mild symptoms controlled initially with H2 receptor antagonists therapy and with minimal esophagitis, histamine receptor antagonists are an acceptable long-term maintenance treatment.

In 2001, Caro et al reviewed the then-published randomized, controlled studies of PPI maintenance therapy.[48] Fifteen studies of omeprazole, lansoprazole, and/or rabeprazole were reviewed. Seven studies compared PPI to placebo, 5 to ranitidine, and 3 were comparisons among PPIs. Follow-up ranged from 6 to 12 months, and efficacy was defined primarily by endoscopic findings. Relapse rates during the first 6 months of therapy were found to be 6% to 42% with PPI, 42% to 69% with ranitidine, and 52% to 100% with placebo. Endoscopic remission rates at 12 months were 87% for PPIs, 40% for ranitidine, and 28% for placebo. While symptoms were generally not the endpoints of the studies, 91% of patients taking omeprazole were asymptomatic at 1 year, compared to 62% of those taking ranitidine.

Since that analysis was published, further studies have shown comparable results. In 2001, Vakil et al evaluated the efficacy of esomeprazole in maintenance therapy.[142] Three-hundred seventy-five patients were randomized to placebo and esomeprazole doses of 10, 20, and 40 mg. Patients were followed for 6 months and were assessed both endoscopically and clinically. Endoscopic healing remained improved compared to placebo, with 88% of patients on 40 mg and 79% on 20 mg maintaining esophageal healing, compared to 29% of those on placebo. Heartburn symptoms were also less in the esomeprazole group when compared to placebo. In 2003, Metz et al published a comparison of varying doses of pantoprazole and BID ranitidine for maintaining healing in 371 patients with grade 0 or 1 esophagitis.[143] After 12 months, 33% of those on ranitidine remained healed versus 82% of those on 40 mg of pantoprazole daily.

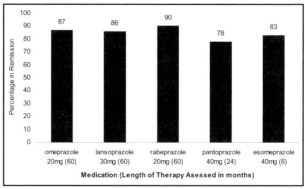

Figure 2-6. Percentage of patients in remission on long-term PPI. References in order: 1) *Gut.* 1995;36:492-498. 2) *Aliment Pharmacol Ther.* 2001;15:1819-1826. 3) *Dig Dis Sci.* 2000;45:845-853. 4) *Aliment Pharmacol Ther.* 1999;13:1023-1028. 5) *Aliment Pharmacol Ther.* 2003;17(Suppl):24-27.

Symptom-free days were 78% for the pantoprazole group versus 48% for those on ranitidine. The use of antacids was also significantly less in the pantoprazole group.

Data beyond the standard 6-12 month maintenance period have also been published (Figure 2-6). Klinkenberg-Knol et al evaluated omeprazole for its long-term efficacy and safety.[144] In a study that included individual follow-up of up to 11 years, only 158 relapse episodes were observed in 1490 treatment years in a study of 230 patients. The average maintenance dose was 20 mg daily, with incremental increases of 20 mg up to 120 mg/day during relapses. Bardhan et al evaluated the safety and efficacy of long-term maintenance therapy with 40 mg of pantoprazole. This 3-year study found remission of 85% at 12 months and 78% at 24 months.[145] Thjodleifsson et al compared maintenance therapy with omeprazole 20 mg to rabeprazole 10 mg and 20 mg in 243 patients with healed grades 2 to 4 esophagitis.[146] One-hundred twenty-three patients were followed for 5 years, and relapses occurred in 11.5%, 9.8%, and 13.3% of patients, respectively. More than 90% of patients reported no or mild heartburn, and antacid use was less than 10%.

Long-term robust suppression of gastric acid may be a double-edged sword. A review of the maintenance literature suggests that patients with erosive esophagitis healed with regular-dose H2 receptor antagonists or cisapride and then were maintained on the initial medication or placebo experience endoscopic relapse rates of less than 23% to 62% after discontinuation of the acute regimen.[147-150] In contrast, when a PPI is used for acute treatment, recurrence rates approximate 70% to 80% in patients receiving placebo maintenance (see Figure 2-5). Whereas some investigators have attributed these high recurrence rates to a selection bias toward refractory patients, it has been suggested that PPIs may induce parietal cell hyperplasia or hypertrophy, with consequent rebound acid hypersecretion when PPI therapy is discontinued.[151,152] These provocative observations suggest that the mode of initial antireflux therapy may affect the agent required to maintain long-term remission. Clinically, for patients treated initially with a PPI, it may be that only a PPI will be effective in maintaining remission.[153-155]

Moreover, robust acid suppression can render patients hypochlorhydric, potentially leading to bacterial proliferation in the proximal portion of the GI tract.[156] In fact, PPI (and H2 receptor antagonists) use was recently associated with an increased risk of community-acquired pneumonia.[157] In addition, increased release of gastrin from antral G cells with associated enterochromaffin-like cell hyperplasia has been reported, although the significance of this remains unclear.[158] Atrophic gastritis has been reported to occur in approximately 30% of patients treated with either long-term omeprazole or lansoprazole. In both cases, an association with *H. pylori* infection seems to be involved,[159,160] although this issue has not been conclusively settled.[161] Despite these concerns, however, long-term evaluations of PPI therapy have not shown any increased incidence of gastric dysplasia or neoplasia.[143-145,162] Thus far, PPIs appear safe.

MAINTENANCE THERAPY WITH PROKINETICS

The use of prokinetics for maintenance therapy has been evaluated since Lieberman suggested that higher LES pressures might play a role in GERD patients who were maintained in remission for more than 2 years as compared with those who experienced a relapse (13.1 versus 4.9 mmHg).[163] Several 6- and 12-month studies were done on prokinetic agents that may increase resting LES pressure to assess long-term maintenance therapy for GERD.[164,165] In a European multicenter study involving 443 patients with grade 1 or 2 esophagitis, 95% of patients who had healed initially with a conventional regimen of an H2 receptor antagonist and 5% with omeprazole, endoscopic recurrence rates at 12 months were significantly lower for those on cisapride, 10 mg BID (34%) and 20 mg at bedtime (32%), than with placebo (51%).[148] In a study comparing single-agent and combination regimens, Italian investigators noted that the combination of ranitidine and cisapride was significantly more effective than ranitidine alone, and the combination of omeprazole plus cisapride showed a trend toward more effective maintenance than seen with omeprazole alone.[86] As noted earlier, however, the use of prokinetics in the treatment of acute GERD symptoms is limited by their side effects and availability; those same limitations certainly apply to chronic maintenance therapy.

COSTS OF MAINTENANCE THERAPY

Although GERD symptoms clearly have a negative impact on patient quality of life, with the exception of an increased risk of esophageal adenocarcinoma, GERD is not a life-threatening disease. Therefore, no discussion of maintenance therapy for GERD would be complete without addressing the costs of long-term treatment. Harris et al compared 3 maintenance strategies in patients with erosive esophagitis after initial healing: lansoprazole 15 mg daily and ranitidine 150 mg and 300 mg BID. This 1997 cost-effectiveness analysis concluded that high-dose H2 receptor antagonists are more costly and less effective than PPI.[166] As summarized by O'Connor et al, several other studies have also supported the use of PPIs over H2 receptor antagonists when a cost analysis is used.[167] A more recent Hong Kong study comparing standard-dose BID H2 receptor antagonists with daily low dose and standard dose omeprazole, lansoprazole, rabeprazole, and pantoprazole also supported the use of standard dose PPI for chronic maintenance therapy based on both an absolute cost-basis and quality of life cost basis.[168] Studies comparing PPI costs are scarce, but a 2001 analysis of maintenance with 20 mg omeprazole, 30 mg lansoprazole, and 20 mg of rabeprazole found that the long-term costs of all 3 were similar ($1414 to $1671), with a cost per symptom recurrence favoring rabeprazole ($1637) over omeprazole ($1968) and lansoprazole ($2439).[169]

Finally, surgical and endoluminal therapies offer an alternative form of chronic maintenance therapy. The long-term data are being presented elsewhere in this text.

Noncontinuous Therapy

As previously noted, GERD symptoms affect 10% to 15% of the US population at least once weekly and up to 7% daily.[170] When evaluated endoscopically, more than 50% of GERD patients have NERD.[171] Despite the negative endoscopic findings, NERD patients often respond to acid suppression therapy,[172] and may require long-term therapy because relapse of symptoms is common.[86] The implications of long-term medication usage and the substantial costs associated with long-term treatment have made alternative treatment regimens attractive.[165] On-demand and intermittent therapy are 2 popular alternatives.

On-demand therapy is based on the idea that many NERD patients who respond to acid suppression can stop their PPI for periods of time and remain asymptomatic. When symptoms recur, they can restart their medications and continue them until symptoms again abate. Studies have shown that this is, in fact, a pattern many patients follow, unbeknown to their physicians.[173,174] This contrasts with intermittent therapy in which patients take their medications for planned periods of time when symptoms start, with on-off treatment regimens determined by their doctor.

On-demand/intermittent therapy has been advocated for several reasons.[175] It is generally accepted, although not absolutely proven, that NERD does not progress to erosive esophagitis in most patients. The potential risks of long-term PPI therapy, such as atrophic gastritis, can be avoided.[157] Patients may actually prefer on-demand regimens to continuous therapy. Finally, several studies have shown that noncontinuous therapy is cost-effective when compared to H2 receptor antagonists therapy and continuous PPI therapy, as well as to several other treatment strategies.[176-178] These studies evaluated not only direct costs, but also quality of life assessments.

Noncontinuous therapy is contraindicated in patients with severe esophagitis and structural complications of GERD such as stricture, Schatzki's ring, and Barrett's esophagus. Patients on PPI therapy for extra-esophageal complications such as cough or asthma, sore throat or hoarseness, or oropharyngeal changes seen on endoscopy/laryngoscopy are also not candidates for on-demand or intermittent therapy.

Lind et al evaluated on-demand therapy in 424 patients 18 and older with endoscopy-negative heartburn who had symptom resolution following short-term treatment with PPI.[179] Patients were randomized to omeprazole 20 mg, 10 mg, or placebo and were followed for 6 months. Upon experiencing symptoms, patients were told to take their medication until symptom relief. Patients were assessed for willingness to continue therapy, quality of life, and dosing of the study drug and supplemental antacids. Eighty-three percent of patients in the omeprazole 20 mg therapy were in remission (willing to continue the study) compared with 69% on omeprazole 10 mg and 56% taking placebo. Quality of life scores were better for those in remission. The amount of medication used in all 3 groups was similar, with antacid use being significantly higher in the placebo group. The actual cost-savings were not assessed in this study.

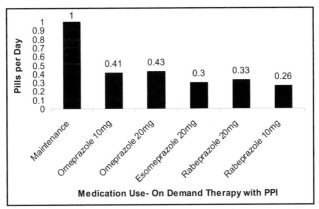

Figure 2-7. PPI use per day in on-demand therapy compared to maintenance therapy. References in order: 1) *Aliment Pharmacol Ther.* 1999;13:907-914. 2) *Aliment Pharmacol Ther.* 2001;15:347-354. 3) *Eur J Gastroenterol Hepatol.* 2002;14:857-863. 4) *Aliment Pharmacol Ther.* 2004;20:181-188. 5) *Dig Dis Sci.* 2004;49:931-936.

Similar 6-month studies found that 86% to 90% of NERD patients were willing to continue on-demand treatment with 20 mg of esomeprazole and more than 94% with rabeprazole 10 mg.[180-182] Ponce et al found a 90% patient satisfaction rate with on-demand therapy.[183] In addition, the authors noted that PPI use averaged 0.3 pills/day. A 6-month comparison, published in abstract form, of continuous and on-demand therapy for patients with NERD or mild-to-moderate GERD showed that mean daily consumption of medication was 0.31 in the on-demand group compared to 0.96 in the continuous therapy group.[184] Symptom relief was higher in the continuous therapy group (86.4% vs. 74.6%) and the withdrawal rate lower (12.3% vs. 18.3%). No study directly comparing the cost-savings of on-demand and continuous therapy has been published to date, although the pills/day in the above-noted studies were 0.3 and 0.31, and 2 further studies noted that patients took PPI on average 1 of every 2 to 3 days over a 6-month period (Figure 2-7).[181,182] Therefore, it certainly stands to reason that the savings might be substantial.[185]

The medical treatment for refractory GERD has improved dramatically in the past 30 years. Prior to the era of acid suppression, short-term symptom relief via antacids and marginal symptom control by recommending lifestyle and medication changes were the medical treatments physicians had to offer. Now, with the advent of histamine receptor antagonists and PPIs, total symptom control is a realistic goal for the majority of patients. Some patients may require multiple doses and/or a combination of different medications; others may be able to take their medications on-demand. The role of *H. pylori* and the use of prokinetics, 5HT4 receptor and GABAB agonists, as well as the considerable costs of controlling GERD symptoms with PPIs, are areas of active debate. Also, the potential implications of long-term acid suppression will need to be followed closely for some time. As these issues are addressed, more effective, efficient management strategies for GERD will evolve.

References

1. Dent J, Brun J, Fendrick AM, et al. An evidence-based appraisal of reflux disease management. The Genval Workshop Report. *Gut.* 1999;44:S1-S16.

2. Inadomi JM, Jamal R, Murata GH, et al. Step-down management of gastroesophageal reflux disease. *Gastroenterology.* 2001;121:1095-1100.

3. Howden CW, Henning JM, Huang B, et al . Management of heartburn in a large, randomized, community-based study: comparison of four therapeutic strategies. *Am J Gastroenterol.* 2001;96:1704-1710.

4. Harvey RF, Gordon PC, Hadley N, et al. Effects of sleeping with the bed-head raised and of ranitidine in patients with severe peptic oesophagitis. *Lancet.* 1987;2:1200-1203.

5. Holloway RH, Hongo M, Berger K, et al. Gastric distension: a mechanism for postprandial gastroesophageal reflux. *Gastroenterology.* 1985;89:779-784.

6. Becker DJ, Sinclair J, Castell DO, et al. A comparison of high and low fat meals on postprandial esophageal acid exposure. *Am J Gastroenterol.* 1989;84:782-786.

7. Murphy DW, Castell DO. Chocolate and heartburn: evidence of increased esophageal acid exposure after chocolate ingestion. *Am J Gastroenterol.* 1988;93:633-636.

8. Castell DO. Medical therapy for reflux esophagitis: 1986 and beyond. *Ann Intern Med.* 1986;104:112-114.

9. Fennerty MB, Castell DO, Fendrick Am, et al. The diagnosis and treatment of gastroesophageal reflux disease in a managed care environment: suggested disease management guidelines. *Arch Intern Med.* 1996;156:477-484.

10. Allen ML, Mellow MH, Robinson MG, et al. The effect of raw onions on acid reflux and reflux symptoms. *Am J Gastroenterol.* 1990;85:377-380.

11. Wendi B, Pfeiffer A, Pehl C, et al. Effect of decaffeination of coffee or tea on gastroesophageal reflux. *Aliment Pharmacol Ther.* 1994;8:283-287.

12. Pehl C, Frommherz M, Wendl B, et al. Gastroesophageal reflux induced by white wine: the role of acid clearance and "rereflux". *Am J Gastroenterol.* 2002;97:561-567.

13. Hamilton JW, Boisen RJ, Yamamoto DT, et al. Sleeping on a wedge diminishes exposure of the esophagus to refluxed acid. *Dig Dis Sci.* 1988;33:518-522.

14. Katz LC, Just R, Castell DO. Body position affects recumbent postprandial reflux. *J Clin Gastroenterol.* 1994;18:280-283.

15. Khoury RM, Camacho-Lobato L, Katz PO, et al. Influence of spontaneous sleep positions on nighttime recumbent reflux in patients with gastroesophageal reflux disease. *Am J Gastroenterol.* 1999;94:2069-2073.

16. Tutuian R, Castell DO. Management of gastroesophageal reflux disease. *Am J Med Sci.* 2003;326:309-318.

17. Wilson LJ, Ma W, Hirschowitz BI. Association of obesity with hiatal hernia and esophagitis. *Am J Gastroenterol.* 1999;94:2840-2844.

18. Pandolfino JE, Kahrilas PJ. Smoking and gastroesophageal reflux disease. *Eur J Gastroenterol Hepatol.* 2000;12:837-842.

19. de Groen PC, Lubbe DF, Hirsch LJ, et al. Esophagitis associated with the use of alendronate. *N Engl J Med.* 1996;335:1016-1021.

20. Weberg R, Berstad A. Symptomatic effect of low dose antacid regimen in reflux oesophagitis. *Scand J Gastroenterol.* 1989;24:401-406.

21. Graham DY, Patterson DJ. Double blind comparison of liquid antacid and placebo in the treatment of symptomatic reflux esophagitis. *Dig Dis Sci.* 1983;28:559-563.

22. Mandel KG, Daggy BP, Brodie DA, et al. Review article: alginate-raft formulations in the treatment of heartburn and acid reflux. *Aliment Pharmacol Ther.* 2000;14:669-690.

23. Fock KM, Talley N, Hunt R, et al. Report of the Asia-Pacific consensus on the management of gastroesophageal reflux disease. *J Gastroenterol Hepatol.* 2004;19:357-367.

24. Paul K, Redman CM, Chen M. Effectiveness and safety of nizatidine, 75 mg, for the relief of episodic heartburn. *Aliment Pharmacol Ther.* 2001;15:1571-1577.

25. Ciociola AA, Pappa KA, Sirgo MA. Nonprescription doses of ranitidine are effective in the relief of episodic heartburn. *Am J Ther.* 2001;8:399-408.

26. Galmiche JP, Shi G, Simon B, et al. On-demand treatment of gastroesophageal reflux symptoms: a comparison of ranitidine 75 mg with cimetidine 200 mg or placebo. *Aliment Pharmacol Ther.* 1998;12:909-917.

27. Simon TJ, Berlin RG, Gardener AH, et al. Self–directed treatment of intermittent heartburn: a randomized, multicenter, double-blind, placebo-controlled evaluation of antacid and low-dose of H2-receptor antagonist (famotidine). *Am J Ther.* 1995;2:304-313.

28. Blum AL. Treatment of acid-related disorders with gastric acid inhibitors; the state of the art. *Digestion.* 1990;47(suppl 1):3-10.

29. Wesdorp E, Bartelsman J, Pape K, et al. Oral cimetidine in reflux esophagitis: a double blind, controlled trial. *Gastroenterology.* 1978;74:821-824.

30. Sontag S, Robinson M, McCallum R, et al. Ranitidine therapy for gastroesophageal reflux disease: results of large double-blind trial. *Arch Intern Med.* 1987;147:1485-1491.

31. Sabesin SM, Berlin RG, Humphries TJ, et al. Famotidine relieves symptoms of Gastroesophageal reflux disease and heals erosions and ulceration. Results of multicenter, placebo-controlled, dose-ranging study. *Arch Intern Med.* 1991;151:2394-2400.

32. Cloud ML, Offen WW, Robinson M. Nizatidine versus placebo in gastroesophageal reflux disease: a 12-week, multicenter, randomized double-blind study. *Am J Gastroenterol.* 1991;86:1735-1742.

33. Tytgat GN, Nio CY, Schotborgh RH. Reflux esophagitis. *Scand J Gastroenterol.* 1990;175:1-12.

34. Pope CE. Acid-reflux disorders. *N Engl J Med.* 1994;331:656-660.

35. Sontag SJ. Rolling review: gastroesophageal reflux disease. *Aliment Pharmacol Ther.* 1993;7:293-312.

36. Chiba N, De Gara CJ, Wilkinson JM, et al. Speed of healing and symptom relief in grade II to IV gastroesophageal reflux disease: a meta-analysis. *Gastroenterology.* 1997;112:1798-1810.

37. Robinson M. Medical management of gastroesophageal reflux disease. In: Castell DO, Richter JE, eds. *The Esophagus.* 3rd ed. Philadelphia: Lippincott, Williams and Wilkins; 1999:447-462.

38. Collen MJ, Lewis JH, Benjamin SB. Gastric acid hypersecretion in refractory GERD. *Gastroenterology.* 1990;98:654-661.

39. Jones R, Bytzer P. Review article: acid suppression in the management of gastroesophageal reflux disease-an appraisal of treatment options in primary care. *Aliment Pharmacol Ther.* 2001;15:765-772.

40. Roufail W, Belsito A, Robinson M, et al. Ranitidine for erosive esophagitis: a double-blind , placebo-controlled study. *Aliment Pharmacol Ther.* 1992;6:597-607.

41. Richardson P, Hawkey CJ, Stack WA. Proton pump inhibitors. Pharmacology and rationale for use in gastrointestinal disorders. *Drugs.* 1998;56:307-335.

42. Klinkenberg-Knol EC, Jansen JM, Festen HP, et al. Double-blind multicentre comparison of omeprazole and ranitidine in the treatment of reflux esophagitis. *Lancet.* 1987;14:349-351.

43. Marks RD, Richter JE, Rizzo J, et al. Omeprazole versus H-2 receptor antagonists in treating patients with peptic stricture and esophagitis. *Gastroenterology.* 1994;106:907-915.

44. Richter JE, Campbell DR, Kahrilas PJ, et al. Lansoprazole compared with ranitidine for the treatment of non-erosive gastroesophageal reflux disease. *Arch Intern Med.* 2000; 160:1803-1809.

45. Brunner G, Creutzfeldt W, Harke U, et al. Efficacy and safety of long term treatment with omeprazole in patients with acid-related diseases resistant to ranitidine. *Can J Gastroenterol.* 1989;3(suppl A):72-76.

46. DeVault KR. Overview of medical therapy for gastroesophageal reflux disease. *Gastroenterol Clin North Am.* 1999;28:831-845.

47. DeVault KR, Castell DO. The Practice Parameters Committee of the American College of Gastroenterology. Updated guidelines for the diagnosis and treatment of gastroesophageal reflux disease. *Am J Gastroenterol.* 1999;94:1434-1442.

48. Caro JJ, Salas M, Ward A. Healing and relapse rates in gastroesophageal reflux disease treated with the newer proton pump inhibitors lansoprazole, rabeprazole and pantoprazole compared with omeprazole, ranitidine and placebo: evidence from randomized clinical trials. *Clin Ther.* 2001;23:998-1017.

49. Tutuian R, Katz PO, Castell DO. A PPI is a PPI is a PPI: lessons from prolonged ambulatory pH monitoring. *Gastroenterology.* 2000;118(suppl 2):A17.

50. Pantoflickova D, Dorta G, Ravic M, et al. Acid inhibition on the first day of dosing: comparison of four proton pump inhibitors. *Aliment Pharmacol Ther.* 2003;17:1507-1514.

51. Inamori M, Togawa J, Takahashi K, et al. Comparison of the effect on intragastric pH of a single dose of omeprazole or rabeprazole: which is suitable for on-demand therapy? *J Gastroenterol Hepatol.* 2003;18:1034-1038.

52. Miner P, Katz PO, Chen Y, et al. Gastric acid control with esomeprazole, lansoprazole, omeprazole, pantoprazole and rabeprazole: a five-way crossover study. *Am J Gastroenterol.* 2003;98:2616-2620.

53. Bell NJ, Burget D, Howden CW, et al. Appropriate acid suppression for the management of gastroesophageal reflux disease. *Digestion.* 1992;51(Suppl 1):59-67.

54. Klok RM, Postma MJ, van Hout BA, et al. Meta-analysis: comparing the efficacy of proton pump inhibitors in short-term use. *Aliment Pharmacol Ther.* 2003;17:1237-1245.

55. Castell DO, Kahrilas PJ, Richter JE, et al. Esomeprazole (40 mg) compared with lansoprazole (30 mg) in the treatment of erosive esophagitis. *Am J Gastroenterol.* 2002;97:575-583.

56. Richter JE, Kahrilas PJ, Johanson J, et al. Efficacy and safety of esomeprazole trial. *Am J Gastroenterol.* 2001;96:656-665.

57. Tutuian R, Castell DO. Management of gastroesophageal reflux disease. *Am J Med Sci.* 2003;326:309-318.

58. Richter JE. Medical management of patients with esophageal or supraesophageal reflux disease. *Am J Med.* 2003;115(Suppl 3A):179-187.

59. Vaezi MF. "Refractory GERD": Acid, nonacid or not GERD? *Am J Gastroenterol.* 2004;99:989-990.

60. Hatlebakk JG, Katz PO, Castell DO. Medical therapy: management of the refractory patient. *Gastroenterol Clin North Am.* 1999;28:847-860.

61. Hatlebakk JG, Katz PO, Kuo B, et al. Nocturnal gastric acidity and acid breakthrough on different regimens of omeprazole 40 mg daily. *Aliment Pharmacol Ther.* 1998;12:1235-1240.

62. Wolfe M. Managing gastroesophageal reflux disease: from pharmacology to the clinical arena. *Gastroenterol Clin North Am.* 2003;32:S37-S46.

63. Hatlebakk JG, Camacho-Lobato L, Katz PO, et al. Omeprazole 20 mg b.i.d. vs lansoprazole 30 mg b.i.d. in control of intragastric acidity. *Am J Gastroenterol.* 1998;93:1636.

64. Inadomi JM, McIntyre L, Bernard L, et al. Step-down from multiple to single-dose proton pump inhibitors (PPIs): a prospective study of patients with heartburn or acid regurgitation completely relieved with PPIs. *Am J Gastroenterol.* 2003;98:1940-1944.

65. Peghini PL, Katz PO, Bracy NA, et al. Nocturnal recovery of gastric acid secretion with twice daily dosing of proton pump inhibitors. *Am J Gastroenterol.* 1998;93:763-767.

66. Peghini Pl, Katz PO, Castell DO. Ranitidine controls nocturnal gastric acid breakthrough on omeprazole: a controlled study in normal subjects. *Gastroenterology.* 1998;115:1335-1339.

67. Xue S, Katz PO, Banerjee P, et al. Bedtime H2 blockers improve nocturnal gastric acid control in GERD patients on proton pump inhibitors. *Aliment Pharmacol Ther.* 2001;15:1351-1356.

68. Katz PO, Anderson C, Khoury R, et al. Gastroesophageal reflux associated with nocturnal gastric acid breakthrough on proton pump inhibitors. *Aliment Pharmacol Ther.* 1998;12:1231-1234.

69. Adachi K, Fujishiro H, Katsube T, et al. Predominant nocturnal acid reflux in patients with Los Angeles grade C and D reflux esophagitis. *J Gastroenterol Hepatol.* 2001;16:1191-1196.

70. Ours TM, Fackler WK, Richter JE, et al. Nocturnal acid breakthrough: clinical significance and correlation with esophageal acid exposure. *Am J Gastroenterol.* 2003;98:545-551.

71. Orr WC, Harnish MJ. The efficacy of omeprazole twice daily with supplemental H2 blockade at bedtime in the suppression of nocturnal oesophageal and gastric acidity. *Aliment Pharmacol Ther.* 2003;17:1553-1558.

72. Fackler WK, Ours TM, Vaezi MF, et al. Long-term effect of H2RA therapy on nocturnal acid breakthrough. *Gastroenterology.* 2002;122:625-632.

73. Castell DO. Nocturnal acid breakthrough in perspective: let's not throw out the baby with the bath water. *Am J Gastroenterol.* 2003;98:517.

74. Ramirez B, Richter JE. Review article: promotility drugs in the treatment of gastroesophageal reflux disease. *Aliment Pharmacol Ther.* 1993;7:5-20.

75. Cohen S, Morris DW, Schoen HJ, et al. The effect of oral and intravenous metoclopramide on human lower esophageal sphincter pressure. *Gastroenterology.* 1976;70:484-487.

76. Albibi R, McCallum RW. Metoclopramide: pharmacology and clinical application. *Ann Int Med.* 1983;98:86-95.

77. Guslandi M, Testoni PA, Passaretti S, et al. Ranitidine versus metoclopramide in the medical treatment of reflux esophagitis. *Hepatogastroenterology.* 1983;30:96-98.
78. Lieberman DA, Keeffe EB. Treatment of severe reflux esophagitis with cimetidine and metoclopramide. *Ann Int Med.* 1986;104:21-26.
79. Ganzini L, Casey DE, Hoffman WF, et al. The prevalence of metoclopramide-induced tardive dyskinesia and acute extrapyramidal movement disorders. *Arch Intern Med.* 1993;153:1469-1475.
80. Jimenez-Jimenez FJ, Garcia-Ruiz PJ, Molina JA. Drug-induced movement disorders. *Drug Saf.* 1997;16:180-204.
81. Phaosawasdi K, Malmud LS, Tolin RD, et al. cholinergic effects on esophageal transit and clearance. *Gastroenterology.* 1981;81:915-920.
82. Thanik KD, Chey WY, Shah AN, et al. Reflux esophagitis: effect of oral bethanachol on symptoms and endoscopic findings. *Ann Int Med.* 1980;93:805-808.
83. Farrell RL, Roling GT, Castell DO. Cholinergic therapy of chronic heartburn. A controlled trial. *Ann Int Med.* 1974;80:573-576.
84. Castell DO, Sigmund C Jr., Patterson D, et al. Cisapride 20mg bid provides symptomatic relief of heartburn and related symptoms of chronic mild to moderate gastroesophageal reflux disease. *Am J Gastroenterol.* 1998;93:547-552.
85. Galmiche JP, Brandstatter G, Evreux M, et al. Combined therapy with cisapride and cimetidine in severe reflux esophagitis. *Gut.* 1988;29:675-681.
86. Vigneri S, Termini R, Leandro G, et al. A comparison of five maintenance therapies for reflux esophagitis. *N Engl J Med.* 1995;333:1106-1110.
87. Champion MC. Prokinetic therapy in gastroesophageal reflux disease. *Can J Gastroenterol.* 1997;11(Suppl B):55B-65B.
88. Smythe A, Bird NC, Troy GP, et al. Does the addition of a prokinetic to proton pump inhibitor therapy help reduce duodenogastro-oesophageal reflux in patients with Barrett's oesophagus? *Eur J Gastroenterol Hepatol.* 2003;15:305-312.
89. Van Rensburg CJ, Bardhan KD. No clinical benefit of adding cisapride to pantoprazole for treatment of gastroesophageal reflux disease. *Eur J Gastroenterol Hepatol.* 2001;13:909-914.
90. Hatlebakk JG, Johnsson F, Vilien M, et al. The effect of cisapride in maintaining symptomatic remission in patients with gastroesophageal reflux disease. *Scand J Gastroenterol.* 1997;32:1100-1106.
91. Poe RH, Kallay MC. Chronic cough and gastroesophageal reflux disease. *Chest.* 2003;123:679-684.
92. Masci E, Testoni PA, Passaretti S, et al. Comparison of ranitidine, domperidone maleate and ranitidine plus domperidone maleate in the short-term treatment of reflux oesophagitis. *Drugs Exp Clin Res.* 1985;11:687-692.
93. Guslandi M, Dell'oca M, Motteni V, et al. Famotidine versus domperidone versus a combination of both in the treatment of reflux esophagitis (abstract). *Gastroenterology.* 1989;96:191.
94. Halter F, Staub P, Hammer B, et al. Study with two prokinetics in functional dyspepsia and GORD: domperidone vs. cisapride. *J Physiol Pharmacol.* 1997;48:185-192.
95. Johanson JF, Wald A, Tougas G, et al. Effect of tegaserod in chronic constipation: a randomized, double-blind, controlled trial. *Clin Gastroenterol Hepatol.* 2004;2:796-805.
96. Kahrilas PJ, Quigley EM, Castell DO, et al. The effects of tegaserod (HTF 919) on oesophageal acid exposure in gastroesophageal reflux disease. *Aliment Pharmacol Ther.* 2000;14:1503-1509.

97. Talley NJ. Update on the role of drug therapy in non-ulcer dyspepsia. *Rev Gastroenterol Disord.* 2003;3:25-30.

98. Mittal RK, Holloway RH, Penagini R, et al. Transient lower esophageal sphincter relaxation. *Gastroenterology.* 1995;109:601-610.

99. Richter JE. Novel medical therapies for gastroesophageal reflux beyond proton-pump inhibitors. *Gastroenterol Clin North Am.* 2002;31:S111-S116.

100. Koek GH, Sifrim D, Lerut T, et al. Effect of the GABA(B) agonist baclofen in patients with symptoms and duodeno-gastro-oesophageal reflux refractory to proton pump inhibitors. *Gut.* 2003;52:1397-1402.

101. Ciccaglione AF, Marzio L. Effect of acute and chronic administration of the GABAB agonist baclofen on 24 hour pH metry and symptoms in control subjects and in patients with gastroesophageal reflux disease. *Gut.* 2003;52:464-470.

102. Zhang Q, Lehmann A, Rigda R, et al. Control of transient lower oesophageal sphincter relaxations and reflux by the GABA(B) agonist baclofen in patients with gastroesophageal reflux disease. *Gut.* 2002;50:19-24.

103. Cange L, Johnsson E, Rydholm H, et al. Baclofen-mediated gastroesophageal acid reflux control in patients with established reflux disease. *Aliment Pharmacol Ther.* 2002;16:869-873.

104. Tonini M, De Giorgio R, De Ponti F. Progress with novel pharmacological strategies for gastroesophageal reflux disease. *Drugs.* 2004;64:347-361.

105. DeVault KR, Castell DO. Updated guidelines for the diagnosis and treatment of gastroesophageal disease. The Practice Parameters Committee of the American College of Gastroenterology. *Am J Gastroenterol.* 1999;94:1434-1442.

106. Beck IT, Champion MC, Lemire S, et al. The second Canadian consensus conference on the management of patients with gastroesophageal reflux disease. *Can J Gastroenterol.* 1997;11:7B-20B.

107. Henry JP, Lenaerts A, Ligny G. Diagnosis and treatment of gastroesophageal reflux in the adult: guidelines recommended by French and Belgian consensus. *Rev Med Brux.* 2001;22:27-32.

108. Wong WM, Lim P, Wong BC. Clinical practice pattern of gastroenterologists, primary care physicians, and otolaryngologists for the management of GERD in the Asia-Pacific region: The FAST survey. *J Gastroenterol Hepatol.* 2004;19(S3):S54-S60.

109. Varanasi RV, Fantry GT, Wilson KT. Decreased prevalence of *H. pylori* infection in gastroesophageal reflux disease. *Helicobacter.* 1998;3:188-194.

110. Martinek J, Pantoflickova D, Hucl T, et al. Absence of nocturnal acid breakthrough in *Helicobacter pylori*-positive subjects treated with twice-daily omeprazole. *Eur J Gastroenterol Hepatol.* 2004;16:445-450.

111. Koike T, Ohara S, Sekine S, et al. *Helicobacter pylori* infection prevents erosive reflux esophagitis by decreasing gastric acid secretion. *Gut.* 2001;1:330-334.

112. Rokkas T, Ladas S, Triantafyllou K, et al. The association between CagA status and the development of esophagitis after the eradication of helicobacter pylori. *Am J Med.* 2001;110(9):703-707.

113. Schwizer W, Thumshirn M, Dent J, et al. *Helicobacter pylori* and symptomatic relapse of gastroesophageal reflux disease: a randomized controlled trial. *Lancet.* 2001;357:1738-1742.

114. Moayyedi P, Bardhan C, Young L, et al. *Helicobacter pylori* eradication does not exacerbate reflux symptoms in gastroesophageal reflux disease. *Gastroenterology.* 2001;121:1120-1126.

115. Laine L, Sugg J. Effect of *Helicobacter pylori* eradication on development of erosive esophagitis and gastroesophageal reflux disease symptoms: a post hoc analysis of eight double blind prospective studies. *Am J Gastroenterol.* 2002;97:2992-2997.

116. Yamamori K, Fujiwara Y, Shiba M, et al. Prevalence of symptomatic gastroesophageal reflux disease in Japanese patients with peptic ulcer disease after eradication of *Helicobacter pylori* infection. *Aliment Pharmacol Ther.* 2004;20(Suppl 1):107-111.

117. Raghunath AS, Hungin AP, Wooff D, et al. The effect of *Helicobacter pylori* and its eradication on gastroesophageal reflux disease in patients with duodenal ulcers or reflux oesophagitis. *Aliment Pharmacol Ther.* 2004;20:733-744.

118. Fallone CA, Barkun AN, Mayrand S, et al. There is no difference in the disease severity of gastroesophageal reflux disease between patients infected and not infected with *Helicobacter pylori.* *Aliment Pharmacol Ther.* 2004;20:761-768.

119. Labenz J, Jaspersen D, Kulig M, et al. risk factors for erosive esophagitis: a multivariate analysis based on the ProGERD study initiative. *Am J Gastroenterol.* 2004;99:1652-1656.

120. Malfertheiner P, Megraud F, O'Morain C, et al. Current concepts in the management of *Helicobacter pylori* infection-M the Maastricht 2-2000 Consensus Report. *Aliment Pharmacol Ther.* 2002;285:2331-2338.

121. Sollano JD. Non-pharmacologic treatment strategies in gastroesophageal reflux disease. *J Gastroenterol Hepatol.* 2004;19:S44-S48.

122. Spechler SJ. Epidemiology and natural history of gastroesophageal reflux: incidence and precipitating factors. *Digestion.* 1992;51:24-29.

123. Achem SR. Endoscopically-negative gastroesophageal reflux disease: the hypersensitive esophagus. *Gastroenterol Clin North Am.* 1999;28:893-904.

124. Drossman DA, Corazziari R, Talley NJ, et al. Rome II. The functional esophageal disorders. In: Drossman DA, ed. *Rome II.* 2nd ed. Lawrence: Allen Press; 2000.

125. Martinez SD, Malagon IB, Garewal, HS, et al. Non-erosive reflux disease (NERD)-M acid reflux and symptom patterns. *Aliment Pharmacol Ther.* 2003;17:537-545.

126. De Vault KR, Castell DO. Guidelines for the diagnosis and treatment of gastroesophageal reflux disease. *Arch Intern Med.* 1995;155:2165-2173.

127. Richter JE, Kovacs TO, Greski-Rose PA, et al. Lansoprazole in the treatment of heartburn patients without erosive oesophagitis. *Aliment Pharmacol Ther.* 1996;13:795-804.

128. Lind T, Havelund T, Carlsson R, et al. Heartburn without oesophagitis: efficacy of omeprazole therapy and features determining therapeutic response. *Scand J Gastroenterol.* 1997;32:974-979.

129. van Pinxteren B, Numans ME, Bonis PA, et al. Short-term treatment with proton pump inhibitor, H2 receptor antagonists and prokinetics for gastroesophageal reflux disease-like symptoms and endoscopy-negative reflux disease. *Cochrane Library.* 2003.

130. Dean BB, Gano AD, Knight K, et al. Effectiveness of proton pump inhibitors in nonerosive reflux disease. *Clin Gastroenter Hepatol.* 2004;2:656-664.

131. Cloud ML, Enas N, Humphries TJ, et al. Rabeprazole in treatment of acid peptic diseases: results of three placebo-controlled dose-response clinical trials in duodenal ulcer, gastric ulcer, and gastroesophageal reflux disease (GERD). *Dig Dis Sci.* 1998;43:993-1000.

132. Richter JE, Bochenek W. Oral pantoprazole for erosive esophagitis: a placebo-controlled, randomized clinical trial. *Am J Gastroenterol.* 2000;95:3071-3080.

133. Bytzer P. Goals for therapy and guidelines for treatment success in symptomatic gastroesophageal reflux disease patients. *Am J Gastroenterol.* 2003;98:S31-S39.

134. Bytzer P, Blum Al. Rationale and proposed algorithms for symptom-based proton pump inhibitor therapy for gastroesophageal reflux disease. *Aliment Pharmacol Ther.* 2004;20:389-398.

135. Hetzel DJ, Dent J, Reed WD, et al. Healing and relapse of severe peptic esophagitis after treatment with omeprazole. *Gastroenterology.* 1988;95:903-912.

136. Hallerback B, Unge P, Carling L, et al. Omeprazole or ranitidine in long-term treatment of reflux esophagitis. *Gastroenterology.* 1994;107:1305-1311.

137. Tytgat GN. Long-term therapy for reflux esophagitis. *N Eng J Med.* 1995;333:1148-1150.

138. Galmiche JP, Bruley VS. Symptoms and disease severity in gastroesophageal reflux disease. *Scand J Gastroenterol Suppl.* 1994;201:62-68.

139. Trimble KC, Douglas S, Pryde A, et al. Clinical characteristics and natural history of symptomatic but not excess gastroesophageal reflux. *Dig Dis Sci.* 1995;40:1098-1104.

140. Koelz HR, Birchler R, Bretholz A, et al. Healing and relapse of reflux esophagitis during treatment with ranitidine. *Gastroenterology.* 1986;91:1198-1205.

141. Hatlebakk JG, Johnsson F, Vilien M, et al. The effect of cisapride in maintaining symptomatic remission in patients with gastroesophageal reflux disease. *Scand J Gastroenterol.* 1997;32:1100-1106.

142. Vakil NB, Shaker R, Johnson DA, et al. The new proton pump inhibitor esomeprazole is effective as a maintenance therapy in GERD patients with healed erosive oesophagitis: a 6-month, randomized, double-blind, placebo-controlled study of efficacy and safety. *Aliment Pharmacol Ther.* 2001;15:927-935.

143. Metz DC, Bochenek WJ. Pantoprazole maintenance therapy prevents relapse of erosive oesophagitis. *Aliment Pharmacol Ther.* 2003;17:155-164.

144. Klinkenberg-Knol EC, Nelis F, Dent J, et al. Long-term omeprazole treatment in resistant gastroesophageal reflux disease: efficacy, safety, and influence on gastric mucosa. *Gastroenterology.* 2000;118:661-669.

145. Bardhan KD, Cherian P, Bishop AE, et al. Pantoprazole therapy in the long-term management of severe acid peptic disease: clinical efficacy, safety, serum gastrin, gastric histology, and endocrine cell studies. *Am J Gastroenterol.* 2001;96:1767-1776.

146. Thjodleifsson B, Rindi G, Fiocca R, et al. A randomized, double-blind trial of the efficacy and safety of 10 or 20 mg rabeprazole compared with 20 mg omeprazole in the maintenance of gastroesophageal reflux disease over 5 years. *Aliment Pharmacol Ther.* 2003;17:343-351.

147. Koelz HR, Birchler R, Bretholz A, et al. Healing and relapse of reflux esophagitis during treatment with ranitidine. *Gastroenterology.* 1986;91:1198-1205.

148. Berlin R, Ebel D, Cook T. Famotidine 20 HS and 40 HS vs placebo in the maintenance therapy of reflux esophagitis: results of a double-blind, multicenter trial. *Gastroenterology.* 1989;96:A39.

149. Toussaint J, Gossuin A, Deruyttere M, et al. Healing and prevention of relapse of reflux oesophagitis by cisapride. *Gut.* 1991;32:1280-1285.

150. Simon TJ, Roberts WG, Berlin RG, et al. Acid suppression by famotidine 20 mg twice daily or 40 mg twice daily in preventing relapse of endoscopic recurrence of erosive esophagitis. *Clin Ther.* 1995;17:1147-1156.

151. Robinson M. Review article: current perspectives on hypergastrinaemia and enterochromaffin-like-cell hyperplasia. *Aliment Pharmacol Ther.* 1999;13 Suppl 5:5-10.

152. Gillen D, Wirz AA, Ardill JE, et al. Rebound hypersecretion after omeprazole and its relation to on-treatment acid suppression and *Helicobacter pylori* status. *Gastroenterology.* 1999;116:239-247.

153. Dent J, Yeomans ND, Mackinnon M, et al. Omeprazole vs ranitidine for prevention of relapse in reflux oesophagitis. A controlled, double-blind trial of their efficacy and safety. *Gut.* 1994;35:590-598.

154. Robinson M, Lanza F, Avner D, et al. Effective maintenance of reflux esophagitis with low-dose lansoprazole. *Ann Intern Med.* 1996;124:859-867.

155. Chiba N. Proton pump inhibitors in acute healing and maintenance of erosive or worse esophagitis: a systematic overview. *Can J Gastroenterol.* 1997;11(Suppl B):66B-73B.

156. Williams C. Occurrence and significance of gastric colonization during acid-inhibitory therapy. *Best Pract Res Clin Gastroenterol.* 2001;15:511-521.

157. Laheij RJ, Sturkenboom MC, Hassing RJ, et al. Risk of community-acquired pneumonia and use of gastric acid-suppressive drugs. *JAMA.* 2004;292:1955-1960.

158. Freston JW. Long-term acid control and proton pump inhibitors: interactions and safety issues in perspective. *Am J Gastroenterol.* 1997;92(4 Suppl):51S-55S; discussion 55S-57S.

159. Kuipers EJ, Landell L, Klinkenberg-Knol EC, et al. Atrophic gastritis and *Helicobacter pylori* infection in patients with reflux oesophagitis treated with omeprazole or fundoplication. *N Eng J Med.* 1996;334:1018-1022.

160. Eissele R, Brenner G, Simon B, et al. Gastric mucosa during treatment with lansoprazole: *Helicobacter pylori* is a risk factor for argyrophil cell hyperplasia. *Gastroenterology.* 1997;112:707-717.

161. Lundell L, Miettinen P, Myrvold HE, et al. Lack of effect of acid suppression therapy on gastric atrophy. *Gastroenterology.* 1999;117:319-326.

162. Geboes K, Dekker W, Mulder CJ, et al. Long-term lansoprazole treatment for gastroesophageal reflux disease: clinical efficacy and influence on gastric mucosa. *Aliment Pharmacol Ther.* 2001;15:1819-1826.

163. Lieberman DA. Medical therapy for chronic reflux esophagitis: long-term follow-up. *Arch Ann Int.* 1987;147:1717-1720.

164. Wiseman LR, Faulds D. Cisapride. An updated review of its pharmacology and therapeutic efficacy as a prokinetic agent in gastrointestinal motility disorders. *Drugs.* 1994;47:116-152.

165. Blum AL, Adami B, Bouzo MH, et al. Effect of cisapride on relapse of esophagitis. A multinational, placebo-controlled trial in patients healed with an antisecretory drug. *Dig Dis Sci.* 1993;38:551-560.

166. Harris RA, Kupperman M, Richter JE. Proton pump inhibitors or histamine-2 receptor antagonists for the prevention of recurrences of erosive reflux esophagitis: cost-effectiveness analysis. *Am J Gastroenterol.* 1997;92:2179-2187.

167. O'Connor JB, Provenzale D, Brazer S. Economic considerations in the treatment of gastroesophageal reflux disease: a review. *Am J Gastroenterol.* 2000;95:3356-3364.

168. You JHS, Lee ACM, Wong SCY, et al. Low-dose or standard-dose proton pump inhibitors for maintenance therapy of gastroesophageal reflux disease: a cost-effectiveness analysis. *Aliment Pharmacol Ther.* 2003;17:785-792.

169. Dean BB, Siddique RM, Yamashita BD, et al. Cost-effectiveness of proton pump inhibitors for maintenance therapy of erosive esophagitis. *Am J Health System Pharm.* 2001;58:1338-1346.

170. Locke GR, Talley NJ, Fett SL, et al. Prevalence and clinical spectrum of gastroesophageal reflux: a population based study in Olmstead County, Minnesota. *Gastroenterology.* 1997;112:1448-1456.

171. Johnsson F, Joelsson B, Gudmundsson K, et al. Symptoms and endoscopic findings in the diagnosis of gastroesophageal reflux disease. *Scand J Gastroenterol.* 1987;22:714-718.

172. Bytzer P. Goals of therapy and guidelines for treatment success in symptomatic gastroesophageal reflux disease patients. *Am J Gastroenterol.* 2003;98;S31-S39.

173. Dent J, Brun J, Fendrick Am, et al. An evidence-based appraisal of reflux disease management – the Genval Workshop report. *Gut.* 1999:44:S1-S16.

174. Fendrick Am, Shaw M, Schachtel B, et al. Self-selection and use patterns of over-the-counter omeprazole for frequent heartburn. *Clin Gastroenterol Hepatol.* 2004;2:17-21.

175. Bytzer P, Blum AL. Rationale and proposed algorithms for symptom-based proton pump inhibitor therapy for gastroesophageal reflux disease. *Aliment Pharmacol Ther.* 2004;20:389-398.

176. Stalhammar NO, Carlsson J, Peacock R, et al. Cost effectiveness of omeprazole and rantidine in intermittent treatment of symptomatic gastroesophageal disease. *Pharmacoeconomics.* 1999;16:483-497.

177. Gerson LB, Robbins AS, Garber A, et al. A cost-effectiveness analysis of prescribing strategies in the management of gastroesophageal reflux disease. *Am J Gastroenterol.* 2000;95:395-407.

178. Wahlqvist P, Junghard O, Higgins A, et al. Cost effectiveness of proton pump inhibitors in gastroesophageal reflux disease without oesophagitis: comparison of on-demand esomeprazole with conventional omeprazole strategies. *Pharmacoeconomics.* 2002;20:267-277.

179. Lind T, Havelund T, Lundell L, et al. On demand therapy with omeprazole for the long-term management of patients with heartburn without oesophagitis-m a placebo-controlled randomized trial. *Aliment Pharmacol Ther.* 1999;13:907-914.

180. Talley NJ, Venables TL, Green JR, et al. Esomeprazole 40 mg and 20 mg is efficacious in the long-term management of patients with endoscopy-negative gastroesophageal reflux disease: a placebo-controlled trial of on-demand therapy for 6 months. *Eur J Gastroenterol Hepatol.* 2002;14:857-863.

181. Talley NJ, Lauritsen K, Tunturi-Hihnala H, et al. Esomeprazole 20 mg maintains symptom control in endoscopy-negative gastroesophageal reflux disease: a controlled trial of 'on-demand' therapy for 6 months. *Aliment Pharmacol Ther.* 2001;15:347-354.

182. Bytzer P, Blum AL, De Herdt D, et al. Six-month trial of on-demand rabeprazole 10 mg maintains symptom relief in patients with non-erosive reflux disease. *Aliment Pharmacol Ther.* 2004;20:181-188.

183. Ponce J, Arguello L, Bastida G, et al. On-demand therapy with rabeprazole in nonerosive and erosive gastroesophageal reflux disease in clinical practice: effectiveness, health-related quality of life, and patient satisfaction. *Dig Dis Sci.* 2004;49:931-936.

184. Bour B, Chousterman M, Labayle D, et al. On-demand therapy with rabeprazole 10 mg: an effective alternative to continuous therapy for patients with frequent gastroesophageal reflux symptomatic relapse. *Gastroenterology.* 2003;A229:S1601.

185. Bytzer P. Rationale and proposed algorithms for symptom-based proton pump inhibitor therapy for gastroesophageal reflux disease. *Aliment Pharmacol Ther.* 2004;20:389-398.

Complications of Gastroesophageal Reflux Disease: Esophageal Stricture, Barrett's Esophagus, and Esophageal Adenocarcinoma

Stuart J. Spechler, MD

The stratified squamous epithelium that normally lines the distal esophagus can be damaged by exposure to the acid, pepsin, and other noxious agents in gastric juice.[1] Consequently, GERD can be complicated by peptic esophageal erosions and ulcerations. It has been estimated that peptic esophageal ulcerations are found in 2% to 7% of patients who have endoscopic examinations for the evaluation of GERD symptoms.[2] Among all patients with esophageal ulcerations, GERD is by far the most common cause. In a recent series of 88 patients with esophageal ulcerations discovered by endoscopy, GERD was the etiology in two thirds of cases, with the remainder caused by a variety of caustic agents and esophageal infections.[3]

Deep peptic ulcerations may penetrate into the blood vessels that supply the esophagus, resulting in esophageal hemorrhage. In a recent series of 7822 patients who had endoscopic examinations to evaluate UGI bleeding, esophageal ulcerations were found in 2.1%.[4] Rarely, peptic esophageal ulcers have perforated into the mediastinum or penetrated into the airway, resulting in esophagotracheal or esophagobronchial fistulae.[5,6] Peptic ulcerations also can stimulate the deposition of fibrous tissue in the wall of the esophagus, resulting in peptic esophageal strictures (Figure 3-1). In one series of 58 patients with peptic esophageal ulcerations, strictures developed in 17%.[3] It has been estimated that 60% to 70% of all benign esophageal strictures in the United States are due to GERD, with the remainder caused by caustic ingestions, radiation, and esophageal infections.[7]

Usually, peptic esophageal ulcerations heal through the regeneration of more stratified squamous epithelial cells. In approximately 10% of patients with GERD, however, esophageal healing occurs through a metaplastic process in which intestinal-type columnar cells replace the reflux-damaged squamous cells.[8] This condition is called Barrett's esophagus (Figure 3-2). Specialized intestinal metaplasia, the abnormal epithelium that characterizes Barrett's esophagus, may be more resistant to GERD than the native squamous mucosa, but the metaplastic cells are predisposed to malignancy. Indeed, GERD and Barrett's esophagus are the major risk factors for esophageal adenocarcinoma, a tumor whose frequency has quintupled over the past few decades among Caucasian men in the United States.[9,10]

Figure 3-1. Endoscopic photograph of an esophageal ulceration associated with an esophageal stricture in a patient with severe GERD. (Reprinted with permission from the Clinical Teaching Project of the American Gastroenterological Association. Spechler SJ, Unit 9. Esophageal Disorders. Used with permission. © American Gastroenterological Association, Bethesda, Md.)

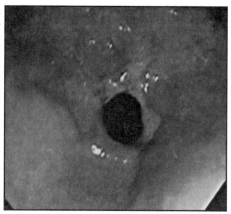

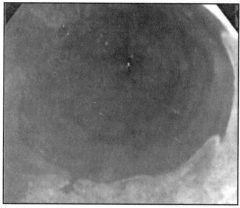

Figure 3-2. This endoscopic photograph shows the characteristic appearance of traditional Barrett's esophagus, with a long segment of columnar epithelium extending well above the GEJ.

There is substantial ethnic variation in the frequency of the esophageal complications of GERD. It has been known for decades that Barrett's esophagus and esophageal adenocarcinoma affect Caucasians predominantly.[11] Although GERD symptoms affect Caucasian and African Americans with similar frequency, erosive esophagitis is twice as common in Caucasians.[12] Peptic esophageal ulcerations and strictures are also found more commonly in Caucasians than in African Americans.[13] Furthermore, studies from Asia have suggested that complicated GERD is rare in Asians.[14]

In one study of 2477 consecutive patients seen in the general endoscopy unit of a Boston hospital, one or more esophageal complications of GERD were found in 267 of 2174 Caucasian patients (12.3%), but in only 7 of 249 African American patients (2.8%) and 1 of 54 Asian patients (1.8%) (Figure 3-3).[15] All of the 50 patients with peptic esophageal strictures were white, as were 61 of the 62 patients with peptic esophageal ulcerations. These data suggest that all of the esophageal complications of GERD have a strong predilection for Caucasians and are uncommon in African Americans and Asians. Consequently, clinicians should be especially cautious about attributing esophageal ulcerations and strictures to GERD in African American and

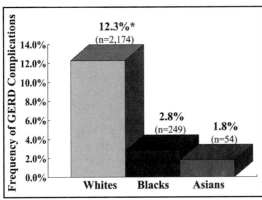

Figure 3-3. Frequency of GERD complications (esophageal ulceration, stricture, Barrett's esophagus) among 2477 patients seen in a general endoscopy unit. *p<0.05 compared to the other groups. (Reprinted with permission from Spechler SJ, Jain SK, Tendler DA, Parker RA. Racial differences in the frequency of symptoms and complications of gastroesophageal reflux disease. *Aliment Pharmacol Ther.* 2002;16:1795-1800.)

Asian patients.[16] Other etiologies (eg, cancer, infection) must be strongly considered and pursued vigorously in these patients.

Peptic Esophageal Erosion and Ulceration

Histologically, esophageal erosions are defined as superficial necrotic defects that do not penetrate the muscularis mucosae, whereas ulcerations extend through the muscularis mucosae into the submucosa. In practice, however, the distinction between an esophageal ulceration and erosion is usually based on a subjective assessment of the depth of the defect found during endoscopic or radiographic evaluation of the esophagus. Clinicians seldom have histological confirmation that the lesions they call "esophageal ulcers" in fact have breached the muscularis mucosae.

A number of systems have been proposed for grading the severity of reflux esophagitis seen on endoscopic examination. One modern system, called the Los Angeles classification, attempts to avoid the problem of distinguishing erosions from ulcerations by referring to both as "mucosal breaks."[17] A mucosal break is defined as an area of slough or erythema with a discrete line of demarcation from the adjacent, more normal-looking mucosa. In the Los Angeles system, esophagitis is graded on a scale of A to D depending on the length and circumferential extent of the mucosal breaks. Los Angeles grades C and D represent severe reflux esophagitis.

Esophageal erosions and ulcerations may result in odynophagia (ie, pain with swallowing), presumably because the ingested bolus stimulates nociceptive nerves exposed by the epithelial injury. Reflux esophagitis also can cause dysphagia, even without any apparent mechanical obstruction of the esophagus.[18] The mechanism underlying this nonobstructive dysphagia is not clear. Heartburn may be the only esophageal symptom noted by most patients with severe reflux esophagitis, and some patients with esophageal ulcerations verified by endoscopic examination have no esophageal symptoms whatsoever.[19]

Endoscopy is the diagnostic procedure of choice to document esophageal erosions and ulcerations. These lesions can be identified by a barium contrast examination as well, but the sensitivity of radiography for detecting reflux esophagitis is only approximately 70% (using endoscopy as the diagnostic gold standard test).[20] Furthermore, lesions identified radiographically usually will require an endoscopic evaluation for confirmation and biopsy sampling.

Only 2 forms of therapy are effective for healing erosive and ulcerative esophagitis: PPIs and antireflux surgery.[21] Histamine H2-receptor antagonists are not reliable agents for patients with such severe reflux disease. PPIs are virtually always effective for healing severe reflux esophagitis provided they are administered in sufficient dosages.[22] A number of studies have demonstrated that antireflux surgery heals the symptoms and signs of severe GERD in the short term, but recent reports have raised questions regarding the long-term efficacy and safety of these operations.[23,24]

Peptic Esophageal Strictures

The precise pathogenetic mechanisms involved in esophageal stricture formation are not known. Deep esophageal ulcerations clearly can result in stricture formation, but it is not known whether ulceration is a necessary step in the pathogenesis of peptic strictures. It is the opinion of some esophagologists that the frequency of peptic esophageal strictures has decreased since 1989 when the first PPI was approved for clinical use in the United States, but definitive data to prove this contention are not available.

Patients with esophageal strictures typically complain of dysphagia for solid foods that progresses slowly (over months to years) in severity. Most patients have no problem swallowing liquids, and they usually experience little or no weight loss. Patients usually perceive that swallowed material sticks at a point that is at or above rather than below the level of the stricture. In one study of 139 patients with dysphagia due to esophageal strictures, for example, the patients' perception of the level of obstruction agreed with the endoscopists' localization of the stricture in 74% of cases.[25] Fifteen percent of patients with a stricture of the distal esophagus localized the obstruction to the proximal esophagus, whereas only 5% of patients with a proximal esophageal stricture perceived the obstruction in the distal esophagus. In clinical practice, therefore, the patient's perception that a swallowed bolus sticks above the suprasternal notch is of little value in localizing an obstruction because this sensation could be caused by a lesion located anywhere from the pharynx to the most distal esophagus. In contrast, patients who localize the obstruction to a point below the suprasternal notch almost always have an esophageal disorder.

Endoscopy generally is the diagnostic procedure of choice if a peptic esophageal stricture is suspected. Although radiography is a sensitive test for esophageal strictures,[26] it is not required for the diagnosis in most cases. Furthermore, strictures identified radiographically usually will require an endoscopic evaluation for confirmation and biopsy sampling. Thus, endoscopy is often the first and only test required for the diagnosis of esophageal strictures. For strictures that are unusually long or tight, a barium swallow can be helpful to delineate the anatomy and to guide the choice among dilators for therapy (see below).

In the era before PPIs, peptic esophageal strictures were widely regarded as fixed, fibrotic lesions that would respond only to dilation therapy aimed at stretching or tearing the fibrous tissue. Medical therapy appeared to have little role in the management of these lesions. Clinical trials that compared histamine H2-receptor antagonists with placebo showed no reduction in the need for esophageal stricture dilation in patients who received medical therapy.[27,28] However, modern studies have shown that PPIs both improve dysphagia and decrease the need for subsequent esophageal dilations in patients with peptic esophageal strictures.[29] These observations indicate that there is a reversible component of reflux esophagitis that contributes to dysphagia in some patients with peptic esophageal strictures.[30]

When dysphagia persists despite treatment with PPIs, patients with peptic esophageal strictures are treated with esophageal dilation. Three major types of dilating devices are commonly used:

1. Mercury filled bougies that are passed blindly through the mouth (eg, Maloney dilators).

2. Polyvinyl bougies that can be passed over a guidewire that is positioned within the stricture using either fluoroscopic or endoscopic guidance (eg, Savary dilators).

3. Balloon dilators that are passed either over a guidewire or through the endoscope.

Guidewires are used routinely if the stricture is unusually long or tight. If bougies are chosen, the physician passes a series of dilators of increasing diameter to stretch the peptic stricture gradually. If a balloon is chosen, it is inflated to its maximal diameter stepwise or all at once. Most patients experience substantial relief of dysphagia when the esophagus is stretched to a diameter between 12 and 18 mm. No study has established the superiority of one type of dilator over another, and serious complications such as perforation and bleeding occur in approximately 0.5% of all esophageal dilation procedures.[31]

Barrett's Esophagus

In Barrett's esophagus, specialized intestinal metaplasia replaces esophageal squamous epithelium that has been damaged by GERD.[1] Specialized intestinal metaplasia is an abnormal epithelium that comprises a variety of columnar cell types, which have gastric, small intestinal, and colonic features (Figure 3-4). The metaplastic mucosa usually shows evidence of DNA damage that presumably underlies the malignant predisposition of Barrett's esophagus.[32,33] The specialized intestinal metaplasia itself causes no symptoms, and the condition usually is discovered when endoscopy is performed to evaluate patients who complain of GERD symptoms.

SCREENING FOR BARRETT'S ESOPHAGUS

For patients with GERD symptoms, there is no clear consensus on when to recommend endoscopy to look for Barrett's esophagus. The Practice Parameters Committee of the American College of Gastroenterology has suggested the following strategy[21]: "If the patient's history is typical for uncomplicated GERD, an initial trial of empirical therapy (including lifestyle modification) is appropriate. Patients in whom empiric therapy is unsuccessful or who have symptoms suggesting complicated disease should have further diagnostic testing (ie, endoscopy)." Symptoms that might suggest complicated disease requiring early endoscopic evaluation include anorexia, weight loss, dysphagia, odynophagia, and bleeding. In another publication dealing specifically with Barrett's esophagus,[34] the Practice Parameters Committee has recommended that, "Patients with chronic GERD symptoms are those most likely to have Barrett's esophagus and should undergo upper endoscopy." These guidelines are merely com-

Figure 3-4. Photomicrograph of specialized intestinal metaplasia in Barrett's esophagus (H&Ex100). Note the villiform surface and the numerous intestinal-type goblet cells.

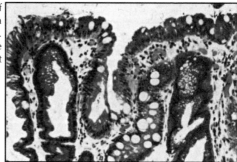

Figure 3-5. Landmarks for the diagnosis of Barrett's esophagus. The squamocolumnar junction (SCJ or Z-line) is the visible line formed by the juxtaposition of squamous and columnar epithelia. The GEJ is the imaginary line at which the esophagus ends and the stomach begins. The GEJ corresponds to the most proximal extent of the gastric folds. When the SCJ is located proximal to the GEJ, there is a columnar-lined segment of esophagus. (Reprinted from *Gastroenterology*, 117, Spechler SJ, The role of gastric carditis in metaplasia and neoplasia at the gastroesophageal junction, 218-228, © 1999, with permission from American Gastroenterological Association.)

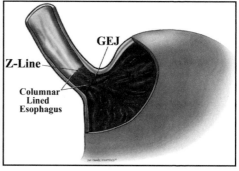

mittee recommendations whose efficacy has not been verified by clinical studies, and some authorities feel that there is insufficient evidence to support the practice of routine endoscopic screening of patients with chronic GERD symptoms.[35]

DIAGNOSIS AND PREVALENCE OF BARRETT'S ESOPHAGUS

Endoscopy is needed to diagnose Barrett's esophagus. Endoscopists recognize columnar epithelium in the esophagus because it has a dull, reddish color that contrasts sharply with the pale, glossy appearance of the squamous epithelium (Figure 3-5). The GEJ, the level at which the esophagus ends and the stomach begins, is recognized endoscopically as the most proximal extent of the gastric folds. Specialized intestinal metaplasia cannot be distinguished from gastric-type columnar epithelia by endoscopic appearance alone, however, and the diagnosis of Barrett's esophagus requires the demonstration of specialized intestinal metaplasia in esophageal biopsy specimens. If specialized intestinal metaplasia extends >3 cm above the GEJ, the condition is called long-segment Barrett's esophagus; <3 cm of esophageal metaplasia is called short-segment Barrett's esophagus.[36]

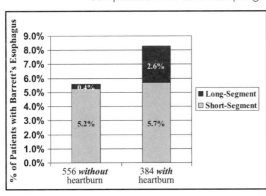

Figure 3-6. Frequency of Barrett's esophagus among patients scheduled for colonoscopy who agreed to have UGI endoscopy performed for research purposes. (Reproduced from *Gastroenterology,* 125, Rex DK, Cummings OW, Shaw M, et al, Screening for Barrett's esophagus in colonoscopy patients with and without heartburn, 1670-1677, © 2003, with permission from American Gastroenterological Association.)

Long-segment Barrett's esophagus is found in 3% to 5% of patients who have endoscopy because of GERD symptoms, whereas 10% to 15% have the short-segment condition.[1] A recent study suggests that Barrett's esophagus is a common condition in the general population as well.[37] Among 961 patients scheduled for elective colonoscopy who agreed to have an UGI endoscopy performed for research purposes, Barrett's esophagus (predominantly short-segment) was found in 6.8%. Among the 556 patients who had no history of heartburn, Barrett's esophagus was found in 5.6%, whereas 8.3% of the 384 colonoscopy patients who complained of heartburn had Barrett's esophagus (Figure 3-6). The difference in the frequency of short-segment Barrett's esophagus between the patients with and without heartburn was not significant.

CANCER RISK AND ENDOSCOPIC SURVEILLANCE FOR BARRETT'S ESOPHAGUS

Published estimates on the annual risk of cancer in patients with Barrett's esophagus have ranged from 0.2% to 2.9%.[38,39] However, there is compelling evidence that the cancer risk in Barrett's esophagus had been overestimated for years because of publication bias (ie, the selective reporting of studies that have positive or extreme results).[39] Modern studies suggest that patients with Barrett's esophagus develop esophageal cancer at the rate of approximately 0.5% per year (ie, 1 cancer per 200 patients per year). Endoscopic surveillance is proposed to identify these neoplasms when they are in an early, curable stage. Although it is not clear that long- and short-segment Barrett's esophagus have the same risk for malignancy, the 2 conditions presently are managed similarly.

There are no randomized controlled trials proving that regular endoscopic surveillance decreases cancer mortality for patients with Barrett's esophagus. Observational studies have demonstrated that endoscopic surveillance can detect curable neoplasms in Barrett's esophagus and that cancers discovered during surveillance are less advanced than those found in patients who present with cancer symptoms like dysphagia and weight loss.[40] Those studies are not definitive, however, because they are subject to a number of biases that can inflate the value of surveillance programs.[41] Computer models also have suggested that screening and surveillance for Barrett's esophagus can prolong life provided certain assumptions are met.[42-44] For example, in one Markov model of 50-year-old patients who had an assumed annual cancer incidence rate of 0.4%, endoscopic surveillance every 5 years was found to be the preferred strategy, costing $98,000 per quality-adjusted life year gained.[44] In another computer model, however, endoscopic surveillance was found to add little to life expectancy, with enormous incremental cost.[42] Whereas these computer models incorporate numerous layers of questionable assumptions, their clinical utility is limited.

DYSPLASIA IN BARRETT'S ESOPHAGUS

Cancers in Barrett's esophagus evolve through a sequence of genetic (DNA) alterations that endow the affected cells with growth advantages.[45] Dysplasia can be viewed as the histological expression of those genetic alterations.[46] Pathologists diagnose dysplasia when they recognize a constellation of characteristic cytological and architectural abnormalities in tissue biopsy specimens (eg, nuclear enlargement, pleomorphism, hyperchromatism, and stratification; atypical mitoses and loss of cytoplasmic maturation; crowding of tubules and villiform surfaces). These abnormalities suggest that the tissue has sustained genetic damage resulting in clonal proliferations of cells with abnormal differentiation and a predisposition to malignancy. Dysplasia is categorized as low-grade or high-grade depending on the degree of histological abnormalities, with more pronounced abnormalities assumed to reflect more severe genetic damage and greater potential for carcinogenesis.

Unfortunately, dysplasia is an imperfect marker for malignancy in Barrett's esophagus for several reasons. Among experienced pathologists, interobserver agreement for the diagnosis of low-grade dysplasia in Barrett's esophagus is less than 50%.[47,48] Biopsy sampling error is another major problem. Cancers (missed because of sampling error) can be found in the resected esophagus of approximately one third of patients who have esophagectomy because of the finding of high-grade dysplasia.[49] The natural history of dysplasia is not well characterized, and published estimates of the 5-year cumulative esophageal cancer incidence for patients with high-grade dysplasia range widely, from 9% to 59%.[50-52] Alternative markers for cancer risk are being studied (eg, abnormalities in p53 expression and flow cytometry) as are endoscopic techniques that enable the endoscopist to identify abnormal tissue for biopsy sampling (eg, chromoendoscopy, endosonography, and fluorescence spectroscopy). Despite the many problems with dysplasia as a biomarker for malignancy, however, endoscopy with biopsy sampling for dysplasia remains the clinical standard for managing patients with Barrett's esophagus. It has been recommended that endoscopists should use a systematic, 4-quadrant biopsy sampling technique designed to maximize the chance of identifying an inconspicuous lesion that may be randomly distributed throughout the Barrett's esophagus. The superiority of this 4-quadrant biopsy technique over other sampling strategies has not been established, however.

There are 4 major management options for patients found to have high-grade dysplasia in Barrett's esophagus:

1. Esophagectomy.
2. Endoscopic ablative therapy.

3. Endoscopic mucosal resection (EMR).

4. Intensive surveillance

Esophagectomy is the only therapy that clearly can prevent the progression from dysplasia to cancer. Unfortunately, esophagectomy has an operative mortality rate of 3% to 20%.[46] The mortality rates for esophagectomy among institutions vary inversely with the frequency with which the operation is performed. In a study of data from the Dutch National Medical Registry, for example, the mortality rates for esophagectomy were 12.1%, 7.5%, and 4.9% at centers performing 1 to 10, 11 to 20, and >50 esophagectomies per year, respectively.[53] Esophagectomy also has a 30% to 50% rate of serious operative complications and substantial long-term morbidity.[46]

Endoscopic ablative therapies use thermal or photochemical energy to destroy the abnormal epithelium (eg, KTP, argon, neodymium:yttrium-aluminum-garnet [Nd: YAG] laser; multipolar electrocoagulation; argon plasma coagulation; photodynamic therapy).[54] The relative merits of the various endoscopic ablative therapies are disputed, and there appears to be a trade-off between the completeness of mucosal ablation and the frequency of complications. Serious side effects (eg, esophageal stricture formation) occur frequently with these treatments, and no study yet has demonstrated that ablative therapy decreases the long-term risk for cancer development in Barrett's esophagus.

In EMR, a diathermy snare or endoscopic knife is used to remove an entire segment of esophageal mucosa down to the submucosa.[55,56] Endoscopic ultrasonography is performed first, and, if there is no ultrasonographic evidence of extension into the submucosa, the endoscopist elevates the mucosal target by injecting fluid into the submucosa (eg, saline, saline with epinephrine, saline with dextrose, hyaluronic acid). For the snare EMR methods, the fluid-elevated mucosa is removed either by a strip biopsy technique using the snare alone or by a "suck and cut" technique in which the mucosa first is suctioned into a cap that fits over the tip of the endoscope and the snare is tightened around the suctioned area. In the endoscopic knife technique, a large segment of mucosa is dissected and removed en bloc. One major advantage of EMR over the endoscopic ablative techniques is that EMR provides large tissue specimens that can be examined by the pathologist to determine the character and extent of the lesion and the adequacy of resection. The results of preliminary studies on EMR for dysplasia in Barrett's esophagus are promising, but as yet too limited to make meaningful conclusions regarding the safety and efficacy of the technique.

Intensive surveillance for high-grade dysplasia involves endoscopic examinations every 3 to 6 months, and invasive therapies are withheld until biopsy specimens show adenocarcinoma. Few published data directly support the safety and efficacy of this practice, however, and published reports suggest that approximately 3% to 10% of cancers discovered in this fashion may be incurable.[52,57,58]

CHEMOPREVENTION FOR BARRETT'S ESOPHAGUS

A number of treatments have been proposed for cancer prevention in Barrett's esophagus. One evidence-based tool that can be used to determine whether the potential benefits of a treatment outweigh its disadvantages is the calculation of the number needed to treat (NNT) using the formula NNT = 1/ARR (ARR is the absolute risk reduction achieved by the treatment). Assume that there is a treatment for Barrett's esophagus that will reduce the risk of cancer development by 50% (ie, from 0.50% to

0.25%) per year. This represents an absolute risk reduction of 0.25%, or 0.0025. In this example, NNT = 1/0.0025 = 400. Thus, 400 patients would need to be treated in order to prevent 1 cancer in 1 year. Such a large NNT can only be acceptable if the treatment is very safe, inexpensive, and convenient.

Indirect evidence suggests that aggressive antisecretory therapy might prevent the development of cancer in Barrett's esophagus. For example, biopsy specimens of specialized intestinal metaplasia maintained in organ culture show hyperproliferation and increased expression of cyclooxygenase-2 (COX-2, a mediator of proliferation) when exposed to acid for 1 hour.[59,60] Brief esophageal acid exposure also activates the mitogen-activated protein kinase (MAPK) pathways that can increase proliferation and decrease apoptosis in Barrett's esophagus.[61] In Barrett's adenocarcinoma cells, acid exposure has been shown to increase COX-2 expression through activation of the MAPK pathways.[62] These observations suggest that acid reflux in patients with Barrett's esophagus might stimulate hyperproliferation, suppress apoptosis, and promote carcinogenesis in specialized intestinal metaplasia.

One group took biopsy specimens from 39 patients with Barrett's esophagus at baseline and after 6 months of therapy with PPIs given only in doses sufficient to eliminate GERD symptoms.[63] The expression of PCNA (a proliferation marker) decreased and the expression of villin (a differentiation marker) increased significantly in biopsy specimens from the 24 patients in whom PPIs normalized esophageal acid exposure, but not in the 15 with persistently abnormal acid reflux during PPI therapy. Another group found no significant change in the proliferative activity of Barrett's esophagus (as assessed by in vitro labeling with 5-bromo-2-deoxyuridine) in 22 patients treated with a PPI for 2 years, whereas proliferative activity increased significantly in 23 patients treated for the same time with an H2RA.[64]

During chronic PPI therapy, most patients develop islands of squamous epithelium within their metaplastic columnar lining.[65] This suggests that acid suppression induces partial regression of specialized intestinal metaplasia. It is not clear that this partial regression is beneficial, however. Biopsy specimens of the squamous islands show underlying intestinal metaplasia in approximately 40% of cases, suggesting that the islands may result from an overgrowth of squamous epithelium rather than a true regression of the metaplastic mucosa.[66] Furthermore, biopsy specimens from the squamous islands frequently exhibit abnormalities in Ki-67 staining (a proliferation marker) and p53 expression that might favor carcinogenesis.[67]

Finally, a recent study of 236 veteran patients with Barrett's esophagus who were followed for a total of 1170 patient-years has found that the use of PPIs is associated with a reduced incidence of dysplasia.[68] In a Kaplan-Meier survival analysis, the 10-year cumulative incidence of dysplasia was 21% for the 155 patients on PPI therapy, compared to 58% for the 81 patients treated with either a histamine H2-receptor antagonist or no antisecretory therapy.

Surgeons have proposed that fundoplication might be better than antisecretory therapy for preventing cancer in Barrett's esophagus.[69] Two small, uncontrolled studies found fewer cases of dysplasia and cancer among patients with Barrett's esophagus who had antireflux surgery than among those who had received medical treatment.[70,71] Some have proposed that antisecretory therapy itself might predispose to malignancy[72,73] and that the increasing use of antisecretory medications might underlie the rising frequency of esophageal adenocarcinoma in Western countries.[74] However, the limited studies that have addressed this issue directly have not found a significant association between esophageal adenocarcinoma and the use of antisecretory agents per se.[75,76]

A report describing the long-term outcome of a randomized trial of medical and surgical therapies for 247 veteran patients with complicated GERD does not support the contention that fundoplication prevents esophageal cancer better than antisecretory therapy.[23] During 10 to 13 years of follow-up, 4 of 165 patients (2.4%) in the medical group and 1 of 82 (1.2%) in the surgical group developed an esophageal adenocarcinoma. The difference between the treatment groups in the incidence of this tumor was not statistically significant but, with such a low observed rate of cancer development, the study did not have sufficient statistical power to detect small differences in the incidence of esophageal cancer. Another report describing the results of a large, Swedish, population-based cohort study also refutes the contention that antireflux surgery prevents cancer.[77] In this study, patients with GERD were followed for up to 32 years. The relative risk for developing esophageal adenocarcinoma (compared to the general population) among 35,274 men who received medical antireflux therapy was 6.3 (95% CI 4.5 to 8.7), whereas the relative risk for 6406 men treated with fundoplication was 14.1 (95% CI 8.0 to 22.8). These studies suggest that antireflux surgery should not be advised solely for cancer prophylaxis for patients with GERD and Barrett's esophagus.

Epidemiological studies suggest that aspirin and other NSAIDs, which inhibit cyclooxygenase (COX), might protect against cancer in Barrett's esophagus.[78] The specialized intestinal metaplasia of Barrett's esophagus exhibits increased expression of COX-2,[79] and inhibition of COX-2 has antiproliferative and proapoptotic effects in Barrett's-associated esophageal adenocarcinoma cell lines.[80] Furthermore, COX-2 inhibitors have been found to prevent the development of esophageal adenocarcinoma in an animal model of Barrett's esophagus.[81] Nevertheless, prospective clinical studies are needed before NSAIDs can be recommended for chemoprevention for patients with Barrett's esophagus in general, and specifically for patients with intestinal metaplasia at the GEJ.

Even if efficacy in cancer prevention could be demonstrated, it is not clear that the high cost and potential cardiovascular risks of the COX-2 selective NSAIDs would be justified for routine clinical use in patients with Barrett's esophagus. Aspirin, an inexpensive, nonselective NSAID that can prevent cardiovascular as well as neoplastic complications, might be a useful drug if its protective effects can be shown to outweigh its risk of GI complications. Presently, a large, controlled trial of aspirin for the chemoprophylaxis of Barrett's esophagus is underway in the United Kingdom.

MANAGEMENT RECOMMENDATIONS

No management strategy for patients with Barrett's esophagus has been proved to prolong life. Some of the controversies regarding the management of this condition were highlighted in a recent, critical review conducted by an 18-member panel of experts (the American Gastroenterology Association [AGA] Chicago workshop).[82] The management strategy that has been endorsed by the American College of Gastroenterology is arguably the most complete and widely followed of the published guidelines for the management of patients with Barrett's esophagus.[83] Their guidelines, with minor modifications, are as follows:

- Patients with Barrett's esophagus should have regular surveillance endoscopy to obtain esophageal biopsy specimens. GERD should be treated prior to surveillance to minimize confusion caused by inflammation in the interpretation of dysplasia.

- For patients who have had 2 consecutive endoscopies that show no dysplasia, surveillance endoscopy is recommended at an interval of every 3 years.

- If dysplasia is noted, another endoscopy should be performed with extensive biopsy sampling (especially from areas with mucosal irregularity) to look for invasive cancer, and the histology slides should be interpreted by an expert pathologist.

- For patients with verified low-grade dysplasia after extensive biopsy sampling, yearly surveillance endoscopy is recommended.

- For patients with verified, multifocal high-grade dysplasia, intervention (eg, esophagectomy) may be considered.

Although not specifically recommended in the practice guidelines, clinicians can consider the use of experimental endoscopic therapies such as photodynamic therapy or EMR for their patients with high-grade dysplasia in Barrett's esophagus, provided the therapy is administered as part of an established, approved research protocol. The use of endoscopic therapies outside of research protocols cannot be condoned at this time.

References

1. Spechler SJ. A 59-year-old woman with gastroesophageal reflux disease and Barrett esophagus. *JAMA.* 2003;289:466-475.
2. Spechler SJ. Epidemiology and natural history of gastro esophageal reflux disease. *Digestion.* 1992;51(suppl 1):24-29.
3. Higuchi D, Sugawa C, Shah SH, Tokioka S, Lucas CE. Etiology, treatment, and outcome of esophageal ulcers: a 10-year experience in an urban emergency hospital. *J Gastrointest Surg.* 2003;7:836-842.
4. Boonpongmanee S, Fleischer DE, Pezzullo JC, et al. The frequency of peptic ulcer as a cause of upper-GI bleeding is exaggerated. *Gastrointest Endosc.* 2004;59:788-794.
5. Cappell MS, Sciales C, Biempica L. Esophageal perforation at a Barrett's ulcer. *J Clin Gastroenterol.* 1989;11:663-666.
6. Diehl JT, Thomas L, Bloom MB, et al. Tracheoesophageal fistula associated with Barrett's ulcer: the importance of reflux control. *Ann Thorac Surg.* 1988;449-450.
7. Marks RD, Shukla M. Diagnosis and management of peptic esophageal strictures. *The Gastroenterologist.* 1996;4:223-237.
8. Spechler SJ. Barrett's esophagus. *N Engl J Med.* 2002;346:836-842.
9. Lagergren J, Bergstrom R, Lindgren A, Nyren O. Symptomatic gastroesophageal reflux as a risk factor for esophageal adenocarcinoma. *N Engl J Med.* 1999;340:825-831.
10. Brown LM, Devesa SS. Epidemiologic trends in esophageal and gastric cancer in the United States. *Surg Oncol Clin N Am.* 2002;11:235-256.
11. Cameron AJ. Epidemiology of columnar-lined esophagus and adenocarcinoma. *Gastroenterol Clin N Am.* 1997;26:487-494.

12. El-Serag HB, Petersen NJ, Carter J, et al. Gastroesophageal reflux among different racial groups in the United States. *Gastroenterology.* 2004;126:1692-1699.

13. Sonnenberg A, Massey BT, Jacobsen SJ. Hospital discharges resulting from esophagitis among Medicare beneficiaries. *Dig Dis Sci.* 1994;39:183-188.

14. Ho KY, Kang JY, Seow A. Prevalence of GI symptoms in a multiracial Asian population, with particular reference to reflux-type symptoms. *Am J Gastroenterol.* 1998;93:1816-1822.

15. Spechler SJ, Jain SK, Tendler DA, Parker RA. Racial differences in the frequency of symptoms and complications of gastroesophageal reflux disease. *Aliment Pharmacol Ther.* 2002;16:1795-1800.

16. Spechler SJ. Esophageal complications of gastroesophageal reflux disease: presentation, diagnosis, management, and outcome. *Clinical Cornerstone.* 2003;5:41-50.

17. Lundell LR, Dent J, Bennett JR, et al. Endoscopic assessment of esophagitis: clinical and functional correlates and further validation of the Los Angeles classification. *Gut.* 1999;45:172-180.

18. Triadafilopoulos G. Nonobstructive dysphagia in reflux esophagitis. *Am J Gastroenterol.* 1989;84:614-618.

19. Knill-Jones RP, Card WI, Crean GP, James WB, Spiegelhalter DJ. The symptoms of gastroesophageal reflux and esophagitis. *Scand J Gastroenterol.* 1984;19 (suppl 106):72-76.

20. Ott DJ. Gastroesophageal reflux disease. *Radiol Clin North Am.* 1994;32:1147-1166.

21. DeVault KR, Castell DO, and The Practice Parameters Committee of the American College of Gastroenterology. Updated guidelines for the diagnosis and treatment of gastroesophageal reflux disease. *Am J Gastroenterol.* 1999;94:1434-1442.

22. Klinkenberg-Knol EC, Nelis F, Dent J, et al. Long-term omeprazole treatment in resistant gastroesophageal reflux disease: efficacy, safety, and influence on gastric mucosa. *Gastroenterology.* 2000;118:661-669.

23. Spechler SJ, Lee E, Ahnen D, et al. Long-term outcome of medical and surgical treatments for gastroesophageal reflux disease. Follow-up of a randomized controlled trial. *JAMA.* 2001;285:2331-2338.

24. Vakil N, Shaw M, Kirby R. Clinical effectiveness of laparoscopic fundoplication in a U.S. community. *Am J Med.* 2003;114:1-5.

25. Wilcox CM, Alexander LN, Clark WS. Localization of an obstructing esophageal lesion. Is the patient accurate? *Dig Dis Sci.* 1995;40:2192-2196.

26. Luedtke P, Levine MS, Rubesin SE, Weinstein DS, Laufer I. Radiologic diagnosis of benign esophageal strictures: a pattern approach. *Radiographics.* 2003;23:897-909.

27. Ferguson R, Dronfield MW, Atkinson M. Cimetidine in treatment of reflux esophagitis with peptic stricture. *Br Med J.* 1979;2:472-474.

28. Farup PG, Modalsli B, Tholfsen JK. Long-term treatment with 300 mg ranitidine once daily after dilatation of peptic esophageal strictures. *Scand J Gastroenterol.* 1992;27:594-598.

29. Smith PM, Kerr GD, Cockel R, et al. A comparison of omeprazole and ranitidine in the prevention of recurrence of benign esophageal stricture. *Gastroenterology.* 1994;107:1312-1318.

30. Dakkak M, Hoare RC, Maslin SC, Bennett JR. Esophagitis is as important as esophageal stricture diameter in determining dysphagia. *Gut.* 1993;34:152-155.

31. Spechler SJ. AGA technical review on treatment of patients with dysphagia caused by benign disorders of the distal esophagus. *Gastroenterology.* 1999;117:233-254.

32. Wong DJ, Paulson TG, Prevo LJ, et al. p16(INK4a) lesions are common, early abnor-malities that undergo clonal expansion in Barrett's metaplastic epithelium. *Cancer Res.* 2001;61:8284-8289.

33. Maley CC, Galipeau PC, Xiaohong L, et al. The combination of genetic instability and clonal expansion predicts progression to esophageal adenocarcinoma. *Cancer Res.* 2004;64:7629-7633.

34. Sampliner RE and The Practice Parameters Committee of the American College of Gastroenterology. Updated guidelines for the diagnosis, surveillance, and therapy of Barrett's esophagus. *Am J Gastroenterol.* 2002;97:1888-1895.

35. Shaheen N, Ransohoff DF. Gastroesophageal reflux, Barrett esophagus, and esopha-geal cancer. *JAMA.* 2002;287:1972-1981.

36. Sharma P, Morales TG, Sampliner RE. Short segment Barrett's esophagus. The need for standardization of the definition and of endoscopic criteria. *Am J Gastroenterol.* 1998;93:1033-1036.

37. Rex DK, Cummings OW, Shaw M, et al. Screening for Barrett's esophagus in colonoscopy patients with and without heartburn. *Gastroenterology.* 2003;125:1670-1677.

38. Drewitz DJ, Sampliner RE, Garewal HS. The incidence of adenocarcinoma in Barrett's esophagus: a prospective study of 170 patients followed 4.8 years. *Am J Gastroenterol.* 1997;92:212-215.

39. Shaheen NJ, Crosby MA, Bozymski EM, Sandler RS. Is there publication bias in the reporting of cancer risk in Barrett's esophagus? *Gastroenterology.* 2000;119:333-338.

40. Corley DA, Levin TR, Habel LA, Weiss NS, Buffler PA. Surveillance and sur-vival in Barrett's adenocarcinomas: a population-based study. *Gastroenterology.* 2002;122:633-640.

41. Shaheen NJ, Provenzale D, Sandler RS. Upper endoscopy as a screening and surveil-lance tool in esophageal adenocarcinoma: a review of the evidence. *Am J Gastroenterol.* 2002;97:1319-1327.

42. Inadomi JM, Sampliner R, Lagergren J, Lieberman D, Fendrick AM, Vakil N. Screening and surveillance for Barrett esophagus in high-risk groups: a cost-utility analysis. *Ann Intern Med.* 2003;138:176-186.

43. Soni A, Sampliner RE, Sonnenberg A. Screening for high-grade dysplasia in gastroesophageal reflux disease: is it cost-effective? *Am J Gastroenterol.* 2000;95:2086-2093.

44. Provenzale D, Schmitt C, Wong JB. Barrett's esophagus: a new look at surveillance based on emerging estimates of cancer risk. *Am J Gastroenterol.* 1999;94:2043-2053.

45. Morales CP, Souza RF, Spechler SJ. Hallmarks of cancer progression in Barrett's esophagus. *Lancet.* 2002;360:1587-1589.

46. Spechler SJ. Dysplasia in Barrett's esophagus: limitations of current management strategies. *Am J Gastroenterol.* 2005;100(4):927-935.

47. Skacel M, Petras RE, Gramlich TL, Sigel JE, Richter JE, Goldblum JR. The diag-nosis of low-grade dysplasia in Barrett's esophagus and its implications for disease progression. *Am J Gastroenterol.* 2000;95:3383-3387.

48. Montgomery E, Bronner MP, Goldblum JR, et al. Reproducibility of the diagnosis of dysplasia in Barrett esophagus: a reaffirmation. *Hum Pathol.* 2001;32:368-378.

49. Collard JM. High-grade dysplasia in Barrett's esophagus. The case for esophagectomy. *Chest Surg Clin North Am.* 2002;12:77-92.

50. Reid BJ, Levine DS, Longton G, Blount PL, Rabinovitch PS. Predictors of progression to cancer in Barrett's esophagus: baseline histology and flow cytometry identify low- and high-risk patient subsets. *Am J Gastroenterol.* 2000;95:1669-1676.

51. Buttar NS, Wang KK, Sebo TJ, et al. Extent of high grade dysplasia in Barrett's esophagus correlates with risk of adenocarcinoma. *Gastroenterology.* 2001;120:1630-1639.

52. Schnell TG, Sontag SJ, Chejfec G, et al. Long-term nonsurgical management of Barrett's esophagus with high-grade dysplasia. *Gastroenterology.* 2001;120:1607-1619.

53. Van Lanschot JJB, Hulscher JBF, Buskens CJ, Tilanus HW, ten Kate FJW, Obertop H. Hospital volume and hospital mortality for esophagectomy. *Cancer.* 2001;91:1574-1578.

54. Sampliner RE. Endoscopic ablative therapy for Barrett's esophagus. *Gastrointest Endosc.* 2004;59:66-69.

55. Soetikno RM, Gotoda T, Nakanishi Y, Soehendra N. Endoscopic mucosal resection. *Gastrointest Endosc.* 2003;57:567-579.

56. Pech O, May A, Gossner L, Rabenstein T, Ell C. Management of pre-malignant and malignant lesions by endoscopic resection. *Best Pract Res Clin Gastroenterol.* 2004;18:61-76.

57. Reid BJ, Blount PL, Feng Z, Levine DS. Optimizing endoscopic biopsy detection of early cancers in Barrett's high-grade dysplasia. *Am J Gastroenterol.* 2000;95:3089-3096.

58. Weston AP, Sharma P, Topalovski M, Richards R, Cherian R, Dixon A. Long-term follow-up of Barrett's high-grade dysplasia. *Am J Gastroenterol.* 2000;95:1888-1893.

59. Fitzgerald RC, Omary MB, Triadafilopoulos G. Dynamic effects of acid on Barrett's esophagus. An ex vivo proliferation and differentiation model. *J Clin Invest.* 1996;98:2120-2128.

60. Shirvani VN, Ouatu-Lascar R, Kaur BS, Omary B, Triadafilopoulos G. Cyclooxygenase 2 expression in Barrett's esophagus and adenocarcinoma: ex vivo induction by bile salts and acid exposure. *Gastroenterology.* 2000;118:487-496.

61. Souza RF, Shewmake K, Terada LS, Spechler SJ. Acid exposure activates the mitogen activated protein kinase pathways in Barrett's esophagus. *Gastroenterology.* 2002;122:299-307.

62. Souza RF, Shewmake K, Pearson S, et al. Acid increases proliferation via ERK and p38 MAPK-mediated increases in cyclooxygenase-2 in Barrett's adenocarcinoma cells. *Am J Physiol.* 2004;287:G743-G748.

63. Ouatu-Lascar R, Fitzgerald RC, Triadafilopoulos G. Differentiation and proliferation in Barrett's esophagus and the effects of acid suppression. *Gastroenterology.* 1999;117:327-335.

64. Peters FT, Ganesh S, Kuipers EJ, et al. Effect of elimination of acid reflux on epithelial cell proliferative activity of Barrett esophagus. *Scand J Gastroenterol.* 2000;35:1238-1244.

65. Srinivasan R, Katz PO, Ramakrishnan A, Katzka DA, Vela MF, Castell DO. Maximal acid reflux control for Barrett's esophagus: feasible and effective. *Aliment Pharmacol Ther.* 2001;15:519-524.

66. Sharma P, Morales TG, Bhattacharyya A, Garewal HS, Sampliner RE. Squamous islands in Barrett's esophagus: what lies underneath? *Am J Gastroenterol.* 1998;93:332-335.

67. Garewal H, Ramsey L, Sharma P, Kraus K, Sampliner R, Fass R. Biomarker studies in reversed Barrett's esophagus. *Am J Gastroenterol.* 1999;94:2829-2833.

68. El-Serag H, Aguirre TV, Davis S, Kuebeler M, Bhattacharyya A, Sampliner RE. Proton pump inhibitors are associated with reduced incidence of dysplasia in Barrett's esophagus. *Am J Gastroenterol.* 2004;99:1877-1883.

69. DeMeester SR, DeMeester TR. Columnar mucosa and intestinal metaplasia of the esophagus. Fifty years of controversy. *Ann Surg.* 2000;231:303-321.

70. McCallum RW, Polepalle S, Davenport K, Frierson H, Boyd S. Role of anti-reflux surgery against dysplasia in Barrett's esophagus. *Gastroenterology.* 1991;100:A121.

71. Katz D, Rothstein R, Schned A, Dunn J, Seaver K, Antonioli D. The development of dysplasia and adenocarcinoma during endoscopic surveillance of Barrett's esophagus. *Am J Gastroenterol.* 1998;93:536-541.

72. Theisen J, Nehra D, Citron D, et al. Suppression of gastric acid secretion in patients with gastroesophageal reflux disease results in gastric bacterial overgrowth and deconjugation of bile acids. *J Gastrointest Surg.* 2000;4:50-54.

73. Kauer WKH, Peters JH, DeMeester TR, Ireland AP, Bremner CG, Hagen JA. Mixed reflux of gastric and duodenal juices is more harmful to the esophagus than gastric juice alone. The need for surgical therapy re-emphasized. *Ann Surg.* 1995;222:525-533.

74. Wetscher GJ, Hinder RA, Smyrk T, Perdikis G, Adrian TE, Profanter C. Gastric acid blockade with omeprazole promotes gastric carcinogenesis induced by duodenogastric reflux. *Dig Dis Sci.* 1999;44:1132-1135.

75. Chow WH, Findkle WD, McLaughlin JK, Frankl H, Ziel HK, Fraumeni JF Jr. The relation of gastroesophageal reflux disease and its treatment to adenocarcinomas of the esophagus and gastric cardia. *JAMA.* 1995;274:474-477.

76. Garrow DC, Vaughan TL, Sweeney C, et al. Gastroesophageal reflux disease, use of H2 receptor antagonists, and risk of esophageal and gastric cancer. *Cancer Causes Control.* 2000;11:231-238.

77. Ye W, Chow WH, Lagergren J, Yin L, Nyren O. Risk of adenocarcinoma of the esophagus and gastric cardia in patients with gastroesophageal reflux diseases and after antireflux surgery. *Gastroenterology.* 2001;121:1286-1293.

78. Corley DA, Kerlikowske K, Verma R, Buffler P. Protective association of aspirin/NSAIDs and esophageal cancer: a systematic review and meta-analysis. *Gastroenterology.* 2003;124:47-56.

79. Wilson KT, Fu S, Ramanujam KS, Meltzer SJ. Increased expression of inducible nitric oxide synthase and cyclooxygenase-2 in Barrett's esophagus and associated adenocarcinomas. *Cancer Res.* 1998;58:2929-2934.

80. Souza RF, Shewmake K, Beer DG, Cryer B, Spechler SJ. Selective inhibition of cyclooxygenase-2 suppresses growth and induces apoptosis in human esophageal adenocarcinoma cells. *Cancer Res.* 2000;60:5767-5772.

81. Buttar NS, Wang KK, Leontovich O, et al. Chemoprevention of esophageal adenocarcinoma by COX-2 inhibitors in an animal model of Barrett's esophagus. *Gastroenterology.* 2002;122:1101-1112.

82. Sharma P, McQuaid K, Dent J, et al. A critical review of the diagnosis and management of Barrett's esophagus: the AGA Chicago Workshop. *Gastroenterology.* 2004;127:310-330.

83. Spechler SJ. The role of gastric carditis in metaplasia and neoplasia at the gastroesophageal junction. *Gastroenterology.* 1999;117:218-228.

Surgical Treatment of Gastroesophageal Reflux Disease

Daniel T. Dempsey, MD, FACS

Introduction

Fundoplication is an effective treatment for severe GERD. Until the early 1990s, this operation was performed through either an upper abdominal or thoracic incision. The ability to perform the identical operation laparoscopically has revolutionized the surgical treatment of GERD. Appropriate patient evaluation, selection, and management by a multidisciplinary team including surgeon, gastroenterologist, and primary care physician will help ensure good outcomes.

Terminology

A Nissen fundoplication is a 360-degree fundic wrap around the lower esophagus and GEJ (Figure 4-1).[1] This is the gold standard operation for reflux. Henceforth, when the term fundoplication is used in this chapter it means a complete 360-degree fundic wrap unless otherwise indicated. The term Nissen-Rossetti is also a complete 360-degree fundic wrap, but the term implies that the fundus has not been completely mobilized from the spleen by division of the short gastric vessels. The Toupet fundoplication is a posterior partial fundoplication (usually about 270 degrees) (Figure 4-2), and the Dor fundoplication is an anterior partial fundoplication (usually about 180 degrees) (Figure 4-3).[2,3] The extent of fundic mobilization with these partial wraps is variable. All these operations are now most commonly performed laparoscopically, and numerous clinical series have shown that all are reasonably effective in decreasing GERD as assessed by both symptom scores and 24-hour pH-metry. We will discuss their relative efficacy below.

The Hill procedure involves suturing the GEJ to the preaortic fascia. This operation can be done laparoscopically and although not widely used, it is an effective antireflux operation in experienced hands. The Belsey-Mark IV operation is a transthoracic antireflux procedure that "inkwells" the lower esophagus into the cardia of the stomach. It is not used much nowadays because it is difficult to perform with

Figure 4-1. Nissen fundoplication (360-degree wrap). Usually implies full fundic mobilization with ligation of short gastric vessels whereas Nissen-Rossetti is 360-degree wrap without division of short gastrics. (Reprinted with permission from Laws HL, Clements RH, Swillie CM. A randomized, prospective comparison of the Nissen fundoplication versus the Toupet fundoplication for gastroesophageal reflux disease. *Ann Surg.* 1997;225(6):647-654.)

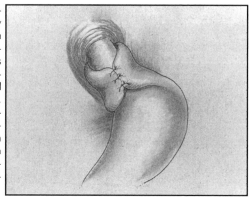

Figure 4-2. Toupet fundoplication, a posterior hemi fundoplication. (Reprinted with permission from Katkhouda N, Khalil MR, Manhas S, et al. Andre Toupet: surgeon technician par excellence. *Ann Surg.* 2002;235(4):591-599.)

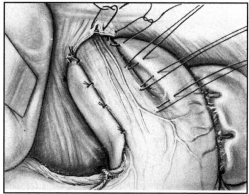

Figure 4-3. Dor anterior hemi-fundoplication, here added to an esophagomyotomy in a patient with achalasia. (Reprinted with permission from Hunter JG, Trus TL, Branum GD, Waring JP. Laparoscopic Heller myotomy and fundoplication for achalasia. *Ann Surg.* 1997;225(6):655-665.)

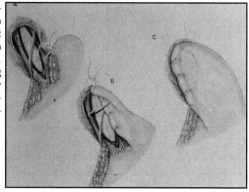

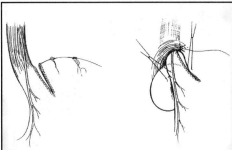

Figure 4-4. Collis gastroplasty "lengthens" a short esophagus by tubularizing gastric cardia. Here, a posterior hemifundoplication is added. (Reprinted with permission from Jobe BA, Horvath KD, Swanstrom LL. Postoperative function following laparoscopic collis gastroplasty for shortened esophagus. *Arch Surg.* 1998;133(8):867-874. © 1998, American Medical Association. All rights reserved.)

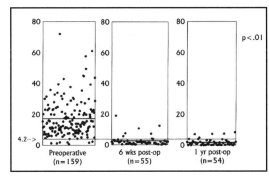

Figure 4-5. Twenty-four hour ambulatory pH study. Laparoscopic fundoplication-controlled pH in 87% of patients studied 6 weeks after operation and 91% of patients studied 1 year after operation. (Reprinted with permission from Hunter JG, Trus TL, Branum GD, Waring JP, Wood WC. A physiologic approach to laparoscopic fundoplication for gastroesophageal reflux disease. *Ann Surg.* 1996;223(6):673-687.)

minimally invasive techniques. The Collis gastroplasty is an esophageal lengthening procedure and fundoplication that may rarely be useful in the event of a "short esophagus" (Figure 4-4),[4] a phenomenon much more commonly written about than encountered clinically. When the above operations are performed for GERD, any concomitant hiatal hernia is repaired.

Pathophysiology of Gastroesophageal Reflux Disease and How Fundoplication Works

A variety of physiologic abnormalities have been described in patients with GERD. These include high esophageal acid exposure, low LES pressure, inappropriate LES relaxation, delayed esophageal clearance of acid, decreased effectiveness of distal esophageal motility, and delayed gastric emptying. Nissen fundoplication (and in some cases partial fundoplication) has been shown to normalize all of these abnormalities.

Distal esophageal acid exposure is normalized by fundoplication (Figure 4-5),[5] as is the pressure profile of the LES (Table 4-1).[6] Following fundoplication, the LES pressure exceeds the intragastric pressure over a very wide range of pressures tested.[7] Fundoplication also minimizes inappropriate LES relaxation (Figure 4-6)[8] and increases the effectiveness of distal esophageal peristalsis (Figure 4-7).[5] Finally, any

Table 4-1

LOWER ESOPHAGEAL SPHINCTER BEFORE AND AFTER FUNDOPLICATION

Characteristic	Before Fundoplication	After Fundoplication	p
Total LES length, mm	23.6 (21.0 to 26.5)	39.0 (34.5 to 42.2)	0.006
Intra-abdominal length, mm	16.1 (15.2 to 19.7)	30/8 (23.1 to 38.1)	0.006
LES pressure, mmHg	9.2 (5.9 to 12.2	14.1 (9.6 to 18.4)	0.03

* Data are given as the median (and interquartile range).

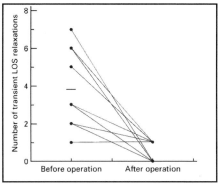

Figure 4-6. Fundoplication decreases the frequency of transient LES relaxations. (Effect of fundoplication on transient lower esophageal sphincter relaxation and gas reflux. Johnsson F, Holloway RH, Ireland AC, Jamieson GG, Dent J. *Br J Surg.* 1997;84(5):686-689. © British Journal of Surgery Society Ltd. Reproduced with permission. Permission is granted by John Wiley & Sons Ltd on behalf of BJSS Ltd.)

preoperative delay in gastric emptying is very likely to be much improved following fundoplication (Table 4-2).[9] This makes a concomitant gastric emptying procedure unnecessary even in most patients with significant preoperative delay in gastric emptying. The mechanisms for this catalogue of beneficial effects are poorly understood. Putative mechanisms explaining the above-described benefits are shown in Table 4-3.

Indications for Operation in Gastroesophageal Reflux Disease

Operation should be reserved for patients with severe GERD (ie, those patients with GERD complications) or those whose disease cannot be adequately managed

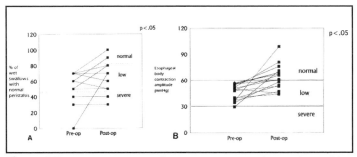

Figure 4-7. In some patients with poor transmission of peristalsis and low amplitude esophageal body pressure, peristalsis and amplitude of pressure waves may improve following fundoplication. (Reprinted with permission from Hunter JG, Trus TL, Branum GD, Waring JP, Wood WC. A physiologic approach to laparoscopic fundoplication for gastroesophageal reflux disease. *Ann Surg.* 1996;223(6):673-687.)

medically.[10] Patients with debilitating typical reflux symptoms requiring continuous high dose PPIs should also be considered for surgical evaluation, especially patients with large hiatal hernia and low LES pressure. Patients presenting with ulcerative esophagitis, Barrett's esophagus, or stricture may benefit from operation too. Patients with symptoms managed well with intermittent use of OTC products should generally not be considered candidates for antireflux operation.

Typical (primary) symptoms of GERD include heartburn, regurgitation, and/or intermittent (usually cervical) dysphagia. Atypical (secondary) symptoms of GERD include chest pain, asthma, laryngitis, and oropharyngeal complaints. In general, patients with heartburn and/or regurgitation do very well with fundoplication, with patient satisfaction above 90%. Patients with secondary symptoms as the chief complaint don't do as well.[11] Amelioration of the chief presenting symptom with high dose PPI is most encouraging that a good response to fundoplication will be achieved. Failure of the GERD patient to respond symptomatically to high-dose PPI is quite concerning and may herald an unsatisfied patient after fundoplication. Operation may still be indicated in these patients if preoperative testing confirms GERD (acid or alkaline) and reasonably normal esophageal function. Whether patients with visceral hypersensitivity (eg, severe symptoms from physiologic amounts of reflux) benefit from fundoplication is unclear. The best results with laparoscopic fundoplication for GERD are achieved by experienced surgeons in patients with typical symptoms and documented acid reflux who respond to PPIs (Table 4-4).[12]

As our society becomes more overweight, an increasing number of patients referred for antireflux surgery are morbidly obese. It should be recognized that a fundoplication might be less durable in a significantly overweight patient. Patients with body mass index (BMI) over 40 and pathologic GERD may be better served with a gastric bypass operation.[13] This procedure (Figure 4-8)[14] creates a small proximal gastric pouch that does not produce much acid. This diminutive pouch is drained into a long Roux limb, which prevents bile from coming into the proximal gastric pouch. Thus, there is only a small amount of acid and no bile to reflux into the esophagus. Although the operative mortality risk of a gastric bypass (0.5% to 1%) is somewhat

Table 4-2

FUNDOPLICATION NORMALIZES GASTRIC EMPTYING IN MANY GASTROESOPHAGEAL REFLUX DISEASE PATIENTS WITH PREOPERATIVE DELAY IN GASTRIC EMPTYING

Gastric Emptying for Solid Food	Normal Preoperative Gastric Emptying (n = 26)			Delayed Preoperative Gastric Emptying (n = 10)		
	Preoperative	Postoperative	P	Preoperative	Postoperative	P
Lag phase (min)	26.2 (11.6	15.1)9.7)	<.01	37.9 (21.6)	17.7 (9.7)	.017
Emptying rate (%/n)	35.2 (8.0)	47.7 (12.6)	<.01	15.2 (7.5)	42.0 (15.0)	<.01
T$_{50}$	115.1 (21.1)	82.7 (24.1)	<.01	390.3 (440.5)	82.3 (29.7)	.05

Values are expressed as means (SD).

Reprinted with permission from Bais JE, Samsom M, Boudesteijn EA, van Rijk PP, Akkermans LM, Gooszen HG. Impact of delayed gastric emptying on the outcome of antireflux surgery. Ann Surg. 2001;234(2):139-146.

Table 4-3

POSSIBLE MECHANISMS OF BENEFICIAL EFFECTS OF FUNDOPLICATION IN GASTROESOPHAGEAL REFLUX DISEASE

Benefit	Possible Mechanisms
Restore LES pressure profile	Maintain lower esophageal/LES in abdomen
	Buttress or reorient gastric sling fibers
	Transmit intragastric pressure to lower esophageal/LES
Decrease inappropriate LES relax	Decrease in fundic distention
	Interfere with intrinsic neural reflex
Improve lower esophageal peristalsis	Decreased mucosal inflammation improves muscle function
	Keep esophagus at optimum length for contraction
Improve gastric emptying	Decrease in fundic compliance
	Interference with accommodation/receptive relaxation

Table 4-4

PREDICTORS OF SUCCESS FOLLOWING LAPAROSCOPIC FUNDOPLICATION

Predictor	Odds Ratio* (95% CI)	Walds's p Value
Positive pH score	8.2 (2.7 to 25)	<0.001
Typical symptom	6.9 (2.4 to 19.6)	<0.001
Good response to medical Rx	4.5 (1.6 to 12.3)	<0.004

*Odds of success compared to not present.

Reprinted from *J Gastrointest Surg*, 3(3), Campos GM, Peters JH, DeMeester TR, et al, Multivariate analysis of factors predicting outcome after laparoscopic Nissen fundoplication, 292-300, © 1999, with permission from Society for the Surgery of the Alimentary Tract.

Figure 4-8. Roux-en-Y gastric bypass. (Reprinted with permission from Higa KD, Boone KB, Ho T, Davies OG. Laparoscopic Roux-en-Y gastric bypass for morbid obesity: technique and preliminary results of our first 400 patients. *Arch Surg.* 2000;135(9):1029-1034. © 2000, American Medical Association. All rights reserved.)

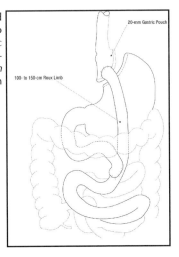

greater than fundoplication (<0.5%), the long-term results—both in terms of reflux symptoms as well as overall health benefit to the patient—may favor the larger operation. Finally, it must be recognized that laparoscopic fundoplication in an already obese patient may be associated with further weight gain as reflux symptoms are eliminated. Redo fundoplication or gastric bypass operation in such a patient who has had a fundoplication is more complicated[15] and potentially less effective (because it may be difficult to create a very small proximal gastric pouch).

Preoperative Evaluation

Is this patient a candidate for antireflux surgery? The answer to this question usually requires an evaluation by an experienced gastroenterologist and surgeon, and sometimes substantial clinical judgment. It may be appropriate for the primary care physician to refer the patient with GERD symptoms and/or complications to an experienced antireflux surgeon in order to discuss the risks and benefits of operation. If, after such discussion, both the patient and surgeon agree that fundoplication is a reasonable consideration, a complete preoperative workup is carried out. This includes upper endoscopy, esophageal motility testing, and usually esophageal pH testing. More commonly in many regions, the patient is seen and managed first by the gastroenterologist who may request surgical consultation in patients with refractory or complicated disease. This team approach is most helpful for the surgeon, especially in difficult preoperative and postoperative patients.

In general, the likelihood of a poor outcome following antireflux operation in well selected and properly evaluated patients is 5% or less, and the operative mortality risk is less than 0.5% (see outcomes below). When evaluating the patient, it should be recognized that healthy patients with typical GERD symptoms and preoperative test results do the best, while unhealthy patients with atypical GERD symptoms and atypical preoperative test results do worse. If the surgeon and gastroenterologist agree—on the basis of symptomatology and/or comorbidities—that the patient is a

Table 4-5

FACTORS ASSOCIATED WITH LONG SEGMENT BARRETT'S ESOPHAGUS

Variable	Odds Ratio (95% CI)	p value
Hiatal hernia		
>4 cm	17.8 (4.1 to 76.6)	<0.001
2 to 4 cm	8.5 (2.3 to 31.7)	0.002
Defective LES	16.9 (1.6 to 181.4)	0.02
Longest reflux episode		
<31.7 min	8.1 (2.8 to 24.0)	<0.001
19.9 to 31.7 min	6.8 (2.3 to 20.1)	0.001

* Baseline values are for short segment Barrett's esophagus. CI indicates confidence interval; LES, lower esophageal sphincter.

Reprinted with permission from Campos GM, DeMeester SR, Peters JH, et al. Predictive factors of Barrett esophagus: multivariate analysis of 502 patients with gastroesophageal reflux disease. *Arch Surg.* 2001;136(11):1267-1273. © 2001, American Medical Association. All rights reserved.

poor candidate for surgery, then there may be no point in completing the preoperative evaluation. Otherwise the preoperative evaluation should be completed and the results reviewed between patient, gastroenterologist, surgeon, and primary physician.

Esophagoscopy is necessary in all preoperative patients, both to rule out confounding diseases (eg, tumor, paraesophageal hernia) and to evaluate the severity of the esophagitis and reflux complications (eg, Barrett's metaplasia, stricture). Mucosal biopsy is usually indicated. It should be recognized that gross esophagitis may respond well to intensive antireflux medication, even though symptoms remain bothersome.[16] Barium swallow is occasionally useful for the surgeon (eg, to judge the size of hiatal hernia, the likelihood of short esophagus, or the location of an esophageal stricture).

Preoperative esophageal motility testing is somewhat controversial because it has been shown (at least in high volume centers) that tailoring the wrap based on this information does not improve results with fundoplication, nor does the information predict outcomes.[17,18] However, we feel that some sort of evaluation of esophageal motor function is necessary in all patients prior to fundoplication. Usually, this is done with esophageal manometry, but esophageal impedance testing may be added or a dedicated contrast esophagography by an experienced radiologist may be substituted in the occasional patient. Although we would admit that this usually does not change our decision for surgery or our operative approach, we continue to find occasional surprises that in the individual patient may have a significant effect. Furthermore, patients with profoundly decreased LES pressures (eg, <8 mmHg) tend to have the most severe disease (Table 4-5) and may benefit most from fundoplication.[19,20]

Relative contraindications to antireflux operation include significant dysmotility in the esophageal body, significantly elevated LES pressure, and/or incomplete LES relaxation. Normal LES pressure or low pressure esophageal peristaltic waves do not contraindicate fundoplication, although if severe (distal peristaltic amplitude <20 mmHg) the latter may indicate partial fundoplication depending on the clinical circumstances.

Esophageal pH testing may be useful as part of the preoperative evaluation. This technique is generally accepted as the gold standard for the diagnosis of GERD (ie, if a patient has normal pH-metry off acid suppressive medication, another diagnosis should be entertained). A diagnosis of GERD made on the basis of symptoms and esophagoscopy may be erroneous one third of the time.[20] Together with manometry, pH testing can define patients at the very tip of the "GERD iceberg" (ie, those at risk for the most severe complications such as stricture and Barrett's esophagus) (Table 4-6).[20] Certainly comparison of preoperative to postoperative pH data may be the best way to evaluate the physiologic function of a wrap in the postoperative patient with persistent or recurrent symptoms. Esophageal pH testing is typically done with a small nasoesophageal pH catheter probe placed under manometric (optimal) or radiologic guidance and left in place for about 24 hours. The number and length of low (<4) pH episodes is integrated into a "DeMeester score." Recently, the Bravo capsule seems to be gaining greater patient and physician acceptance. This device is endoscopically attached to the distal esophageal mucosa and transmits pH data to an extracorporeal recorder before it falls off 48 hours later.[21] These tests are most useful to the surgeon when performed with the patient off all antisecretory agents. Unfortunately, a gastroenterologist sometimes performs them with the patient on medication to assess whether acid suppression is optimal, and the patient and/or the insurance company is loath to repeat the test off medication preoperatively. In the occasional patient, assessment of duodenogastroesophageal reflux may be helpful.[22] This can be done with a nasoesophageal probe that detects bilirubin, or with scintigraphy at an experienced center.

GI scintigraphy may be useful in selected patients. The routine addition of a gastric emptying procedure to fundoplication in patients with significantly delayed gastric emptying is unnecessary and mettlesome.[9,23] However, if the patient referred for antireflux operation has a preponderance of epigastric symptoms, nausea, and/or vomiting, we continue to recommend a gastric emptying scan because this may lead to useful baseline information and/or facilitate the informed consent discussion prior to operation. This test should certainly be considered in all patients with a suboptimal result following antireflux operation and in all patients being considered for reoperation. Pre-existing idiopathic gastroparesis or postvagotomy gastroparesis may compromise the clinical outcome after fundoplication. Further testing of vagal integrity (eg, serum pancreatic polypeptide response to sham feeding) may be necessary to prove the latter diagnosis. The experienced nuclear medicine physician may use a variant of the HIDA biliary scan to provide the gastroenterologist or surgeon with useful semiquantitative information on duodenogastroesophageal (ie, alkaline) reflux.[24] Other occasionally useful scintigraphic tests in the GERD patient include esophageal transit and GER scans.

Table 4-6

HIGHER ACID REFLUX ON pH MONITORING INDICATES SEVERE DISEASE

	Group B1 (score <70; 430 patients)	Group B2 (score ≥ 70; 145 patients)	p
Age (year)	49 ± 15	51 ± 13	NS
Symptom duration	85 ± 102	113 ± 112	0.006
Heartburn (% patients)	80	94	0.001
Hiatal hernia (% patients)	34	41	0.001
Grade III esophagitis (% patients)	8	19	0.001
LES pressure (mmHg)	11 ± 5	8 ± 5	0.001
NSEMD (% patients)	45	64	0.001
pH 5 cm above LES			
Reflux episodes (N)	133 ± 73	244 ± 143	0.001
Time pH <4 (total) (%)	10 ± 4	33 ± 16	0.001
Time pH <4 (upright) (%)	11 ± 6	29 ± 16	0.001
Time pH <4 (supine) (%)	7 ± 6	38 ± 22	0.001
Acid clearance (min)	0.8 ± 1.2	1.8 ± 4.4	0.001
pH 20 cm above LES			
Reflux episodes (N)	35 ± 37	52 ± 46	0.001
Time pH <4 (total) (%)	2 ± 2	5 ± 10	0.001
Time pH <4 (upright) (%)	2 ± 3	3 ± 5	0.001
Time pH <4 (supine) (%)	1 ± 3	6 ± 10	0.001
Acid clearance (min)	1.2 ± 1.1	3.3 ± 6.6	0.001

LES = lower esophageal sphincter; NSEMD = nonspecific esophageal motility disorder (based on amplitude, duration, velocity, and morphology of peristaltic waves).

Reprinted with permission from Patti MG, Diener U, Tamburini A, Molena D, Way LW. Role of esophageal function tests in diagnosis of gastroesophageal reflux disease. *Dig Dis Sci.* 2001;46(3):597-602.

Choice of Operation

Laparoscopic fundoplication is the procedure of choice for the large majority of surgical candidates with severe GERD. Most surgical experts favor a complete 360-degree wrap (a floppy 2-cm wrap) in the majority of patients because experience suggests that this is a more durable and dependable barrier to reflux in the typical surgical patient.[5,25] This remains controversial (see below). In the occasional patient with profound esophageal hypomotility (eg, scleroderma or achalasia), partial fundoplication is the preferred surgical antireflux option. Reduction and repair of hiatal hernia is an essential part of any antireflux operation. Laparoscopic fundoplication is performed under general anesthesia usually with 5 laparoscopic ports. Fundoplication can be performed laparoscopically in 98% of patients who have not had previous upper abdominal surgery. Even in this latter group, laparoscopic fundoplication is likely to be accomplished by an experienced surgeon.

The essential technical aspects of fundoplication are generally agreed upon.[5] The stomach should be nasally or orally intubated and decompressed if it is at all distended at the beginning of the operation. Distal esophageal mobilization ensures that at least 3 cm of distal esophagus rests comfortably in the abdomen. Together with posterior crural repair using nonabsorbable suture (ie, reconstituting a normal-sized diaphragmatic esophageal hiatus by suturing the right and left crural pillars together posterior to the esophagus), this fixes the sliding hiatal hernia in nearly all patients. Adequate fundic mobilization ensures a tension-free floppy wrap that does not distort the GEJ. The diaphragmatic esophageal hiatus is reconstituted by suturing the right and left crural pillars together posterior to the esophagus (posterior crural repair), care being taken to avoid constricting the esophagus. The "shoe-shine" maneuver ensures that the correct fundic flaps have been chosen to make the wrap, that there is no twisting, and that there is adequate length between flaps to easily encircle a 52 French dilator. The wrap must be short, floppy, and anchored to the distal esophagus. It must lay easily in the abdomen; some surgeons anchor the wrap to the crural diaphragm with sutures. Routine postoperative nasogastric intubation is unnecessary.

Outcomes With Antireflux Operation

Fundoplication is a very safe operation with an operative mortality risk of <0.5% (Table 4-7).[26] There are many series (published and unpublished) of several hundred operations without a perioperative death. Serious complications are rare and include intraoperative perforation of the esophagus, stomach, or bowel; pneumothorax; hemorrhage (1% of fundoplication patients require a transfusion); splenectomy; and pancreatitis. Other more common complications include atelectasis and ileus. Most patients experience no significant complication and can be discharged home on a liquid diet within 24 hours of operation. Some surgeons (including the author) continue to perform a limited upper GI study in the early postoperative period. This is admittedly unnecessary unless the recovery is complicated by signs and symptoms that suggest a problem (eg, leak, total obstruction of the distal esophagus, acute herniation of the wrap). However, the information gained from this test assures the surgeon of a good anatomic result and provides a baseline for future studies should the patient develop symptoms months or years in the future. In this era of early hospital discharge, it is also reassuring to know that both the esophagus and stomach empty easily and that there is no unrecognized leak.

Table 4-7

COMPLICATIONS OF LAPAROSCOPIC FUNDOPLICATION
N = 2453

Parameter	Number	Percent (%)
Mortality	4	0.2
Conversion	143	5.8
Early dysphagia	500	20
Late dysphagia	114	5.5
Reoperation for dysphagia	18	0.9

Reprinted with permission from Perdikis G, Hinder RA, Lund RJ, Raiser F, Katada N. Laparoscopic Nissen fundoplication: where do we stand? *Surgical Laparoscopy & Endoscopy.* 1997;7(1):17-21.

Patients are discharged home on antisecretory medication (we continue whatever medications the patient was taking preoperatively) and a liquid diet (no carbonation). Narcotic analgesia in decreasing amounts should be needed only for about 3 to 5 days. Some dysphagia and early satiety are extremely common for the first few days or weeks after fundoplication. Frequent communication and reassurance are helpful for many patients; the surgeon and staff must understand and welcome this. The diet is advanced slowly (every few days a change can be made) as tolerated, first to soft food then to regular food. The patient must be instructed to eat slowly and chew food thoroughly. Antisecretory agents are tapered after the first postoperative month.

It is very common for the patient to lose 5% of body weight postoperatively, with the nadir reached at 10 to 14 days. We ask our patients to record weekly weights for the first month. This information is helpful in assessing the significance of postoperative complaints. Because most postoperative complaints resolve spontaneously in 2 to 3 months and because most patients do not have problems with excessive perioperative weight loss and dehydration, it is extremely important that early unnecessary dilation or reoperation be avoided. We have seen several patients who had dilations of the wrap 1 month postoperatively (despite the fact that they were tolerating a soft diet with stable weight) and then at 3 months had recurrent reflux symptoms presumably from loosened or disrupted wrap. On the other hand, severe early dysphagia associated with rapid weight loss and dehydration is an indication for contrast radiography and EGD and may necessitate early dilation or reoperation. Early reoperation (within the first week) is clearly preferred if there is an identifiable radiographic or endoscopic anatomic abnormality. Failure of the patient to tolerate a liquid diet after endoscopic dilation is another indication for early reoperation. Reoperation becomes much more difficult technically during the period 2 to 6 weeks after the initial operation.

The true durability of fundoplication is unknown, but probably at best it is around 90% at 10 years. That is, if one performs 100 wraps and follows those 100 patients for

Table 4-8

Open Fundoplication vs Medical Treatment for Gastroesophageal Reflux Disease: Long-Term Follow-Up

Outcome During 140 Months	Surgical	Medical	RBR (95% CI)[†]	NNH (CI)[†]
Survival	60%	72%	20% (0.5 to 33)	7 (5 to 283)
Outcomes at Mean 10 year			RRR (CI)	NNT (CI)
Any antireflux medication	62%	92%	33% (17 to 50)	4 (3 to 7)
PPI use	32%	64%	49% (21 to 70)	4 (3 to 9)
Histamine 2 receptor blocker use	41%	65%	37% (8.7 to 60)	5 (3 to 20)

RBR = relative benefit reduction.
[†] Calculated using Cox proportional-hazards data.

10 years, close to 90 patients will still have a functioning wrap. In a series of 100 open fundoplications, DeMeester et al reported the 10-year actuarial percentage of patients with intact functioning wraps as 90%.[27] This may be overly optimistic. Spechler et al recently provided 10-year follow-up on a randomized prospective multicenter Veterans Administration trial comparing open fundoplication to medical therapy for GERD and noted that most patients in both groups were currently taking antisecretory medication (Table 4-8).[28] Interestingly, the 10-year actuarial patient survival was lower in the surgical group. The initial report clearly showed that fundoplication was significantly better than H2 receptor antagonist treatment in patients with severe symptomatic reflux.[29] At 1 year, another randomized prospective trial strongly favored laparoscopic fundoplication over PPIs.[30] Substantial 10-year follow-up data on laparoscopic fundoplication is not yet available.

Table 4-9

ANATOMIC FINDINGS IN REDO FUNDOPLICATION

Operative Findings	Internal Primary Fundoplication n = 54	External Primary Fundoplication n = 187
Hiatal hernia	61	47
Wrap disruption	6	7
Slipped wrap	13	11
Crural stenosis	0	2
Twisted wrap	2	5*
Misplaced wrap	2†	11
Other‡	0	1‡
Unknown	17	17

* Inadequate fundus mobilization.
† p <0.05.
‡ Foreign body removal.

Reprinted with permission from Smith CD, McClusky DA, Rajad MA, Lederman AB, Hunter JG. When fundoplication fails: redo? *Ann Surg.* 2005;241(6):861-871.

Reoperative Fundoplication

It can be anticipated that 3% to 5% of patients will require repeat fundoplication for new or recurrent symptoms, usually within the first 2 years following the original fundoplication.[31] Redo fundoplication should only be performed in symptomatic patients with documented physiologic abnormalities (eg, positive pH-metry) and/or anatomic defects (eg, wrap herniation). It is important to understand that new or recurrent symptoms may not indicate recurrent reflux or a dysfunctional wrap.[32] Thus, thorough re-evaluation is important prior to any consideration of reoperation. The most common indications for redo fundoplication are dysphagia, GERD, and paraesophageal hernia. At reoperation, at least 50% of the patients will have some sort of hiatal herniation and 25% will have a slipped or misplaced wrap (Table 4-9). Most redo operations can be completed successfully laparoscopically in experienced hands, but the operative risk is about double the initial operation and long-term patient satisfaction is less (about 75%). It must be recognized that occasionally redo fundoplication can be a very difficult operation. Intraoperative damage to the distal esophagus and/or cardia may rarely necessitate esophagogastrectomy. Obviously, this should be avoided unless the patient's symptoms are severe. The logic of performing esophagogastrectomy to treat a hiatal hernia in the patient without severe symptoms

Figure 4-9. Following laparoscopic fundoplication in patients with Barrett's esophagus, some investigators have noted much more regression than progression in the disease. (Reprinted with permission from Oelschlager BK, Barreca M, Chang L, Oleynikov D, Pellegrini CA. Clinical and pathologic response of Barrett's esophagus to laparoscopic antireflux surgery. *Ann Surg.* 2003;238(4):458-464; discussion 464-466.)

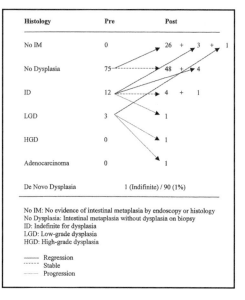

is suspect because part of the stomach will still be in the mediastinum following reconstruction.

Controversies

Although randomized clinical trials suggest that laparoscopic fundoplication is at least as good as PPIs for severe GERD (Figure 4-9),[29,30] there are several controversial areas with which the clinician should be familiar. A recent review is helpful.[33]

PARTIAL VS COMPLETE WRAP

Most experts feel that complete fundoplication is a more effective antireflux operation than partial wrap and, therefore, prefer the former operation in the large majority of surgical patients with GERD. However, partial fundoplication performs quite favorably when compared to Nissen wrap in clinical trials and is the preferred operation in patients with profound esophageal hypoperistalsis (eg, scleroderma, achalasia). In fact, level 1 data from randomized clinical trials suggest that total and partial fundoplication are comparable operations in terms of clinical outcomes and patient satisfaction.[1,33-39] There is evidently a trade-off, with most studies showing a higher incidence of recurrent reflux but less dysphagia and side effects with partial fundoplication. The anterior hemifundoplication (Dor) seems to present the least resistance at the GEJ and thus appears least likely to cause dysphagia but more likely to predispose to recurrent reflux.[37] Currently, most antireflux surgeons in the United States still prefer the total fundoplication in the routine patient coming to antireflux surgery.

FUNDIC MOBILIZATION

There continues to be debate about the need to routinely fully mobilize the fundus by ligating the short gastric vessels in all fundoplication operations. The advantage to such an approach is that it decreases the likelihood of both an overly tight wrap and distortion of the GEJ. The disadvantage of routine fundic mobilization is that it may predispose to postoperative hiatal herniation (nothing tethering the fundus in the abdomen). It may also lead the inexperienced surgeon to choose the incorrect fundic flaps to make the wrap, leading to an anatomically distorted and dysfunctional fundoplication. In randomized prospective studies, full fundic mobilization with division of the short gastric vessels has never been shown to be better than partial mobilization[40-42] and may predispose to "wind-related" side effects. Clearly some patients require full fundic mobilization to construct a proper functional fundoplication.

ESOPHAGEAL LENGTHENING PROCEDURE

Rarely, the GEJ cannot be brought into the abdomen despite aggressive mediastinal esophageal mobilization. If a fundoplication is performed in this situation, the wrap will usually reside in the lower mediastinum and proper function may be problematic. The Collis-Nissen gastroplasty, an interesting and appealing maneuver, adds 2 to 3 cm of tabularized cardia to the distal esophagus and then performs a wrap.[4] While this allows the wrap to sit comfortably in the abdomen and probably decreases the chance of wrap herniation, reflux symptoms may persist because of the acid-secreting tabularized stomach above the wrap. The important question, for which there is no answer, is as follows: Would the patient be better off with a standard wrap in the lower mediastinum, a Collis-Nissen gastroplasty, or no operation at all? What is clear is that the true incidence of short esophagus is low (<2% in most series of fundoplications) and that aggressive mediastinal mobilization of the esophagus can usually bring the GEJ comfortably into the abdomen. Liberal use of esophageal lengthening procedures should be avoided, and the somewhat unusual problem of truly short esophagus should be anticipated and discussed preoperatively.

DOES ANTIREFLUX SURGERY ALTER THE NATURAL HISTORY OF BARRETT'S ESOPHAGUS?

The most objective answer to this question based on the currently available data is "perhaps." One small randomized prospective study suggested less inflammation in those patients with Barrett's esophagus treated with fundoplication compared to PPIs.[43] Adenocarcinoma did not develop in either group, but high-grade dysplasia developed in 2 of 43 patients in the PPI group and 2 of 58 patients in the fundoplication group. A careful endoscopic study by Pellegrini and colleagues suggests regression of Barrett's metaplasia in some patients treated with fundoplication[44]; however, whether fundoplication decreases the risk of death from esophageal cancer in patients with Barrett's esophagus is entirely unknown. Therefore, fundoplication cannot be recommended (yet) for the purpose of decreasing cancer risk. Furthermore, patients with Barrett's metaplasia undergoing fundoplication should be counseled to continue lifelong endoscopic surveillance. Although initially a concern, most endoscopists feel that fundoplication does not compromise their ability to adequately evaluate and monitor Barrett's esophagus.

*WHAT IS THE ROLE OF ENDOSCOPIC MANAGEMENT
OF GASTROESOPHAGEAL REFLUX DISEASE?*

This question is beyond the scope of this chapter. However, it is important to consider whether previous attempts at endoscopic management of GERD (Stretta procedure, endoscopic suturing techniques, or RFA) might make subsequent fundoplication more difficult, more risky, and/or less effective. Although there are only anecdotal data in this regard, the consensus at this time is that the answer to all 3 of these questions is no. Clearly further experience and more data are needed.[45-47]

References

1. Laws HL, Clements RH, Swillie CM. A randomized, prospective comparison of the Nissen fundoplication versus the Toupet fundoplication for gastroesophageal reflux disease. *Ann Surg.* 1997;225(6):647-654.

2. Katkhouda N, Khalil MR, Manhas S, et al. Andre Toupet: surgeon technician par excellence. *Ann Surg.* 2002;235(4):591-599.

3. Hunter JG, Trus TL, Branum GD, Waring JP. Laparoscopic Heller myotomy and fundoplication for achalasia. *Ann Surg.* 1997;225(6):655-665.

4. Jobe BA, Horvath KD, Swanstrom LL. Postoperative function following laparoscopic collis gastroplasty for shortened esophagus. *Arch Surg.* 1998;133(8):867-874.

5. Hunter JG, Trus TL, Branum GD, Waring JP, Wood WC. A physiologic approach to laparoscopic fundoplication for gastroesophageal reflux disease. *Ann Surg.* 1996;223(6):673-687.

6. Mason RJ, DeMeester TR, Lund RJ, et al. Nissen fundoplication prevents shortening of the sphincter during gastric distention. *Arch Surg.* 1997;132(7):719-726.

7. Farrell TM, Smith CD, Metreveli RE, Richardson WS, Johnson AB, Hunter JG. Fundoplications resist reflux independent of in vivo anatomic relationships. *Am J Surg.* 1999;177(2):107-110.

8. Johnsson F, Holloway RH, Ireland AC, Jamieson GG, Dent J. Effect of fundoplication on transient lower esophageal sphincter relaxation and gas reflux. *Br J Surg.* 1997;84(5):686-689.

9. Bais JE, Samsom M, Boudesteijn EA, van Rijk PP, Akkermans LM, Gooszen HG. Impact of delayed gastric emptying on the outcome of antireflux surgery. *Ann Surg.* 2001;234(2):139-146.

10. DeVault KR, Castell DO. American College of Gastroenterology. Updated guidelines for the diagnosis and treatment of gastroesophageal reflux disease. *Am J Gastroenterol.* 2005;100(1):190-200.

11. Johnson WE, Hagen JA, DeMeester TR, et al. Outcome of respiratory symptoms after antireflux surgery on patients with gastroesophageal reflux disease. *Arch Surg.* 1996;131(5):489-492.

12. Campos GM, Peters JH, DeMeester TR, et al. Multivariate analysis of factors predicting outcome after laparoscopic Nissen fundoplication. *J Gastrointest Surg.* 1999;3(3):292-300.

13. Perry Y, Courcoulas AP, Fernando HC, Buenaventura PO, McCaughan JS, Luketich JD. Laparoscopic Roux-en-Y gastric bypass for recalcitrant gastroesophageal reflux disease in morbidly obese patients. *Journal of the Society of Laparoendoscopic Surgeons.* 2004;8(1):19-23.

14. Higa KD, Boone KB, Ho T, Davies OG. Laparoscopic Roux-en-Y gastric bypass for morbid obesity: technique and preliminary results of our first 400 patients. *Arch Surg.* 2000;135(9):1029-1034.

15. Raftopoulos I, Awais O, Courcoulas AP, Luketich JD. Laparoscopic gastric bypass after antireflux surgery for the treatment of gastroesophageal reflux in morbidly obese patients: initial experience. *Obes Surg.* 2004;14(10):1373-1380.

16. Desai KM, Frisella MM, Soper NJ. Clinical outcomes after laparoscopic antireflux surgery in patients with and without preoperative endoscopic esophagitis. *J Gastrointest Surg.* 2003;7(1):44-52.

17. Heading RC. Should abnormal esophageal motility in gastro-esophageal reflux disease (GORD) influence decisions about fundoplication? *Gut.* 2002;50(5):592-593.

18. Fibbe C, Layer P, Keller J, Strate U, Emmermann A, Zornig C. Esophageal motility in reflux disease before and after fundoplication: a prospective, randomized, clinical, and manometric study. *Gastroenterology.* 2001;121(1):5-14.

19. Campos GM, DeMeester SR, Peters JH, et al. Predictive factors of Barrett esophagus: multivariate analysis of 502 patients with gastroesophageal reflux disease. *Arch Surg.* 2001;136(11):1267-1273.

20. Patti MG, Diener U, Tamburini A, Molena D, Way LW. Role of esophageal function tests in diagnosis of gastroesophageal reflux disease. *Dig Dis Sci.* 2001;46(3):597-602.

21. Pandolfino JE, Schreiner MA, Lee TJ, Zhang Q, Boniquit C, Kahrilas PJ. Comparison of the Bravo wireless and Digitrapper catheter-based pH monitoring systems for measuring esophageal acid exposure. *Am J Gastroenterol.* 2005;100(7):1466-1476.

22. Sarela AI, Hick DG, Verbeke CS, Casey JF, Guillou PJ, Clark GW. Persistent acid and bile reflux in asymptomatic patients with Barrett esophagus receiving proton pump inhibitor therapy. *Arch Surg.* 2004;139(5):547-551.

23. Pellegrini CA. Delayed gastric emptying in patients with abnormal gastroesophageal reflux. *Ann Surg.* 2001;234(2):147-148.

24. Jurgens MJ, Drane WE, Vogel SB. Dual-radionuclide simultaneous biliary and gastric scintigraphy to depict surgical treatment of bile reflux. *Radiology.* 2003;229(1):283-287.

25. Swanstrom LL. Partial fundoplications for gastroesophageal reflux disease: indications and current status. *J Clin Gastroenterol.* 1999;29(2):127-132.

26. Perdikis G, Hinder RA, Lund RJ, Raiser F, Katada N. Laparoscopic Nissen fundoplication: where do we stand? *Surgical Laparoscopy & Endoscopy.* 1997;7(1):17-21.

27. DeMeester TR, Bonavina L, Albertucci M. Nissen fundoplication for gastroesophageal reflux disease—Evaluation of primary repair in 100 consecutive patients. *Ann Surg.* 1986;204(9):9-20.

28. Spechler SJ, Lee E, Ahnen D, et al. Long-term outcome of medical and surgical therapies for gastroesophageal reflux disease: follow-up of a randomized controlled trial. *JAMA.* 2001;285(18):2331-2338.

29. Spechler SJ. Comparison of medical and surgical therapy for complicated gastroesophageal reflux disease in veterans. *N Engl J Med.* 1992;326:786-792.

30. Mahon D, Rhodes M, Decadt B, et al. Randomized clinical trial of laparoscopic Nissen fundoplication compared with proton-pump inhibitors for treatment of chronic gastro-esophageal reflux. *Br J Surg.* 2005;92(6):695-699.

31. Smith CD, McClusky DA, Rajad MA, Lederman AB, Hunter JG. When fundoplication fails: redo? *Ann Surg.* 2005;241(6):861-871.

32. Galvani C, Fisichella PM, Gorodner MV, Perretta S, Patti MG. Symptoms are a poor indicator of reflux status after fundoplication for gastroesophageal reflux disease: role of esophageal functions tests. *Arch Surg.* 2003;138(5):514-519.

33. Catarci M, Gentileschi P, Papi C, et al. Evidence-based appraisal of antireflux fundoplication. *Ann Surg.* 2004;239(3):325-337.

34. Baigrie RJ, Cullis SN, Ndhluni AJ, Cariem A. Randomized double-blind trial of laparoscopic Nissen fundoplication versus anterior partial fundoplication. *Br J Surg.* 2005;92(7):819-823.

35. Ludemann R, Watson DI, Jamieson GG, Game PA, Devitt PG. Five-year follow-up of a randomized clinical trial of laparoscopic total versus anterior 180 degrees fundoplication. *Br J Surg.* 2005;92(2):240-243.

36. Watson DI, Jamieson GG, Lally C, et al. International Society for Diseases of the Esophagus—Australasian Section. Multicenter, prospective, double-blind, randomized trial of laparoscopic Nissen vs anterior 90 degrees partial fundoplication. *Arch Surg.* 2004;139(11):1160-1167.

37. Hagedorn C, Jonson C, Lonroth H, Ruth M, Thune A, Lundell L. Efficacy of an anterior as compared with a posterior laparoscopic partial fundoplication: results of a randomized, controlled clinical trial. *Ann Surg.* 2003;238(2):189-196.

38. Watson DI, Jamieson GG, Pike GK, Davies N, Richardson M, Devitt PG. Prospective randomized double-blind trial between laparoscopic Nissen fundoplication and anterior partial fundoplication. *Br J Surg.* 1999;86(1):123-130.

39. Lundell L, Abrahamsson H, Ruth M, Rydberg L, Lonroth H, Olbe L. Long-term results of a prospective randomized comparison of total fundic wrap (Nissen-Rossetti) or semifundoplication (Toupet) for gastro-esophageal reflux. *Br J Surg.* 1996;83(6):830-835.

40. O'Boyle CJ, Watson DI, Jamieson GG, Myers JC, Game PA, Devitt PG. Division of short gastric vessels at laparoscopic Nissen fundoplication: a prospective double-blind randomized trial with 5-year follow-up. *Ann Surg.* 2002;235(2):165-170.

41. Chrysos E, Tzortzinis A, Tsiaoussis J, Athanasakis H, Vasssilakis J, Xynos E. Prospective randomized trial comparing Nissen to Nissen-Rossetti technique for laparoscopic fundoplication. *Am J Surg.* 2001;182(3):215-221.

42. Watson DI, Pike GK, Baigrie RJ, et al. Prospective double-blind randomized trial of laparoscopic Nissen fundoplication with division and without division of short gastric vessels. *Ann Surg.* 1997;226(5):642-652.

43. Parrilla P, Martinez de Haro LF, Ortiz A, et al. Long-term results of a randomized prospective study comparing medical and surgical treatment of Barrett's esophagus. *Ann Surg.* 2003;237(3):291-298.

44. Oelschlager BK, Barreca M, Chang L, Oleynikov D, Pellegrini CA. Clinical and pathologic response of Barrett's esophagus to laparoscopic antireflux surgery. *Ann Surg.* 2003;238(4):458-464; discussion 464-466.

45. Schiefke I, Zabel-Langhennig A, Neumann S, et al. Long-term failure of endoscopic gastroplication (EndoCinch). *Gut.* 2005;54(6):752-758.

46. Galmiche JP, Bruley des Varannes S. Endoluminal therapies for gastro-esophageal reflux disease. *Lancet.* 2003;361(9363):1119-1121.

47. Mahmood Z, McMahon BP, Arfin Q, et al. Endocinch therapy for gastro-esophageal reflux disease: a one year prospective follow up. *Gut.* 2003;52(1):34-39.

Endoscopic Treatment of Gastroesophageal Reflux Disease

Annapurna Korimilli, MD; Mark Lee, BS; and Larry S. Miller, MD

Introduction

GERD is a common GI disorder. In fact, it is the fourth most prevalent GI disease in the United States. More than one fourth of adults in the United States use antisecretory medications at least 3 times per month, resulting in a large economic burden. It has been estimated that almost $2 billion is spent in the United States each year on OTC antacids and histamine-2 receptor antagonists, and another $10 billion is spent on prescription histamine-2 receptor antagonists and PPIs.

Current methods for the pharmacological treatment of GERD include antacids, promotility agents, histamine receptor blockers, and PPIs. Surgical barrier methods (Nissen fundoplication) are most often performed laparoscopically. Lifestyle changes may help to diminish some of the symptoms associated with GERD. Although medical therapy has been shown to be effective, the inconvenience and cost of long-term drug therapy has led to the consideration of alternative methods of treatment. Surgical therapy has its drawbacks, in that many patients may require continued medical therapy after surgery and the fundoplication may eventually breakdown.

Introduction to Endoscopic Methods of Treating Gastroesophageal Reflux Disease

Traditional treatments for GERD include drug therapy, lifestyle changes, or invasive surgery. A number of endoscopic methods of treatment have been developed in recent years, have been FDA approved, and are in clinical use. The following 5 endoscopic methods are in use today:

1. Endoscopic Suturing (EndoCinch [Bard, Inc, Bellerica, Mass]) (approved by the FDA in March 2000).

2. Injection Therapy (ENTERYX [Boston Scientific Corp, Natick Mass]) (approved by the FDA in April 2003, voluntary recall by the company in September 2005).

3. Radio frequency ablation (Stretta procedure [Curon Medical, Freemont, Calif]) (approved by the FDA in April 2000).

4. Endoscopic Plicator (NDP Surgical, Mansfield, Mass) (approved by the FDA in April 2000).

5. Gatekeeper Reflux Repair System (Medtronic, Minneapolis, Minn) (not approved by the FDA).

Endoscopic treatments for GERD focus on altering the structure of the gastroesophageal segment by directly modifying the GEJ in a minimally invasive manner. These methods rely on the augmentation of the natural barriers to reflux. New evidence shows that these endoscopic methods target the gastric sling fibers and TLESRs. The endoluminal therapies for GERD theoretically offer the advantage of reducing symptoms caused by both acid and nonacidic reflux. Three endoscopic modalities of therapy are in common use today (endoscopic suturing, injection of a bulking agent, and radiofrequency scarring of the distal esophagus and cardia). The Endoscopic Plicator is also FDA approved, but there is less clinical experience with this device. The Gatekeeper device has not yet been FDA approved in the United States.

In general, the mechanisms of endoscopic antireflux therapies are as follows. The EndoCinch procedure involves placing stitches into the proximal folds of the gastric cardia to create a mucosal cardioplasty. In preliminary studies, it was found that the EndoCinch plications replace the absent pressure profile from abnormal gastric sling fibers. ENTERYX (polyvinyl alcohol with tantalum dissolved in dimethyl sulfoxide [DMSO]) is injected directly into the muscle layer of the esophagus to cause bulking and fibrosis of the muscle at the GEJ. Stretta (radiofrequency scarring of the high-pressure zone) involves scarring of the region of the cardia and distal esophagus. The endoscopic plicator places a full-thickness plication at the area of the gastric cardia, mechanically impeding GER. Finally, the Gatekeeper Reflux Repair System encompasses a submucosal injection of a hydrogel that expands after implantation into the distal esophagus.

ENDOCINCH

Background

Swain and Mills first described the concept and technology of endoscopic suturing or sewing in 1986.[1] Subsequent animal and cadaver studies documented that endoscopic placement of sutures in the cardia of the stomach was feasible. Early manometric reports demonstrated manometrically that the technique increased the overall length of the LES, its intra-abdominal length, and/or its pressure depending on the configuration of the suture placement.[2-4] Initial use in humans with GERD was first described in 2001.[5] Two endoscopic suturing devices are currently available (EndoCinch and Sew-Right Device [Wilson-Cook Medical, Inc, Winston Salem, NC]). Only EndoCinch, however, is FDA approved for use as therapy in patients with GERD at the present time.[6]

Technique

The system used to place the plications is the Bard EndoCinch Suturing System. EndoCinch is a commercial system used to permit suturing in GI tract using 2 flexible endoscopes. One endoscope is used to place the sutures and the other to secure

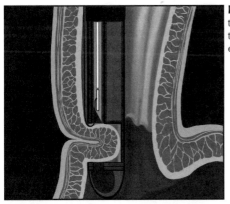

Figure 5-1. The needle penetrating the mucosa within the capsule and the suture tag captured in the distal end of the capsule.

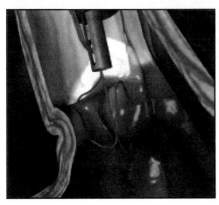

Figure 5-2. The suture-securing device is poised to secure the sutures and then cut the sutures.

the sutures in place. An overtube is placed into the esophagus over a savory dilator. The endoscope, with the EndoCinch suturing device, is placed through the overtube. A capsule, present at the end of the endoscope, is positioned against the tissue to be sutured. Suction is applied to bring a fold of tissue into the capsule. A needle is then activated, which drives a suture with a suture tag through the tissue (Figure 5-1). Once the sutures are placed at the appropriate site, suction is turned off to release the fold, and the endoscope is withdrawn from the esophagus. The suture tag is then reloaded, and the scope is reinserted to place a second stitch adjacent to the first one. A suture-securing device is actuated through a second endoscope in order to cinch and cut the suture, and a plication is thus formed (Figure 5-2). Three or more plications are usually placed in a patient in a spiral fashion starting at approximately 2 cm below the GEJ and moving proximally up in a circumferential manner to just below the GEJ (Figure 5-3). The number, location, orientation, and technique of placement of the plications vary from center to center and investigator to investigator.

Clinical Studies

Endoscopic suturing techniques were first described in the United Kingdom in the 1980s by Swain.[1] Later, this group reported their initial results on 102 patients who

Figure 5-3. There are 3 completed plications in this picture.

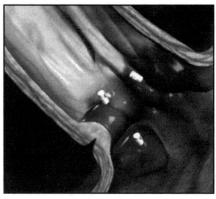

were followed for 4 years. Suturing resulted in a significant improvement in the mean values for the length of the LES, basal LES pressure, 24-hr esophageal pH exposure, GERD symptom score, and use of antisecretory therapy.

Filipi et al[5] reported the results from a multicenter trial of 64 GERD patients treated by endoscopic suturing. Heartburn severity and frequency as well as regurgitation showed significant improvement from baseline. Twenty-four-hour esophageal acid exposure also showed improvement from baseline at 6-month follow-up but percentage of time pH <4 was still in the abnormal range. At 6 months, there was no significant change in the LES pressure measurement, and erosive esophagitis had healed in 25% of patients. Antisecretory medication use decreased in 62% of patients. One patient had a self-contained suture perforation that was successfully treated with antibiotics.

Mahmood et al[7] found that 22 of 26 patients treated with endoscopic suturing were available for assessment at 1 year. Significant reduction in heartburn and regurgitation scores was seen. Use of PPIs was reduced by 64% at 12 months. Quality of life scores showed significant improvement. However, there was no reduction in the total time during which the esophageal pH was less than 4. Reported complications included bleeding in 2 patients (one patient required transfusion) and a gastric tear in another.

Rothstein et al[8] evaluated 2-year follow-up data on 39 patients from 3 different institutions. Thirty-three of the 39 patients were followed for a mean of 25 months. Significant reduction in heartburn severity and frequency scores was found, but regurgitation scores did not show significant improvement. Two years after the procedure, 25% of patients were completely off antisecretory medications, 40% were on full-dose medications, and 6% failed the procedure and required antireflux surgery.

Rothstein and colleagues[9] presented data from the EndoCinch sham randomized controlled trial at the Digestive Disease Week meeting in 2004. Patients were randomized to either 4 endoscopic gastric plications or a sham procedure. Of the 17 patients enrolled in each arm, 16 were evaluable at 3 months, which represented the endpoint for the primary measures. There was a statistically significant improvement in frequency of GERD symptoms, in need for PPIs, in intraesophageal acid exposure (12.5% normalized), and in quality of life. There were no significant differences in

GERD symptom severity, regurgitation scores, or percentage of patients discontinuing PPI use. This study indicates that the procedure was effective for well-selected patients with GERD.

Mechanism of Action

Miller et al[10] performed a study to define the mechanism of action of endoscopic-plication in the treatment of GERD. High-frequency endoscopic ultrasound (HFUS) and simultaneous manometry were used to evaluate 10 GERD patients during breath holding with a machine pull-through of a simultaneous ultrasound and manometry catheter assembly before and after endoscopic plication. Pull-throughs were repeated before and after intravenous administration of atropine in order to ablate the intrinsic sphincter components of the GEJ high-pressure zone. For each pull-through, the axial location of the margin of the right crural diaphragm was located on the ultrasound image and used as a reference point. It was found that 8 of the 10 patients (80%) had significant clinical benefit after endoscopic-plication. From prior studies, it was shown that in normal volunteers the difference between the pre- and postatropine pressure profiles (the intrinsic sphincter components) displayed 2 peaks (sling fibers and LES). The distal pressure peak (gastric sling fibers) was missing in the pre-EndoCinch patients with GERD. Post-EndoCinch, the distal pressure peak was established in the GERD patients at the same axial location as the distal pressure peak in normal volunteers. It was concluded that GERD patients lack the pressure profile due to the gastric sling fibers and that endoscopic plications re-establish this distal pressure profile (Figure 5-4).

Tam et al[11] performed a study to determine the impact of endoscopic suturing of the GEJ on LES function in patients with GERD. In 15 patients with GERD, 2 plications were performed circumferentially 1 cm below the GEJ. Endoscopy and combined postprandial esophageal manometry and pH monitoring were performed before and 6 months after treatment. Twenty-four-hour ambulatory pH monitoring and symptom assessment were also performed before treatment and at 6 and 12 months after treatment. It was found that 6 months after treatment, the rate of TLESRs was decreased by 37% (p<0.05) and basal LES pressure had increased from 4.3 ± 2.2 mmHg to 6.2 ± 2.1 mmHg (p<0.05). The rate of postprandial reflux events and acid exposure time were not altered. Endoscopic suturing significantly reduced 24-hr esophageal acid exposure from 9.6% (9.0 to 12.1) to 7.4% (3.9 to 10.1) at 6 months due predominantly to a reduction in upright acid exposure. The reduction in total 24-hr acid exposure was sustained to 12 months. Seven patients (47%) remained off medications at 6 and 12 months follow-up. The investigators concluded that in patients with GERD, endoscopic suturing of the GEJ resulted in a reduction in the rate of TLESRs and an increase in basal LES pressure.

Summary

To date, the 5 published studies show that heartburn severity and frequency improve significantly from baseline. Antisecretory medication use is decreased at 6 months between 40% and 65%. Quality of life scores showed significant improvement. Most of the available data are uncontrolled, short duration (6 months or less), and retrospective. Rothstein[12] has reviewed the clinical data on EndoCinch, in more than 5000 patients. This uncontrolled trial data indicated a consistent improvement in symptoms and intraesophageal acid exposure. At 2 years postprocedure, approximately 25% to 50% of treated patients remain off of GERD medications.[13]

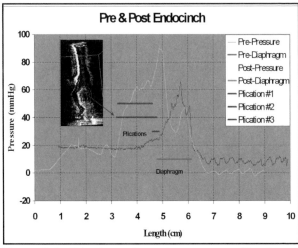

Figure 5-4. This picture shows the pressure profiles through the gastroesophageal junction high pressure zone pre- and post EndoCinch in a patient with GERD referenced to the right crural diaphragm. Note that the darker color curve represents the pre-EndoCinch pressure profile, while the lighter color curve represents the post-EndoCinch pressure profile. The horizontal lines represent the locations of endoscopic plications (top, middle and bottom lines), and the right crural diaphragm (two horizontal lines above the word "diaphragm") located from the ultrasound images.

Side Effects and Complications

There have been no reported deaths with the use of EndoCinch. However, there have been a number of complications reported. These include a contained perforation requiring antibiotic therapy, a number of episodes of GI bleeding, and a gastric tear.[6]

Indications

Indications include patients who desire an alternative therapy for their GERD symptoms. The optimal patient appears to be the one with mild-to-moderate physiologic or anatomic derangement and who responds to PPI therapy.[6]

Contraindications

Relative contraindications for endoscopic suturing are patients with bleeding dyscrasia and/or severe comorbidities, patients with gastric or esophageal varices, and patients with a large hiatal hernia.[6]

Duration of Therapeutic Effect

The duration of therapeutic effect of endoscopic suture therapy is unknown. Most studies have only 6-month follow-up. Zabel-Langhennig and colleagues[14] conducted a single-center, prospective, observational study to evaluate the long-term effectiveness of this device in 33 patients. At 18 months, 26 of 33 patients had a return of their heartburn, 12 of 33 again reported regurgitation, and 91% of patients required regular medical therapy for GERD symptoms. Rothstein et al[8] noted that 25% to 50% of patients treated remained off GERD medication for 2 years.

ENTERYX

Background

ENTERYX is an injectable method of treating GERD. ENTERYX material consists of 8% ethylene vinyl alcohol copolymer labeled with tantalum for radiographic visualization dissolved in DMSO. The dimethyl sulfoxide diffuses away upon injection into tissue, causing precipitation of the polymer.[15]

Technique

The ENTERYX vial is agitated for 10 minutes to suspend the tantalum in the biopolymer solution before use. The injection is performed during endoscopy using special syringes and catheters that do not dissolve in DMSO. The Z line is identified, and the endoscope is positioned in the distal esophagus just above the GEJ. The preloaded injection needle and catheter are advanced into the lumen of the esophagus, and a site for injection is identified. The needle is advanced into the esophageal wall. The ENTERYX is injected into the muscularis propria at a rate of 1 mL per min under combined fluoroscopic and endoscopic guidance. Heat is generated in the exothermic reaction as the DMSO dissipates and the ethyl vinyl alcohol solidifies. A total of 1 to 2 mL at each site is injected. After the injection at the site is complete, the needle is kept in place for 20 seconds, allowing the material to stabilize and solidify and avoid leakage through the injection site.[15]

On September 23, 2005, Boston Scientific voluntarily initiated a recall of all ENTERYX procedure kits and ENTERYX single pack injectors. The company has found that the technique used to inject the materials is critical in achieving appropriate results. Recently, there have been instances in which injections have been made transmurally that went undetected during the procedure and resulted in adverse events. The company considers the risk of undetected transmural injections unacceptable and, therefore, has chosen to voluntarily recall these products. The recall is indefinite and the company has notified the FDA of their actions.

STRETTA PROCEDURE

The Stretta procedure is an endoluminal therapy during which radiofrequency energy is delivered to the esophagogastric junction. Radiofrequency has been used in surgical practice since 1921.[16] The Stretta system is a monopolar radiofrequency energy device. There is an active electrode (needles) and a dispersive electrode (grounding pad). Heating occurs at the active electrode as radiofrequency current flows between the needle and the surrounding tissue because of inductive and frictional heating of water molecules. The power density is inversely related to the surface area of tissue in contact with the electrodes, thereby being highest at the needle electrode and insignificant at the skin to which the dispersive electrode is applied.

Radiofrequency energy is delivered in a more controlled manner with constant tissue temperature monitoring and automated modulation of radiofrequency power output. A thermocouple (electrical thermometer) is incorporated into the active electrode to provide constant tissue temperature feedback. A target temperature is preselected

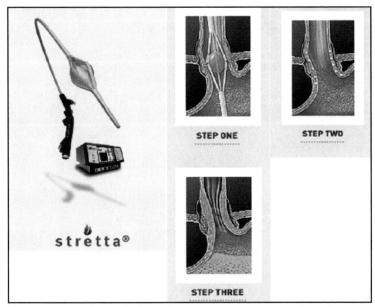

Figure 5-5. The Stretta device and the three steps used to perform the Stretta procedure. In step one the balloon is distended and the radiofrequency needles are deployed. The tissue is then heated at various levels through the distal esophagus and proximal cardia. The last picture shows the area of fibrosis. (Courtesy of Curon Medical, Freemont, Calif.)

(ie, 85°C) on the temperature-control system, and the power is automatically modulated to achieve but not exceed the prescribed temperature. Maintaining lesion temperatures below 100°C prevents vaporization, high tissue impedance, or tissue desiccation and facilitates the formation of a spherical thermal lesion. Collagen contraction occurs immediately upon exposure to 65°C, resulting in tissue shrinkage.[17]

Materials and Methods

The Stretta System (Figure 5-5) consists of a 4-channel radiofrequency generator and single-use radiofrequency energy catheters. The generator delivers pure sine-wave energy, 465 kHz, 2 to 5 watts per channel, and 80 volts maximum at 100 to 800 Ohms. A dispersive electrode is applied to the midback of the patient and connected to the radiofrequency generator. The delivery device (catheter) comprises balloon-basket assembly, 4 electrode delivery sheaths positioned radially at 90-degree increments around the balloon, suction, and irrigation. A curved nickel-titanium needle electrode (25 gauge, 5.5 mm length) with a thermocouple at the tip and base is contained within each delivery sheath. The catheter is positioned and the needles are deployed into the wall of the distal esophagus or gastric cardia, and radiofrequency energy is delivered to each electrode to achieve a temperature of 85°C at the electrode tip. Irrigation through the catheter maintains mucosal temperature below 50°C. This causes a thermal lesion in the tissue surrounding the tip of the electrode with relatively intact overlying mucus.[18]

Technique

Stretta treatments are typically performed in endoscopy or ambulatory surgery units with patients under conscious sedation. Endoscopy is performed, noting the distance from the squamocolumnar junction to the incisors. A coated stiff guidewire (0.035 to 0.039 inch) is passed into the duodenum, and the endoscope is removed. The Stretta assembly is then passed over the guidewire into the stomach and withdrawn to a position 1 cm proximal to the squamocolumnar junction by using the centimeter markings on the catheter shaft, which are referenced to the position of the electrodes. The guidewire is then removed, suction and irrigation lines are connected, and the device is ready to begin treatment.

Each application of radiofrequency energy requires the following sequence of steps: the balloon at the end of the Stretta assembly is inflated, the electrodes are deployed, the generator is turned on for a specified period of time, the electrodes are withdrawn, and the balloon is then deflated. Electrode contact with tissue is evidenced by a reduction in the electrode impedance displayed on the generator monitor. After completing a lesion at each axial level, the catheter is then rotated 45 degrees and a second set of lesions is made, thereby making a ring of 8 radial lesions at that axial location. The current manufacturer's recommendation[18] is to inflate the balloon to 2.5 psi before electrode deployment. The generator is activated for 90 seconds with each deployment to create rings of lesions in the following sequence: 1 cm above the squamocolumnar junction, 0.5 cm above the squamocolumnar junction, at the squamocolumnar junction, and 0.5 cm distal to the squamocolumnar junction. Two additional rings of 3 sets each are created in the gastric cardia by positioning the catheter in the stomach, inflating the balloon to 25 mL for the first set and 22 mL for the second, retracting the assembly against the hiatus until resistance is felt, and deploying the electrodes. The final result is 4 rings of 8 lesions each in the distal esophagus and 2 pullback rings of 12 lesions each in the gastric cardia. This requires 14 repetitions of the radiofrequency energy application sequence and a total of 21 minutes of active radiofrequency energy delivery.

Proposed Mechanisms of Action

Two potential mechanisms of action have been proposed for Stretta treatment of the GEJ in GERD patients: scarring of the GEJ and neurolysis in the region of the GEJ. Neurolysis in the region of the GEJ could potentially destroy sensory or motor nerve endings. The destruction of chemosensitive or mechanosensitive nerve endings could potentially reduce the sensitivity of the esophagus to noxious stimuli. Destruction of vagal afferents in the region of the gastric cardia or decreased compliance of the gastric cardia could potentially reduce the occurrence of TLESRs, thereby reducing the number of reflux events.

Utley et al[19] published longitudinal animal studies to elucidate the mechanism of action and effect of Stretta as it relates to LES physiology and histopathology. In these studies, radiofrequency elevated the LES pressure and gastric yield pressure in a porcine model of botulinum toxin-induced LES hypotension.

Thickening of the LES after radiofrequency delivery has been demonstrated using histopathological evaluation and endoscopic ultrasound. Additionally, using a canine model[20] of triggered TLESRs, Stretta procedure significantly reduced the frequency of TLESRs and reflux events. Histological data were also obtained from the canine study. The experimental animals showed marked hypertrophy as well as fibrosis within the muscle. Measurements of the gastric cardia showed a highly significant (63%) increase in thickness.

No histopathological data demonstrating neurolysis exist. What data do exist in the pig[19] and dog[21] indicate no macroscopic or microscopic damage to the vagus nerves. Thus, evidence supporting the concept of neurolysis is based on physiologic measurements, and because there are currently no data available on chemosensitivity or mechanosensitivity in man or animals, these data focus on the elicitation of TLESRs, LES pressure, and esophageal acid exposure.

Tam et al,[20] in a human trial including 20 patients, found that the postprandial TLESRs rate diminished from 6.8 (5.7 to 8.1) to 5.2 (4.2 to 5.8) per hour during 3-hour postprandial recordings. In each trial, there was also a reduced total number of acid reflux events, from 34 to 21 in the dogs and from 202 to 131 in the patients.

Studies

Triadafilopoulos et al[22] performed a large, multicenter prospective clinical trial of the Stretta procedure. This study investigated the long-term (12-month) safety and efficacy of radiofrequency energy delivery for the treatment of GERD. One hundred eighteen patients with chronic heartburn and/or regurgitation who required antisecretory medication daily and had demonstrated pathologic esophageal acid exposure, a sliding hiatal hernia ($\leq$2 cm), and esophagitis ($\leq$grade 2) were studied. Seventy-two men and 46 women were treated. At 12 months, 94 patients were available for follow-up. There were improvements after 12 months in the median heartburn score (4 to 1, p = 0.0001), GERD score (27 to 9, p = 0.0001), satisfaction (1 to 4, p = 0.0001), and quality of life (mental SF-36, 46.3 to 55.4, p<0.0001; physical SF-36, 40.9 to 53.1, p = 0.0001); PPI requirement fell from 88.1% to 30% of patients. Esophageal acid exposure improved significantly (10.2% to 6.4%, p = 0.0001). There were 10 (8.6%) complications, none of which required therapeutic intervention.

Corley et al[23] published a randomized, double blind, sham-controlled, multicenter clinical trial. When compared to the sham group (n = 30) at 6 months, the patients who underwent the Stretta procedure (n = 34) showed a significant decrease in heartburn (p<0.01) and improvement in quality of life scores (p<0.001). However, there was no significant difference in the use of antisecretory medications between the treatment and sham groups.

Houston et al[24] prospectively evaluated 41 patients undergoing the Stretta procedure. Patients were studied pre- and post-Stretta with esophageal manometry, 24-hr pH testing, quality of life SF12 surveys, and GERD-specific questionnaires (QOLRAD). The quality-of-life scores were significantly improved at 6 months: QOLRAD score increased from 3.7 $\pm$ 0.2 to 5.1 $\pm$ 0.2 (p = 0.002), SF12 mental score increased from 44.3 $\pm$ 2.0 to 51.8 $\pm$ 1.7 (p = 0.001), and SF12 physical score increased from 26.2 $\pm$ 2.4 to 33.1 $\pm$ 3.8 (p = 0.001). There was a significant decrease in esophageal acid exposure time (8.4 $\pm$ 0.9% to 4.4 $\pm$ 1.3%, p = 0.03) and Johnson-DeMeester score (32.8 $\pm$ 4.6 to 22.9 $\pm$ 5.3, p = 0.04). There was no significant change in mean LES pressure (25.3 $\pm$ 2.4 mmHg to 26.8 $\pm$ 2.6 mmHg, p = 0.63). Twenty of 31 patients (65%) available for 6-month follow-up were completely off PPIs.

Wolfsen and Richards[25] studied surveys of 558 patients (33 institutions, mean follow-up of 8 months). After treatment, onset of GERD relief was less than 2 months (68.7%) or 2 to 6 months (14.6%). The median drug requirement improved from PPIs twice daily to antacids as needed (p<0.0001). The percentage of patients with satisfactory GERD control (absent or mild) improved from 26.3% at baseline (on drugs) to 77.0% after Stretta (p<0.0001). Median baseline symptom control on drugs was 50% compared with 90% at follow-up (p<0.0001). Baseline patient satisfaction on drugs was 23.2%, compared with 86.5% at follow-up (p<0.0001). Subgroup analysis (<1 year vs >1 year of follow-up) showed a superior effect on symptom control and drug use in those patients beyond 1 year of follow-up, supporting procedure durability.

Stretta treatment is associated with no significant change in the severity of esophagitis and no change in LES pressure. Data on esophageal acid exposure[22,26] as measured by 24-hr esophageal pH show a significant numerical reduction in percent acid exposure, averaging 3.7% in the uncontrolled trial and no change in the sham-controlled trial.[27] Esophageal acid exposure was normalized in fewer than half of the individuals treated in the uncontrolled trial because the post-treatment median acid exposure value was 6.4%. The only controlled trial, currently reported in abstract form, suggests that although PPI usage was reduced, it was reduced to a similar degree among sham-treated individuals. The one consistent observation in all trials has been of a significant reduction in the severity of heartburn among treated individuals followed for a period of up to 12 months. A second effect convincingly demonstrated was of a slight reduction in the frequency of TLESRs both among patients and dogs.

Food and Drug Administration Approval and Safety

The FDA approved the Stretta System on April 18, 2000 as follows[27]: "the Stretta System is intended for general use in the electrosurgical coagulation of tissue and intended specifically for use in the treatment of GERD." Patients tolerate the Stretta treatment of GERD well without general anesthesia, with shorter hospital stay, and with less recovery time compared to published reports on fundoplication. Thus, the clinical data show that the Stretta device is safe and effective for treatment of GERD, and the risk-benefit profile is substantially equivalent to that of fundoplication surgery.

Indications

The patients with GERD enrolled in the Stretta trials that showed substantial clinical improvement were those patients with suboptimal heartburn resolution on PPIs, absent or low grade esophagitis, and minimal hiatal hernia.

Contraindications

Contraindications for Stretta treatment are circumstances in which there has been no demonstration of clinical efficacy: high-grade esophagitis, Barrett's metaplasia, management of extraesophageal manifestations of GERD, or management of any GERD symptom other than heartburn.

Complications

Post market surveillance data on Stretta can be found in the MAUDE database[28] on the FDA website. There are 15 significant complications found on that website including 5 perforations and 2 deaths. Most of these occurred within the first 6 months after FDA approval. Only one complication of any severity has been reported to that website since November 27, 2001, and that involved a patient being burned at the site of the dispersing electrode pad. The only complication related to Stretta was a case of gastroparesis 10 days postoperatively that resolved completely.

Figure 5-6. The plicator device. (Courtesy of NDP Surgical, Mansfield, Mass.)

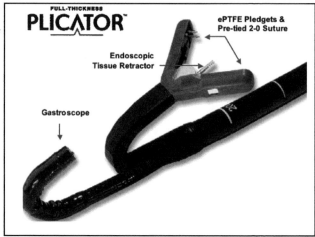

ENDOSCOPIC PLICATOR

Background

The endoscopic plication system is designed to fixate stomach tissue approximately 1 cm distal to the GEJ with serosa-to-serosa apposition. The device consists of a reusable instrument and a single-use, suture-based implant (Figure 5-6). In addition, a helical tissue retractor and standard overtube are used to perform the endoscopic full-thickness plication procedure.

Technique

The endoscopic plication system is a reusable instrument that passes 2 needles through tissue at the desired location to place an implant for tissue approximation, plication, and fixation. Controls on the instrument handle actuate the distal end of the device and allow for retroflexion of the distal end, opening and closing of the instrument arms, and delivering the implant. The instrument contains 2 dedicated channels: one for insertion of the tissue retractor, the other for passage of the endoscope.

The endoscopic tissue retractor is designed to engage the deep gastric wall, allowing for creation of the serosa-to-serosa plication. The tissue retractor is configured in a helical fashion and includes a protective outer sheath to stabilize gastric mucosa while engaging the wall. Typically, the retractor is inserted 1 cm distal to the GEJ. This allows the gastric wall to be drawn into the arms of the instrument before deployment of the implant.

The implant, which allows for fixation of the transmural plication, consists of a pre-tied suture, 2 bolsters, and 2 titanium retention bridges. The suture is standard United States Pharmacopeia (USP) size 2-0 polypropylene and is pretied and pre-threaded onto the retention bridges. The suture bolsters are made of soft, flexible, expanded polytetrafluoroethylene.

Clinical Studies

A multicenter study involving 64 patients who underwent endoscopic full-thickness plication was just completed.[29] All patients received a single, endoscopic full-thickness plication in the gastric cardia within 2 cm of the GEJ. No retreatments were performed. One year postplication, the median off-meds GERD-HRQL scores improved 65% and were superior when compared to the patients baseline on-meds HRQL scores. Twenty-four hour pH-metry studies at 6 months postprocedure demonstrated a 31% decrease in median time pH <4 with 30% of patients experiencing a normalization of pH at 6 months. At 1-year postprocedure, 70% of patients remained off daily PPI therapy. The most common adverse event was sore throat in 41% of patients that resolved spontaneously. It was concluded that a single full-thickness plication placed at the GEJ reduced symptoms, medication use, and esophageal acid exposure associated with GERD.

Mechanism of Action

The mechanisms of action are thought to be a decrease in TLESRs and an alteration in the compliance of the GEJ.

Indications

Patients who desire an alternative therapy for their GERD symptoms are indicated.

Side Effects and Complications

The most common adverse event was sore throat in 41% of patients that resolved spontaneously. Abdominal pain occurred in 20%, chest pain in 17%, GI disorder in 17%, eructation in 14%, dysphagia in 11%, and nausea in 6%. One patient experienced a gastric perforation, which was closed with endoclips. One patient experienced a pneumothorax.

Contraindications

Patients with large hiatal hernias, Barrett's esophagus, or severe esophagitis were excluded from the multicenter study cited above.

Duration of Therapeutic Effect

In the multicenter trial, 65% patients were able to discontinue antisecretory therapy at 6 months.

THE GATEKEEPER REFLUX REPAIR SYSTEM

Background

The Gatekeeper Reflux Repair System is a form of injectable endoscopic therapy for GERD. It consists of expandable hydrogel prostheses that are placed within the lumen of the GEJ. The hydrogel prostheses are made from a soft pliable material that expands to 90% in 6 hours, is radio opaque, and is removable.

Figure 5-7. The 5 sequential steps in performing the Gatekeeper procedure. The first step is to stabilize the device. The next step is to create space to inject. The next step is to access the space. The next step is delivering the Gatekeeper hydrogel product.

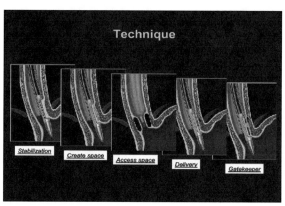

Technique

The hydrogel material is injected into the submucosal layer of the esophagogastric junction using an overtube suction device during endoscopy (Figure 5-7).

Clinical Studies

Fockens et al[30] presented the results of the European multicenter trial assessing the safety and efficacy of this device. This trial involved 68 patients who were treated with up to 6 hydrogel prosthetic implants, with 10 patients undergoing a second elective procedure. At 6 months, GERD-related quality-of-life scores were significantly improved, with a decrease in esophageal acid exposure and an increase in LES pressure. One definite advantage of the Gatekeeper Reflux Repair System over the other endoscopic treatments currently being developed is its reversibility. Studies are still limited and long-term data unknown.

Side Effects and Complications

Two patients suffered adverse events. One patient had a pharyngeal perforation on introduction of the overtube. Another patient complained of nausea 1 week postprocedure; the prosthesis was removed endoscopically at 3 weeks.

Duration of Therapeutic Effect

Fockens et al[30] have shown efficacy at 6 months after the procedure. Long-term studies are needed to determine the duration of therapeutic effect.

Summary

Endoscopic therapy for GERD is an exciting area with a great deal of potential. However, a number of questions remain concerning these new innovative therapies.

The first question regards the mechanism of action. How do these endoscopic therapies work? Good progress has been made in describing the mechanism of action within the last year. Miller et al[10] showed that the area of the gastric sling fibers is bolstered with the EndoCinch device. Tam et al[11] showed a decrease in the number of TLESRs. These 2 mechanisms are consistent with each other in that bolstering the gastric sling fibers would decrease the compliance of the cardia and decrease the number of TLESRs by decreasing the distensibility of the cardia. Most investigators seem to think that all of the endoscopic treatments work by similar mechanisms.

Questions to be answered include: What is the cost effectiveness of these procedures? What is the optimal technique to apply these devices? Who are the optimal patients to receive these procedures? What is the long-term durability of these devices? Finally, what is the long-term safety of these procedures? As these questions are answered, the true place for these endoscopic therapies will be determined.

References

1. Swain CP, Mills TN. An endoscopic sewing machine. *Gastrointest Endosc.* 1986;32:36-38.

2. Swain CP, Kadirkamanathan SS, Gong F, et al. Knot tying at flexible endoscopy. *Gastrointest Endosc.* 1994;40:722-729.

3. Kadirkamanathan SS, Evans DF, Gong F, Yazaki E, Scott M, Swain CP. Antireflux operations at flexible endoscopy using endoluminal stitching techniques: an experimental study. *Gastrointest Endosc.* 1996;44:133-143.

4. Martinez-Serna T, Davis RE, Mason R, et al. Endoscopic valvuloplasty for GERD. *Gastrointest Endosc.* 2000;52:663-670.

5. Filipi CJ, Lehman GA, Rothstein RI, et al. Transoral, flexible endoscopic suturing for treatment of GERD: a multicenter trial. *Gastrointest Endosc.* 2001;53:416-422.

6. Fennerty BM. Endoscopic suturing for treatment of GERD. *Gastrointest Endosc.* 2003;7:390-395.

7. Mahmood Z, McMahon BP, Arfin Q, et al. EndoCinch therapy for gastroesophageal reflux disease: a one year prospective follow up. *Gut.* 2003;52:34-39.

8. Rothstein RI, Pohl H, Grove M, et al. Endoscopic gastric plication for the treatment of GERD. Two-year follow-up results. *Am J Gastroenterol.* 2001;96:S35.

9. Rothstein RI, Hynes ML, Grove M, Pohl H. Endoscopic gastric plication (EndoCinch) for GERD: a randomized, sham controlled, blinded single center study. *Gastrointest Endosc.* 2004;59(5):AB679.

10. Miller LS, Dai Q, Dimitriou J, Schiffer B, Brasseur J. Endoscopic plication (EndoCinch) repairs a physiologic defect in patients with gastroesophageal reflux disease (GERD): absent pressure profile due to the gastric sling fibers. *Gastroenterology.* 2004;126(suppl 2):A-330.

11. Tam WCE, Holloway RH, Dent J, Rigda R, Schoeman MN. Impact of endoscopic suturing of the gastroesophageal junction on lower esophageal sphincter function and gastroesophageal reflux in patients with reflux disease. *Am J Gastroenterol.* 2004;99(2):195-202.

12. Rothstein RI. Sutures and clips for GERD. In: ASGE Clinical Symposium—Endoscopic Therapy for GERD. Program and abstracts of Digestive Disease Week 2004; May 15-20, 2004; New Orleans, Louisiana.

13. Fennerty B. Endotherapy for GERD—what a difference a year makes. Available at: http://www.medscape.com/viewarticle/480235?src. Accessed December 30, 2005.

14. Zabel-Langhennig A, Schiefke I, Neumann S, Gundling F, Moessner J, Caca K. Endoscopic gastroplication (EndoCinch) as an alternative option in treatment of GERD—an 18-month follow up. *Gastroenterology.* 2004;126(suppl 2):A-330.

15. Edmundowicz SA. Injection therapy of the lower esophageal sphincter for the treatment of GERD. *Gastrointest Endosc.* 2004;59(4):545-552.

16. Cosman BJ, Cosman ER. *Guide to Radiofrequency Lesion Generation in Neurosurgery. Radionics Procedure Technique Series Monographs.* Burlington, Mass: Radionics; 1974.

17. Gustavson KH. *The Chemistry and Reactivity of Collagen. The Contraction of Collagen, Particularly Hydrothermal Shrinkage and Cross-linking Reactions.* New York: Academic Press; 1956:211-223.

18. Curon Medical Inc. The Stretta procedure. Endoluminal delivery of temperature-controlled radio frequency energy for the treatment of gastroesophageal reflux disease. Procedure summary, patient selection, clinical data. Version August 15, 2002.

19. Utley DS, Kim M, Vierra MA, Triadafilopoulos G. Augmentation of lower esophageal sphincter pressure and gastric yield pressure after radio frequency energy delivery to the GEJ: a porcine model. *Gastrointest Endosc.* 2000;52:81-86.

20. Tam W, Shoeman MN, Zhang Q, et al. Delivery of radio frequency energy to the lower esophageal sphincter inhibits transient LES relaxations in patients with gastroesophageal reflux disease (GERD): 12 months follow-up. *Gut.* 2003;52(4):479-485.

21. Kim MS, Holloway R, Dent J, Utley DS. Radiofrequency energy (RFe) delivery to the gastric cardia inhibits triggering of transient lower esophageal sphincter relaxations and gastroesophageal reflux in dogs. *Gastrointest Endosc.* 2003;57:17-22.

22. Triadafilopoulos G, DiBaise J, Nostrant IT, et al. The Stretta procedure for the treatment of GERD: 6 and 12-month follow-up of the U.S. open label trial. *Gastrointest Endosc.* 2002;55:149-156.

23. Corley DA, Katz P, Wo J, et al. Temperature-controlled radio frequency energy delivery to the GEJ for the treatment of GERD (the Stretta procedure): a randomized, double-blind, sham-controlled, multi-center clinical trial. *Gastrointest Endosc.* 2002;55:AB19.

24. Houston H, Khaitan L, Holzman M, et al. First experience of patients undergoing the Stretta procedure. *Surg Endosc.* 2003;17(3):401-404.

25. Wolfsen HC, Richards WO. The Stretta procedure for the treatment of GERD, a registry of 558 Patients. *J Laparoendosc Adv Surg Tech.* 2002;12(6):395-402.

26. Triadafilopoulos G, Dibaise J, Nostrant RR, et al. Radiofrequency energy delivery to the GEJ for the treatment of GERD. *Gastrointest Endosc.* 2001;53:407-415.

27. U.S. Food and Drug Administration. Center for Devices and Radiological Health. Available at: www.fda.gov/cdrh.

28. U.S. Food and Drug Administration. Center for Devices and Radiological Health. Available at: www.accessdata.fda.gov/scripts/cdrh/cfdocs/cfMAUDE/search.cfm.

29. Pleskow D, Rothstein R, Lo S, et al. Endoscopic full-thickness plication for the treatment of GERD: 12-month follow-up for the North American open-label trial. Gastrointest Endosc. 2005;61(6):643-649.

30. Fockens P, Bruno MJ, Gabbrielli A, et al. Endoscopic augmentation of the lower esophageal sphincter in the treatment of gastroesophageal reflux disease: Multicenter study of the gatekeeper reflux repair system. *Endoscopy.* 2004;36(8):682-689.

Peptic Ulcer Disease

M. Michael Wolfe, MD; Jonathan T. Simon, MD;
and Robert C. Lowe, MD

Introduction

Peptic ulcer disease (PUD) comprises ulcers in the stomach or duodenum resulting from the digestive action of the gastric secretions on the mucosal surface when the latter is rendered susceptible to their actions.[1] While much has been learned about the causative factors that increase mucosal susceptibility, such as NSAIDs and *H. pylori*, gastric acid still remains the most important of these. Moreover, because acid-reducing medication continues to constitute the mainstay of therapy, it is safe to affirm that Schwarz's dictum stated almost 100 years ago of "no acid, no ulcer" remains applicable.[2] This chapter aims to discuss the pathophysiology of PUD and the manner in which it relates to the clinical presentation, diagnosis, and management of the condition.

Epidemiology

Despite the discovery nearly 20 years ago of *H. pylori* and its association with gastroduodenal ulceration, PUD remains a significant public health problem.[3] The prevalence in the community of PUD has been estimated to be 4% to 10%.[4] More than 10% of residents in the United States have a history of PUD and approximately one third of these have had an active ulcer within the previous year.[5] Moreover, greater than 20% of those with PUD experienced a decline in their functional status, and over 30% complained of somatic and psychological symptoms.[6] The estimated cost attributable to recent ulcers, including the direct costs of health care and indirect costs of lost productivity, amounted to $4.92 to $5.65 billion per year, not including the cost of antisecretory medications.[6] One must keep in mind, however, that PUD is associated with numerous other conditions, including chronic obstructive pulmonary disease (COPD), chronic liver disease, pancreatitis, arthropathies, and arthritis, all of which could contribute to a decreased quality of life.[7,8] It is also unclear how the widespread treatment of *H. pylori* and the addition of the safer NSAIDs (eg, selective COX-2 inhibitors) will affect these statistics.

Despite the enormity of the problem, numerous epidemiologic studies indicate that the prevalence of PUD is declining.[5,9-13] Based on data from the National Hospital Discharge Survey from 1992 to 1999, hospitalizations for PUD declined from 205 to 165 cases per 100,000 patient.[12] Data from the National Diseases Therapeutic Index showed a marked decline in visits for duodenal ulcers (DUs) between 1958 and 1995, while visits for gastric ulcers (GUs) were relatively unchanged.[10] Although these numbers are encouraging, there were still more than 4 million annual physician visits for PUD, and the decrease in prevalence may be a consequence of changes in age demographics. One must also keep in mind that the declining incidence of PUD might be associated with deleterious consequences. A number of studies have suggested that the eradication of *H. pylori* may be contributing to an increase in both GERD and adenocarcinoma of the esophagus.[11,13-16]

Normal Physiology

Because gastric acid plays a critical role in the development of PUD, an understanding of normal gastric acid secretion is essential. The stomach possesses the ability to secrete large quantities of concentrated hydrochloric acid,[17] which creates a sterile intragastric milieu while also aiding in the initiation of digestion. However, under certain conditions, this acid environment can lead to gastroduodenal injury and ultimately ulcer formation.[17] Parietal cells are located in the gastric antrum gastric corpus and fundus and are able to secrete hydrogen ions against the concentration gradient via H+/K+ ATPase. Stimulation of the parietal cell occurs via 3 mechanisms: paracrine, neurocrine, and endocrine (Figure 6-1). The neurotransmitter acetylcholine is released from vagal postganglionic neurons and stimulates muscarinic receptors on the basolateral surface of the parietal cell, leading to acid release. The endocrine stimulus comes from gastrin, which is released by antral G cells and stimulates hydrogen ion formation both directly and indirectly. The indirect mechanism involves gastrin-induced release of histamine from enterochromaffin-like (ECL) cell (often referred to as "controller" cell), which provides the primary paracrine stimulus for acid secretion.[18] Histamine binds to H2 receptors on the basolateral surface of the parietal cell and induces H+ ion generation and secretion. As the principal action of gastrin is mediated via histamine release, it appears that histamine is the more dominant stimulus.[18,19] Coordination among these 3 stimuli leads to the promotion of acid secretion.

Acid secretion is initiated by the release of acetylcholine from the vagus nerve upon the sight, smell, taste, and (most importantly) thought of food. This cephalic phase accounts for 30% to 35% of the total acid output in response to a meal and also accounts for basal and nocturnal acid secretion.[17] Antral distention leads to the initial release of the polypeptide hormone gastrin. Stimulation by gastric distention, however, is transient, and the principal stimuli for the release of gastrin are the pH and protein content of the ingested meal.[17] Moreover, pH constitutes the primary regulation of acid secretion via a negative feedback loop involving gastrin. Once circulating gastrin levels begin to increase after a meal, the intraluminal pH eventually decreases, inducing the release of somatostatin from neighboring antral D cells that then inhibits gastrin release via a paracrine mechanism to prevent post prandial acid hypersecretion. Pyloric glands located in the stomach produce mucus, which protects the gastric mucosa from normal levels of gastric acid and other digestive enzymes.

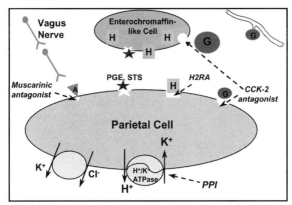

Figure 6-1. Schematic representation of the factors influencing gastric acid secretion by the parietal cell, depicting neurocrine (acetylcholine and other neurotransmitters from vagal efferent neurons), paracrine (somatostatin from D cells and histamine from gastric enterochromaffinlike cells), and endocrine (circulating gastrin) factors. Dashed arrows indicate potential sites of pharmacologic inhibition of acid secretion (in italics), either via receptor antagonism or via inhibition of H+/K+ ATPase. A = acetylcholine and other neurotransmitters, H = histamine, H2RA = H2-receptor antagonist, G = gastrin, CCK-2 = cholecystokinin-2 (gastrin) receptor antagonist, PG = prostaglandin, S = somatostatin, PPI = proton pump inhibitor.

Pathophysiology

As previously stated, PUD develops when the mucosa of the UGI tract becomes susceptible to corrosive forces, the most important of which is gastric acid. The DU patient is an acid hypersecretor.[17] In a study comparing acid secretion among DU patients with age-matched controls, meal-stimulated gastric acid secretion was approximately 70% higher, while night (basal) secretion was approximately 150% higher.[20] The presence of food appears to protect the gastric mucosa against the meal-induced hyperchlorhydria. At night, however, the increased quantity of acid is left to bathe the "bare" gastroduodenal mucosa.[21] Furthermore, duodenal bicarbonate secretion appears to be impaired in DU patients.[22] While acid and pepsin are clear aggressors, other factors clearly play a role in the pathogenesis of ulcers because only 30% of patients with DUs and very few with GUs are actually hyperchlorhydric.[17]

It is helpful to regard factors associated with PUD as either protectors of the gastric mucosa or aggressors (Figure 6-2). When the balance between protective factors (eg, prostaglandins, mucus secretion, and nitric oxide) and aggressive factors (eg, gastric acid, pepsin, and bile salts) is disrupted, mucosal injury may ensue.[17] The 3 main factors that contribute to disturbing this balance are *H. pylori* infection, NSAID use, and smoking. A meta-analysis of risk factors for PUD reported 89% to 95% of cases are attributable to these 3 risk factors.[23]

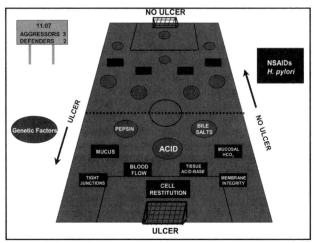

Figure 6-2. Pathogenesis of peptic ulcer modeled as an imbalance between aggressive and defensive factors within the gastroduodenal mucosa. Ulcers form when aggressive factors (eg, acid and pepsin) overwhelm the defensive mechanisms normally present within the mucosa. In most instances, acid and pepsin secretion is not increased, but rather mucosal resistance is diminished by factors such as NSAID ingestion or *H. pylori* infection.

HELICOBACTER PYLORI (H. PYLORI)

H. pylori is a gram-negative, spiral, flagellated, urease-positive bacterium that has the ability to colonize the gastroduodenal mucosa and cause inflammation.[3] By virtue of its ability to split urea into bicarbonate and ammonia, the organism is able to buffer H+ ions before the intracellular pH drops below 5, allowing it to survive in the acidic environment of the stomach and adhere to specific receptors on the gastric epithelial cell.[24] Once attached, the organism causes mucosal damage by various mechanisms. Ammonia may itself cause mucosal injury, and there is also a disruption in gastric acid control because those with *H. pylori* infection have been shown to have a reduced number of somatostatin secreting D cells, thereby disrupting the negative feedback control of gastrin release and subsequently acid secretion.[25-27] This disruption leads to an increase in postprandial acid secretion as the inhibition of gastrin release is attenuated.[21] The principal virulence factors inherent to *H. pylori*, however, appear to be 2 identified proteins, vacuolating cytotoxin A (VacA) and cytotoxin-associated gene (CagA), that are present in some strains of the bacteria.

VacA induces vacuolization of epithelial cells in vitro and induces epithelial cell damage in mice. It is endocytosed by epithelial cells, and the low intragastric pH subsequently activates the toxin, leading to vacuolization and ultimately cell death.[28,29] Different variants of the cytotoxin with differing potencies have been identified, with the more aggressive forms being associated with PUD and the more benign forms being associated with asymptomatic gastritis.[30]

No specific function has been identified for CagA, and the gene product is actually a marker found within an island of approximately 30 genes sometimes referred to as the "CagA pathogenicity island" (cagA PAI). Within the cagA PAI are genes involved in stimulating the production of various proinflammatory cytokines, in particular IL-8,24,31,32, which leads to the migration of neutrophils and the release of proteases and other digestive enzymes, with subsequent mucosal damage. Approximately 60% of isolates from western countries are CagA positive, and epidemiological evidence suggests that this strain confers a higher level of risk than CagA negative strains, as well as a decreased risk of esophageal diseases (ie, GERD and adenocarcinoma of the esophagus).[11,13-16] Other virulence factors have been identified, including CagD and E, urease, neutrophil activating protein, and superoxide dismutase; however, CagA and VacA remain the most important.[31,32]

NONSTEROIDAL ANTI-INFLAMMATORY DRUGS AND COXIBS

NSAIDs produce topical mucosal injury due to their acidic nature,[33] with additional damage due to the biliary secretion and subsequent duodenogastric reflux of active NSAID metabolites.[34,35] The principal toxicity of NSAIDs, however, occurs as a result of their systemic ability to impair prostaglandin synthesis.[33,36] This contention is supported by the fact that enteric-coated aspirin preparations or parenteral delivery of NSAIDs does not protect against PUD.[36-38] Endogenous prostaglandins protect the gastric mucosa through various mechanisms. They promote the production of mucus, which traps H+ ions and permits bicarbonate secreted by epithelial cells to effectively titrate acid. In addition, prostaglandins increase mucosal blood flow to augment delivery of oxygen, nutrients, and bicarbonate and remove toxic metabolites ("alkaline tide"). They maintain intracellular tight junctions to prevent penetration of H+ ions and promote epithelial renewal (ie, cell restitution), enabling the mucosa to repair itself following injury.[17,39-41] It is clearly evident that the elimination of these defense mechanisms would render the gastric mucosa susceptible to even normal amounts of acid, pepsin, and bile salts, as well as to the added insult of the acidic NSAID preparation itself.

As stated above, the main action of NSAIDs is through the inhibition of the cyclooxygenase enzyme that is responsible for the generation of prostaglandins from arachidonic acid (Figure 6-3).[33] Inhibition of this enzyme, not only attenuates the synthesis of proinflammatory cytokines, but also those that protect the GI tract. Approximately 15 years ago came the discovery that the cyclooxygenase enzyme has two related, yet distinct, isomers, designated cyclooxygenase-1 and -2, respectively (COX-1 and COX-2).[42,43] Although structurally similar, they are encoded by 2 distinct genes and are distributed and expressed differently.[44,45] COX-1 is expressed constitutively and is responsible for the production of the protective prostaglandins, whereas COX-2 is nearly undetectable in most tissues under normal physiologic conditions but can be induced by inflammatory stimuli.[46] It has been postulated that the "protective" prostaglandins are mediated by COX-1 activity, while the pro-inflammatory prostaglandins are produced via the induction of COX-2.[43,46] Therefore, by developing COX-2 specific inhibitors, it was postulated that one should be able to achieve an adequate anti-inflammatory effect while avoiding GI toxicity. Early studies have indicated that this hypothesis may in fact be the case.[47-51] These agents, however, are expensive and may promote thrombotic events, and their widespread use may thus not be cost-effective. Furthermore, studies have suggested that other mechanisms, such as increased neutrophil adherence leading to the release of proteases and oxygen-derived free radicals, may be at least partly responsible for the GI toxicity of NSAIDs.[52-54]

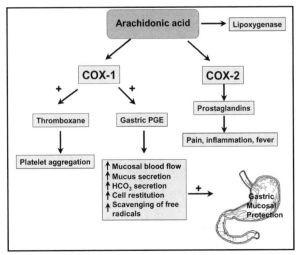

Figure 6-3. Arachidonic acid, derived from membrane phospholipids, is the precursor of prostaglandins, which is catalyzed by the 2 cyclooxygenase enzymes. The gene for cyclooxygenase-1 is expressed constituitively and maintains the homeostasis of organs, which includes the integrity of the gastric mucosa. The COX-2 gene is inducible and is responsible for the production of inflammatory prostaglandins. COX-1 = cyclooxygenase-1, COX-2 = cyclooxygenase 2, PGE = prostaglandin, HCO3 = bicarbonate. (Reprinted with permission from Wolfe, Lichtenstein, Sing. Medical progress: gastrointestinal toxicity of nonsteroidal antiinflammatory drugs. *N Eng J Med.* 1999;340:1888-1899. Copyright © 1999. Massachusetts Medical Society. All rights reserved.)

CIGARETTES

Cigarette smoking has also been considered an aggressive factor in the development of PUD. Smoking adversely affects many of the natural mucosal protective mechanisms and enhances aggressive factors, such as stimulating pepsin release and increasing the production of free radicals.[55] Smoking has no clear effect on acid secretion, although the response to H2-receptor antagonists (H2RAs) in smokers is impaired, and cigarettes relax the pyloric sphincter, allowing the reflux of duodenal contents into the stomach.[55] Over time, smoking leads to a decrease in the amount of gastric mucus produced and to a decrease in the levels of protective prostaglandins.[55-57] It has been demonstrated that immediately after smoking, there is a transient decrease in both pancreatic bicarbonate secretion and acid-stimulated duodenal mucosal bicarbonate secretion, leading to a lower duodenal pH and consequently a reduction in the capacity to buffer gastric acid.[58-60]

Smoking also appears to increase the risk and virulence of *H. pylori*.[55] In one study of patients with normal endoscopy, 50% of smokers versus 36% of nonsmokers were found to be infected with *H. pylori*.[61] Nicotine can induce mucosal cell vacuolization on its own and, in the presence of *H. pylori*, has been shown to potentiate the actions of the vacuolating toxin. Smoking does not, however, have an effect on ulcer recurrence and does not impair ulcer healing after successful treatment of *H. pylori*.[62-64]

Hypersecretory States

In a minority of patients, the balance between protective and aggressive factors is disrupted simply because of the overproduction of acid due to a hypersecretory state. Although the conditions that cause acid hypersecretion are relatively uncommon, they should be ruled out in cases of PUD without typical risk factors (ie, *H. pylori*, NSAIDs) or in those who fail to respond to standard treatments. The most noteworthy of these conditions is Zollinger-Ellison syndrome (ZES), in which a gastrin-secreting tumor stimulates acid production that is not subject to the normal feedback inhibition of acid. Other rare causes of hypersecretory states are systemic mastocytosis, antral G-cell hyperplasia, and extensive small bowel resection.

The true incidence and prevalence of ZES are unknown; however, in the United States, the frequency of ZES is one per million, with most patients presenting in the sixth decade of life.[65,66] ZES can either be due to a sporadic gastrinoma or be part of the Multiple Endocrine Neoplasia I syndrome (MEN 1), an autosomal dominant disorder characterized by parathyroid hyperplasia, peripancreatic endocrine tumors, and pituitary adenomas.[66] ZES is the most common pancreatic neuroendocrine tumor among MEN 1 patients, being present in 10% to 48% of cases, but sporadic tumors account for 62% to 80% of all gastrinoma cases. The overproduction of acid will eventually lead to symptomatic PUD in greater than 90% of individuals with ZES. Other symptoms characteristic of ZES include diarrhea and severe GERD.

Presentation

RISK FACTORS

Because there is generally a paucity of physical findings in patients with uncomplicated PUD, it important to determine those individuals at risk for the disease. Historically, it has been reported that PUD occurs predominantly in men, although more recent studies indicate that the prevalence in men and women is more even than originally thought. The National Health Interview Survey reported that patients with lower levels of education or socioeconomic status were more likely to have had an ulcer,[67] which may be related to higher levels of *H. pylori* infection among lower socioeconomic classes. Genetic factors may be relevant, as well as those with the Lewis blood group phenotype Le (A+ B-). Men with the O or A phenotype, in the ABO blood group, have been found to have a significantly higher lifetime prevalence of PUD.[68] The role of other environmental factors, such as the intake of sugar, alcohol, and caffeine, remains controversial. However, it appears in some studies that there are stronger associations with these environmental stimuli among patients who are genetically susceptible to PUD.[69] Irrespective of these genetic factors, the 3 most important risk factors for PUD are smoking, active *H. pylori* infection, and NSAID use, with the latter 2 being more predictive.[70-73]

SMOKING

As previously stated, smoking adversely affects many of the natural gastric protective mechanisms and enhances the aggressive factors. It is, therefore, no surprise that numerous epidemiological studies have shown that smokers are more likely to develop a peptic ulcer, have ulcers that are difficult to heal, and are more likely to relapse.[55,74-78] It is interesting to note, however, that in the National Health Interview Survey of 41,500 randomly selected individuals in 1989, smokers did not have a higher incidence of PUD than nonsmokers and there was no association between the amount smoked and the incidence of PUD.[67] This discrepancy is likely related to greater PPI use and the treatment of *H. pylori*.

H. pylori

H. pylori infection is present in more than 50% of the world population, but in most individuals, it represents an asymptomatic infection. The bacterium is transmitted via a fecal-oral or oral-oral route and, therefore, is predominantly associated with lower socioeconomic status in which people may live in close quarters and in less than sanitary conditions. In developing countries, up to 90% of the population is infected, with most being infected by other children at a very young age. In contrast, in developed countries, the prevalence is only 5% to 20% in patients under age 40.[24] *H. pylori* infection was initially thought to be associated with up to 95% of PUD; recent studies, however, suggest it may be responsible for as few as 32% of ulcers in nonreferral-based populations.[23]

Nonsteroidal Anti-Inflammatory Drugs

More than 70 million prescriptions for NSAIDs and more than 30 billion over-the-counter NSAID tablets are sold annually in the United States.[79] With these medications being so widely used, it has become important to determine those at greatest risk for developing gastroduodenal ulcer complications while taking NSAIDs (Table 6-1). Various studies have shown that 15% to 20% of chronic NSAID users develop PUD, with the highest risk associated with individuals over age 65, a prior history of PUD, concomitant use of steroids or anticoagulants, higher drug doses or using more than one NSAID, and serious coexisting conditions.[52,80-90]

CLINICAL FEATURES/SYMPTOMS

While the hallmark symptom of PUD is nonradiating epigastric abdominal pain, the disorder can present in a variety of different ways. The pain may be described as burning, "a hunger pang," or cramping and the pain may be associated with nausea and is usually relieved with antacids or food intake. A typical DU patient complains of mid-epigastric pain approximately 2 to 4 hours after eating or in the middle of the night, coincident with a circadian increase in basal acid secretion. Initially, food acts as a buffer, but gastric acid is still secreted after food has traversed the stomach into the small intestine, leaving the ulcer "exposed." Eating typically exacerbates GU pain and this response to a meal had been considered a means of distinguishing gastric from DUs. However, all individuals do not report these "textbook" complaints. In one study of 360 patients with dyspepsia, only 20% of those ultimately found to have DUs reported relief of abdominal pain with eating and only 70% reported their symptoms awakened them from sleep.[91] Other studies have demonstrated that while

Table 6-1

RISK FACTORS FOR PELVIC ULCER DISEASE IN NONSTEROIDAL ANTI-INFLAMMATORY DRUG USERS

Established Risk Factors

- Advanced age >65.
- History of ulcer.
- Concomitant use of corticosteroids.
- Higher doses of NSAIDs or more than one NSAID.
- Concomitant administration of anticoagulants.
- Serious systemic disorder.

Possible Risk Factors

- Concomitant infection with *H. pylori.*
- Cigarette smoking.
- Consumption of alcohol.

the midepigastrium is the most typical location of ulcer pain, patients may complain of pain in other locations in the abdomen.[92] Other nonspecific complaints are also common and include nausea and vomiting in up to 60% of patients. Confounding the problem of such nonspecific clinical complaints is the significant number of asymptomatic patients. As many as 50% to 60% of patients with hemorrhage from NSAID-induced GU report no antecedent GI complaints.[52,80,93-95]

CLINICAL FEATURES/COMPLICATION AND PHYSICAL FINDINGS

Unfortunately, the physical exam is largely unrevealing in PUD patients unless complications, such as a visceral perforation, hemorrhage, or obstruction, have developed. Some patients may experience epigastric tenderness to deep palpation or have guaiac (occult-positive) positive stools; however, no positive physical finding will be found in the vast majority of patients with uncomplicated disease.

Hemorrhage

Upper GI bleeding is responsible for about 250,000 hospitalizations annually,[96] with PUD being the most common cause, accounting for 45% to 78% of episodes.[82,97-99] More recent studies, however, suggest these figures may overstate the true prevalence of ulcer-induced hemorrhage.[100] Patients presenting with GI bleeding may complain of melena or hematemesis, and as many as 10% of patients with an UGI source of blood loss will present with frank hematochezia. It is important to remember that 50% to 60% of patients taking NSAIDs will have no antecedent symptoms before presenting with GI bleeding.[52,80,93-95]

Perforation

Perforation of a GU or DU occurs most commonly in the fifth or sixth decade, with an approximate incidence of 3 to 10 cases per 100,000 persons per year.[101,102] Particular attention should be paid to NSAIDs because their use is associated with a high risk of ulcer complications, which is further increased by concomitant steroid use. The most common presenting symptom is the sudden onset of severe abdominal pain predominantly in the epigastrium initially. In addition, the pain may become more diffuse with radiation to the back, the lower quadrants, or to the shoulders from diaphragmatic irritation. Nausea and vomiting may be present, and 10% to 15% of cases will have concomitant GI bleeding.

Obstruction

The incidence of gastric outlet obstruction form from PUD has been reported to be 6% to 21.5% in several studies,[103] but the incidence is declining with the availability of more potent anti-secretory therapies. Patients generally have a long-standing history of abdominal pain, and the onset of obstruction is usually marked by nausea and vomiting. Other symptoms include early satiety, bloating, and a sense of fullness in the epigastrium. If the process occurs gradually, patients may complain of weight loss and may have signs of dehydration and/or electrolyte abnormalities.

Evaluation

Perhaps the most difficult aspect of the diagnosis of PUD is differentiating it from nonulcer dyspepsia. Dyspepsia is defined as a constellation of symptoms that include midepigastric pain or discomfort that is intermittent or constant and that may be associated with nausea, vomiting, or any symptom perceived to be emanating from the GI tract.[104] Obviously, not everyone with dyspepsia will have PUD. Other diseases to consider are GERD, gastric cancer, or dysmotility syndromes; however, the vast majority of patients will have no identifiable organic cause for their symptoms and will accordingly be labeled as having nonulcer dyspepsia.[105] Determining who to refer for more invasive testing (ie, endoscopy) and who to manage conservatively is a key element of a physician's approach to a patient with dyspepsia.

HISTORY AND PHYSICAL

The initial evaluation of a patient with suspected PUD should start with a history and physical. Although not all patients present with the "textbook" complaint of nonradiating midepigastric pains that improves with eating and antacids, worsens 2 to 4 hours after eating, and occurs during the middle of the night, the presence of these complaints is suggestive of PUD. Because patient complaints will vary, it is helpful to obtain information that may be suggestive of other potential disease processes. The presence of warning signs, such as bleeding (melena, rectal bleeding, and hematemesis), weight loss, or dysphagia, may be worrisome and should prompt the physician to exclude the possibility of gastric or esophageal malignancy and should trigger a more prompt referral for endoscopic evaluation. A family history for GI malignancies is also helpful, and the presence of other tumors in the family may provide a hint to an underlying hypersecretory state in rare cases (ie, MEN 1).

A thorough medication history should also be obtained. A potentially helpful piece of information is any remedy the patient may have self-administered to relieve pain, such as antacids, H2RAs, or over-the-counter PPIs. Furthermore, aggravating medications should also be sought with particular attention to NSAIDs, including aspirin. Ten percent to 20% of patients will experience dyspepsia while on NSAIDs,[52,93] but most people are unaware or are not concerned with potential GI complications caused by NSAIDs.[80] Also, most would expect some type of warning sign prior to the development of serious GI complications; however, as stated above, only a minority of patients who develop serious GI complications report any antecedent dyspepsia.[94,95] Other medications that might increase the risk of complicated PUD in patients taking NSAIDs include anticoagulants and glucocorticoids. Some medications (such as certain antibiotics) may not contribute to the development of PUD, but they may still be responsible for the patient's symptoms. In addition, some drugs (eg, sulfa-containing preparations and azathioprine) can cause pancreatitis, which may help guide the evaluation.

Although the physical exam is largely unrevealing, certain findings may be helpful, especially in the setting of complications. Signs of bleeding can be assessed by a rectal exam, during which time it is more important that the color of the stool be evaluated rather then the presence of fecal occult blood, which could be coming anywhere from the GI tract. A patient may also have signs of anemia, such as orthostasis or pallor. Patients with a perforation may have a low-grade fever, tachycardia, and tachypnea, as well as a tender abdominal exam including (on occasion) peritoneal signs of guarding, rebound tenderness, or rigidity. A patient with gastric outlet obstruction may have abdominal distension and signs of weight loss, and a "succussion splash" may be heard over the epigastrium when the abdomen is shaken from side to side. Lymphadenopathy (ie, "Sister Mary Joseph node" or "Virchow node") and cachexia could be indicative of gastric cancer. The liver may be enlarged from metastases or an abdominal mass may be palpated. All of these findings are nonspecific, but their presence should prompt more thorough evaluation if clinically appropriate.

ROUTINE LAB EVALUATION

The initial evaluation should start with the least invasive test and proceed with more invasive testing as necessary. It is reasonable to begin with a laboratory evaluation; however, in most patients with dyspepsia and no GI warning signs, routine lab testing is unlikely to be helpful. If the patient has signs and symptoms of anemia, a complete blood count should be obtained, as well as iron studies and B_{12} and folate levels if the patient is truly anemic. A rectal exam is indicated to evaluate for the presence of melena or frank hematochezia; however, checking for fecal occult blood in a patient with dyspeptic symptoms is not routinely necessary. Liver enzymes, amylase, and lipase are not routinely recommended in the evaluation of dyspepsia but may reveal another source of symptoms, such as biliary colic or pancreatitis, and thus should be obtained if these conditions are suspected. Obtaining a fasting serum gastrin level may also be helpful if a hypersecretory state is suspected (see below), but one must keep in mind that patients on PPIs may have a false positive value as a result of disruption of the normal negative feedback inhibition of gastrin secretion by acid. As stated above, epidemiologic studies have shown that PUD is more likely to develop in those with blood group O or in patients that are nonsecretors of their blood group antigens.[68] However, such testing has not been shown to be helpful in characterizing individual risk for PUD and is not recommended for guiding management.[106]

Table 6-2

AVAILABLE TESTS FOR *H. PYLORI*

Test	Advantage	Disadvantage
Steiner's stain of gastric biopsy	Considered the gold standard	Invasive/expensive
Rapid urease test	Rapid result, allows for confirmation of cure	Reduced sensitivity with acid suppression or active bleeding Invasive
Culture	Permits antimicrobial sensitivity testing	Requires experienced laboratory and time
Serology (ELISA; lab based)	Accurate and convenient for initial infection	Titers may remain positive after 1 year; therefore, can't use to test for cure
Serology (ELISA; office based)	Fast, convenient, and inexpensive	Less accurate
H. pylori stool antigen	Relatively convenient if available	Sensitivity reduced with active bleeding
String test	Allows for retrieval of viable organisms without endoscopy	Less accurate than biopsy
Urine ELISA	Greater patient acceptance and convenience; not affected by bleeding	Not yet widely available
Saliva ELISA	Greater patient acceptance and convenience; not affected by bleeding	Not yet widely available

NONINVASIVE TESTS FOR H. PYLORI

The gold standard for diagnosing *H. pylori* is the demonstration of the organism in a biopsy specimen of the stomach obtained during endoscopy. Recently, however, several easily available, noninvasive ways of determining the presence of *H. pylori* infection have been developed. These include serum serology against bacterial antigens, breath testing, stool antigen testing, and a string test, each of which has its advantages and disadvantages (Table 6-2).

The string test obtains a specimen for culture by having the patient partially swallow a highly adsorbent polymer string, which is then manually removed.[107] It is less reliable than the other methods[108] and while less invasive than an endoscopy, it is more difficult than obtaining a blood test and is less acceptable to patients than breath testing, which is the reason the test is not widely used.

Serum serology takes advantage of the fact that *H. pylori* is a chronic infection that induces a systemic immune response that results in increased antibody (IgG) titers that will decline slowly after treatment.[109] One potential disadvantage is that this serologic test demonstrates only exposure to the organism, which may not necessarily represent an active infection. On the other hand, it is accurate, is relatively inexpensive, is not affected by acid suppression medication, and does not require patient fasting.[109]

Another noninvasive means of checking for *H. pylori* infection is the 13C-urea breath test, which utilizes the urease-producing capacity of *H. pylori* to determine if active infection is present. Following an overnight fast, the patient is given 13C-labeled urea. Breath samples are then analyzed using an isotope ratio mass spectrometer to measure the amount of radiolabeled $13CO_2$ that is produced compared with what would be expected at baseline. Using a discriminatory value of 6 atom percentage excess over baseline will yield a sensitivity and specificity of 95% to 99% and 94% to 99%, respectively.[110] Patients need to be off PPI therapy for approximately 2 weeks to avoid false-negative results, and the test may be less accurate in postgastrectomy patients.[111]

Stool and urine antigen tests for *H. pylori* are currently being tested and will soon be available for widespread use. The advantages of the stool tests are that they are simple, inexpensive, reliable, and can be used in post-treatment follow-up.[112] However, they have been demonstrated to give a significant number of false positives in patients who are bleeding.[113] This problem may be circumvented by a urine-based antigen test, which represents another simple, inexpensive, and reliable method of detecting *H. pylori*.[114] It may also be more accurate in postgastrectomy patients, is not affected by PPI or bismuth therapy, and is easier to obtain in children or uncooperative patients.[114] Other more invasive ways to test for *H. pylori* are available, such as a rapid urease testing or biopsy, which will be addressed below.

It has been suggested that in certain patient populations with dyspeptic symptoms, it may be reasonable to test for *H. pylori* and empirically treat this infection rather than refer all patients for an endoscopy. While this seems to be a reasonable approach, it raises several questions. In what situations is it acceptable to apply a test-and-treat strategy without further evaluation? Should every patient with *H. pylori* infection be treated? What are the long-term costs and epidemiologic implications (ie, a possible increase in adenocarcinoma of the esophagus)[11,13-16] of such a practice? Moreover, as discussed below, the practice of treating *H. pylori* infection has not been shown to reliably alleviate dyspepsia,[115-117] and widespread antibiotic use may contribute to the serious worldwide problem of antimicrobial resistance.

Whom to Test

Although opinions vary considerably, a simple guideline is that any patient with GI warning signs should not be appropriate for a test-and-treat strategy. These warning signs include weight loss, any sign of GI bleeding, and dysphagia, all of which require more prompt and aggressive diagnostic intervention because they may be indicative of more significant pathology. Furthermore, the new onset of symptoms in patients over age 45 should also be investigated more thoroughly. For the large group of younger dyspeptic patients with no risk factors, the test-and-treat strategy has been the subject

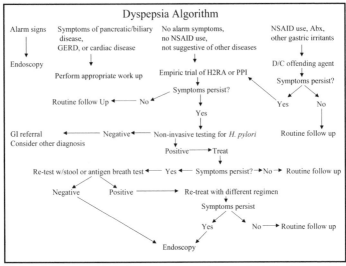

Figure 6-4. Approach to the management of dyspepsia defined as a pain or discomfort in the midepigastrium that is intermittent of persistent for more than 4 weeks. GERD = gastroesophageal reflux disease, NSAIDs = nonsteroidal anti-inflammatory medications, Abx = antibiotics, H2RA = histamine 2 receptor antagonist, PPI =proton pump inhibitor.

of ongoing debate. In a study by Sharma et al of 155 patients with positive *H. pylori* serology and urea breath tests who underwent upper endoscopy, no statistically significant relationship with symptoms and endoscopic diagnoses was detected.[118] Although a 2-week course of antibiotics may seem innocuous, several points bear mentioning. First, there is no clear relief of symptoms in patients with nonulcer dyspepsia after treatment for *H. pylori*.[115-117] Moreover, 2 weeks of antibiotic therapy is expensive, is at times difficult to tolerate, and may lead to antibiotic resistance by not only *H. pylori* but other organisms as well.

It has been suggested that determining the strain of *H. pylori*, with particular attention to the VacA gene and the Cag PAI, may be helpful in predicting which patients with *H. pylori* will have or will develop PUD. There does appear to be a strong correlation between infection with a CagA+ *H. pylori* strain and PUD,[15,119,120] although not all studies have demonstrated this relationship.[121] Moreover, in some patient populations, the percentage of CagA positivity in *H. pylori* strains is significant, precluding the use of this test for population screening.[119] As more is learned about the different strains of *H. pylori*, the clinical use of this information may become clearer, but at present there appears to be no role for these virulence factors in the diagnosis or management of PUD.

In summary, while the definitive answers regarding the appropriate situations in which to test and treat for *H. pylori* have not been elucidated, a role for such testing in the evaluation of young, otherwise healthy, dyspeptic patients without GI warning signs has been recommended by some authorities. An algorithm for evaluation strategies for *H. pylori* testing and treatment is presented in Figure 6-4.

Table 6-3

HIGH RISK PATIENTS FOR PEPTIC ULCER DISEASE

- New-onset dyspepsia in individuals over age 50.
- Dyspepsia associated with dysphagia and/or weight loss.
- Those with evidence of GI bleeding.
- Those who have not responded to an appropriate trial of empiric therapy.
- Those patients using NSAIDs or other ulcerogenic agents.
- Those with signs of UGI tract obstruction.

  Those with ethnic and or racial backgrounds associated with increased risk for UGI malignancies or other significant disease states.

IMAGING

Several radiologic tests can be used in the diagnosis of PUD. However, advances in endoscopy have significantly reduced their role in diagnosis. Unless complications have developed, which may be obvious on physical exam, a KUB (abdominal x-ray) is generally unhelpful. A UGI series may reveal the presence of an ulcer as well as GER or a gastric mass. In the past, it was believed that a UGI series was as accurate as an endoscopic exam when performed by an experienced radiologist.[122] Numerous studies, however, have disproved this contention, with as many as 40% of active DUs and up to 50% of active GUs missed on barium study.[123,124] Furthermore, superficial mucosal lesions are easily missed, and it is difficult to differentiate an active ulcer from a depressed scar.[125] For these reasons, it is recommended that if the resources are available and if the patient is able to tolerate conscious sedation, the preferred test for the evaluation of dyspepsia is an upper endoscopy.

ENDOSCOPY

Endoscopy has replaced barium-based radiographic studies as the gold standard for diagnosing or excluding PUD. In addition to its diagnostic superiority over barium studies, it is easy and safe to perform, is generally well tolerated, and allows for the ability to take biopsies and perform therapeutic interventions if necessary. Any patient who is deemed high risk (Table 6-3) should be referred for endoscopy. Endoscopy should also be performed in any patient who has had no response to empiric acid suppression therapy, who experiences a recurrence of symptoms after completion of therapy, or in whom symptoms progress while on treatment.[126]

Endoscopy also permits definitive testing for *H. pylori*, which should be performed once the diagnosis of PUD is established.[127] This testing may be done by biopsy and sending tissue for histology or via the performance of a rapid urease test (eg, CLO-test [Kimberly-Clark/Ballard Medical Products, Draper, Utah]). The rapid urease test again takes advantage of the ability of the organism to degrade urea. It involves placing a gastric mucosal sample in a well containing urea and a pH-sensitive color indicator in which the color changes when the urea is degraded and the pH increases. It is important to note that PPI therapy can interfere with the test result[127] as can the presence of blood.[128] In such cases, biopsies from the gastric antrum and body should be sent for histologic examination; if both are negative, other tests for *H. pylori* (eg, serology) should be obtained.[127] In addition to searching for *H. pylori* at the time of endoscopy, it may also be necessary to biopsy the edges of the ulcer crater itself if a GU is present. Such biopsies not only evaluate for the presence of *H. pylori* but can also exclude an underlying gastric malignancy.

EVALUATION OF COMPLICATIONS

Bleeding

The presence of melena is a very reliable indicator for an UGI source of blood loss. A nasogastric (NG) tube can be helpful during the assessment of UGI bleeding; however, it should be noted that up to 15% of patients with active UGI bleeding will have a negative NG aspirate, especially if the patient is bleeding from a DU. An NG aspirate may be more helpful to rule out an UGI source of blood loss in the case of a patient with frank hematochezia. If melena is present, an upper endoscopy should be performed promptly to determine the presence of PUD, as well as to exclude other causes of bleeding and for the performance of definitive treatment.

Perforation

If a perforation is suggested by the physical findings, its presence should be confirmed with a plain film of the chest and the abdomen to look for free air under the diaphragm. It is recommended that patients remain upright or in the decubitus position for 10 to 15 minutes prior to obtaining these films to allow air to rise to its highest point. If the diagnosis is still in doubt, a CT scan with oral contrast or an UGI series with water-soluble contrast material (eg, Gastrograffin [Bristol-Myers-Squibb, Princeton, NJ]) may be helpful.

Obstruction

The diagnosis of a gastric outlet obstruction can be made by barium contrast radiography, which will demonstrate a markedly dilated stomach and a lack of emptying of contrast into the duodenum. While an endoscopy is not urgent in this case, it will ultimately need to be performed to rule out a malignant cause for the obstruction.

HYPERSECRETORY STATES

In a relatively small number of patients, a hypersecretory state may be responsible for PUD, and it is important to know when to suspect such a condition and the appropriate diagnostic evaluation. The diagnosis is often missed and several clinical clues should trigger appropriate testing (Table 6-4). These include a lack of typical ulcer risk factors, difficult to control symptoms with standard doses of anti-secretory treatment, multiple duodenal and postbulbar or jejunal ulcers, a family history of PUD and hypercalcemia, a personal history of nephrolithiasis, and PUD associated with chronic diarrhea. It is interesting to note that diarrhea appears to be less frequent among those with ZES associated with MEN 1 than in those with sporadic gastrinomas.[129]

Table 6-4

CLINICAL FEATURES CONSISTENT WITH A HYPERSECRETORY STATE*

- Postbulbar duodenal ulcer
- Multiple duodenal and/or jejunal ulcers
- PUD in association with chronic diarrhea
- PUD refractory to medical therapy
- History of PUD and nephrolithiasis
- Recurrent PUD in the absence of *H. pylori*
- Family history of PUD and hypercalcemia

* eg, ZES.

If ZES is suspected, several tests can be obtained to confirm the diagnosis. A fasting serum gastrin should be obtained initially. It is important to note that patients must be off PPI therapy, which can lead to a falsely elevated serum gastrin level. The diagnosis is certain when the fasting plasma gastrin is >1000 pg/mL and the basal acid output is greater than 15 mmol per hour in patients with intact stomachs or greater than 5 mmol per hour in patients with a history of prior gastric surgery.[65] If positive, somatostatin receptor scintigraphy (eg, Octreoscan [Mallinckrodt, Inc, St. Louis, Mo]) should be performed as the initial test to attempt to localize the tumor. Endoscopic ultrasonography also may help localize the tumor. Ultimately, however, surgical exploration may be necessary by an experienced surgeon to locate the tumor.

It is important to exclude MEN 1 when ZES is diagnosed and equally important to exclude ZES when MEN 1 is found. This distinction is true not only because of the severe gastric acid secretion that may lead to complications, but also because 60% to 90% of gastrinomas will be malignant.[66] It is also important to establish a diagnosis of MEN 1 because the management differs in a number of areas, including the surgical approach,[130,131] the need to evaluate for the presence of other endocrinopathies,[132] the difficulty in controlling the acid secretion (as hypercalcemia can stimulate gastrin release),[133,134] the need for family screening,[132] and the risk of development of other endocrine cell tumors.[66,132] It is important to note that patients with ZES associated with MEN 1 are not amenable to long-term surgical cure.[129,130]

Treatment of Pelvic Ulcer Disease

The goals of therapy should be symptom relief, ulcer healing, and the prevention of complications and recurrence.[135] These goals can be achieved by eliminating aggressive factors and augmenting the protective ones. The discovery of *H. pylori* has dramatically changed the approach to therapy. Because successful eradication results in significantly lower rates of recurrence, the determination of *H. pylori* infection is critical in our approach to management. If the infection is not present, an alternative etiology for PUD should be sought, including the use of NSAIDs, ZES, Crohn's disease, vascular insufficiency, viral infection, radiation treatment, or chemotherapy. Regardless of the etiology, acid suppression remains the cornerstone of therapy.[21]

ACID SUPPRESSION AND OTHER NONSYSTEMIC APPROACHES

Topical Agents

Sucralfate and Antacids

Antacids were first shown to be effective in healing PUD compared with placebo in a study by Peterson et al in 1977.[136] However, they need to be taken in multiple doses throughout the day (at least 4 and up to 7 times daily) and have a high frequency of side effects, including altered bowel movements, electrolyte abnormalities, and decreased absorption of other medications.[137,138] In an attempt to avoid these side effects, sucralfate, an aluminum octasulfate preparation, was introduced in Japan in 1968 and was approved for use in the United States in 1981. This agent has been shown to be effective in healing ulcers[139]; however, it also must be administered 4 times per day to achieve healing. With the advent of potent antisecretory agents, the use of sucralfate in PUD has waned considerably.

ANTISECRETORY AGENTS

H2-Receptor Antagonists

In 1970, it was shown that the selective inhibition of the histamine H2 receptor suppresses acid production,[140] and in 1977, cimetidine, the first commercially available H2RA, was released in the United States, revolutionizing the treatment of acid-related disorders.[141] As a class, H2RAs are more effective in inhibiting acidity during the basal state, which is greatest during the night.[142] Although DU healing is directly proportional to the degree of 24-hr acid suppression, it is also proportional to nocturnal acid reduction. As a result, H2RAs should be ideally administered to patients with DUs between the evening meal and bedtime. Furthermore, it has been shown that a single evening dose (with an equivalent total daily dose) is at least as effective in promoting healing as twice daily dosing.[143] H2RAs promote healing in 70% to 80% of patients after 4 to 6 weeks compared with placebo healing rates of 20% to 45%.[21] No controlled trials have demonstrated the superiority of one H2RA over another at equivalent doses. Based on studies of ulcer healing rates, treatment for 4 weeks for DU and 8 weeks for GU is recommended (Table 6-5).[21,144,145]

Proton Pump Inhibitors

The identification of H+K+ ATPase (the acid or proton pump) as the final common pathway of acid secretion allowed for the development of potent inhibitory agents (PPIs). Ultimately, after several modifications to reduce toxicity and to optimize stability, omeprazole was synthesized in 1979 and introduced in Europe in 1988. The percentage of time that intragastric pH is greater than 3 is significantly greater after administration of a PPI compared with an H2RA.[146,147] Furthermore, studies suggest that PPIs heal gastroduodenal ulcers[148-150] more rapidly than H2RAs. Finally, because

Table 6-5

EQUIVALENT DRUG DOSAGE AND DURATION OF TREATMENT

Medication	Equivalent Dose	Healing Rate
Antacids	>200 mEq of neutralizing capacity	70% to 80% at 4 weeks
Sucralfate	I g four times a day (QID)	70% to 80% at 4 weeks
H2RAs	Famotidine 40 mg every hour as needed (qhs)	
	Ranitidine 300 mg qhs	70% to 80% at 4 weeks
	Nizatidine 300 mg qhs	87% to 94% at 8 weeks
	Cimetidine 800 to 1200 mg qhs	
PPIs	Omeprazole 20 mg every morning (QAM)	80% to 100% at 4 weeks
	Lansoprazole 30 mg by mouth (PO) QAM	
	Rabeprazole 20 mg QAM	
	Pantoprazole 40 mg QAM	
	Esomeprazole 20 mg po QAM	

PPIs are commonly used in *H. pylori* eradication regimens and can heal ulcers in patients continuing to take NSAIDs, they have become first line agents in the treatment of PUD.[135]

Only small differences in healing rates and symptom relief have been reported in controlled trials among the different PPIs.[151-153] Therefore, when initiating treatment, the choice of PPI is not nearly as important as the method of administration. PPIs are prodrugs (ie, they require activation prior to exerting their primary pharmacologic effect). PPIs are converted to an active form, the thiophillic sulfenamide, by an acid-catalyzed conversion almost exclusively within the highly acidic parietal cell secretory canaliculus.[21] Patients are therefore instructed to take PPIs 15 to 30 minutes prior to eating breakfast,[21] which allows time for the medication to be absorbed and taken up by the parietal cell, where stimulation of the cell by meal-induced gastrin, histamine, and acetylcholine release will trigger H+ ion generation, leading to activation of the drug. It is also important that a patient not take concomitant H2RAs or other agents that inhibit acid secretion (eg, anticholinergic agents, prostaglandins, and somatostatin analogs) because such agents can blunt the response by decreasing parietal cell activation.[21,154]

The thiophillic sulfenamide irreversibly binds to the proton pump so that a new enzyme must be created before the drug effect can be overcome. Thus, once daily dosing is generally effective for most patients. A number of patients may complain of breakthrough symptoms, which should be managed individually. For example, if the patient is having symptoms toward the latter part of the day, twice daily dosing may be necessary. If a patient has primarily nocturnal symptoms, he or she may benefit from

---

Table 6-6

INDICATIONS FOR MAINTENANCE ANTISECRETORY THERAPY

- History of ulcer complications
- Patients with frequent ulcer recurrence who are *H. pylori* negative
- Failure to eradicate *H. pylori* infection despite appropriate therapy

---

high-dose H2RA therapy at bedtime to better control unstimulated acid secretion. The recommended dose of PPIs by the US FDA is 40 mg per day of omeprazole for 8 weeks for GU and 20 to 40 mg daily for DU healing. Owing to their unique pharmacology, steady state acid inhibition will not be achieved for 3 to 5 days, and it may therefore be helpful to administer PPIs twice daily for the first 2 to 3 days.[21]

MAINTENANCE THERAPY

The use of maintenance acid suppression after treatment of PUD has been significantly influenced by *H. pylori* eradication. As previously mentioned, the relapse rate is much higher in those treated with antisecretory therapy without therapy for *H. pylori*.[155-160] Therefore, only a subset of high-risk patients require maintenance acid suppression (Table 6-6). This group includes patients with a prior history of complicated PUD, those with frequent recurrences, those who are *H. pylori* negative, and those who fail to clear the infection despite treatment. If *H. pylori* infection is cured, however, maintenance may not be necessary, even in those with a history of complications.[161-163]

H. PYLORI

Once the presence of *H. pylori* is detected, the infection should be eradicated.[127] Although the resolution of nonulcer dyspepsia following *H. pylori* eradication remains an unresolved issue,[115-117] treatment is clearly indicated in PUD because annual recurrence rates of 50% to 80% will be seen when anti-secretory therapy is used alone.[164] While evidence is accumulating that the eradication of the organism might be linked to the rising rate of adenocarcinoma of the esophagus,[11,13-16] infection remains a known risk factor for gastric adenocarcinoma, as well as gastric mucosa-associated lymphoid tissue (MALT) lymphomas. Thus, some authorities advocate the treatment of any active infection.

TREATMENT REGIMENS

Several different antibiotic regimens in combination with antisecretory agents have been demonstrated to be effective in the treatment of *H. pylori*. Acid inhibition is effective because the organism prefers an acidic environment, and acid inhibition augments the effectiveness of antibiotic therapy. The highest eradication rates are seen with the following regimens:

Table 6-7

ERADICATION REGIMENS FOR *H. PYLORI*

- PPI + amoxicillin 1000 mg + clarithromycin 500 mg (twice daily for 2 weeks).
- PPI + metronidazole 500 mg + clarithromycin 500 mg (twice daily for 2 weeks).
- RBC 400 mg + clarithromycin 500 mg + amoxicillin 1000 mg OR metronidazole 500 mg OR tetracycline 500 mg (twice daily for 2 weeks).
- Bismuth subsalicylate 525 mg QID + metronidazole 500 mg TID + tetracycline 500 mg QID + PPI (ea. at indicated frequency for 2 weeks).
- Bismuth subsalicylate 525 mg QID +metronidazole 250 mg QID + tetracycline 500 mg + H2RA (ea. at indicated frequency and H2RA continued for a further 2 weeks).

PPI: omeprazole 30 mg, lansoprazole 30 mg, esomepazole 20 mg, rabeprazole 20 mg, pantoprazole 40 mg; RBC: ranitidine bismuth citrate; TID: 3 times a day; QID: 4 times a day

- A PPI, clarithromycin, and either amoxicillin or metronidazole for 2 weeks.
- Ranitidine bismuth citrate; clarithromycin; and either amoxicillin, metronidazole, or tetracycline for 2 weeks.
- A PPI, bismuth, metronidazole, and tetracycline for 1 to 2 weeks.[127]

Other regimens are listed in Table 6-7. It is recommended that each drug be given twice per day for 2 weeks because of enhanced eradication for this period of time using PPI-based regimens.[165,166] Combination regimens are essential to maximize the rate of eradication and to decrease the chance of resistance.[127] Factors to consider when choosing a regimen include the likelihood of adverse events, patient compliance, and resistance patterns seen in different patient populations. Metronidazole resistance has been reported to be as high as 54% in parts of the United States,[108] and resistance to clarithromycin is emerging.[167] Resistance to amoxicillin is rare,[108] and resistance to tetracycline has not been documented.[127] It has been demonstrated that specific polymorphisms in the interleukin 1 beta gene and the cytochrome p450 gene are determinants of successful eradication because they influence intragastric pH and the metabolism of PPIs, respectively.[168-170] While these genetic tests are not routinely performed, there is evidence that implementing these tests into clinical practice may be cost effective.[168] The use of probiotics is controversial; however, they may have a role as adjunctive agents in the treatment of *H. pylori* with evidence increasing that they may improve eradication rates as well as decrease the incidence of side effects.[171]

FOLLOW-UP EVALUATION

Routine follow-up to ensure *H. pylori* eradication is not required, although this recommendation may change when inexpensive, noninvasive tests become more widely available.[127] It is important, however, to determine *H. pylori* status after treatment if the patient has experienced an ulcer complication to plan further long-term management and give an accurate prognosis. In addition, patients with persistent symptoms despite treatment should also have their *H. pylori* status reassessed. If the infection has not been eradicated, retreatment with an alternate regimen should be attempted. A urea breath test or a stool/urine antigen test, if available, is usually the test of choice unless a repeat endoscopy is required for other reasons, in which case a biopsy may be performed.[108,127] Patients will need to discontinue PPI therapy for 2 weeks prior to testing in order to avoid false-negative results.[172] Serology testing is not practical because it may take more than 1 year for the serology to revert to negative, although a negative test is indicative of successful treatment.[108]

NONSTEROIDAL ANTI-INFLAMMATORY DRUGS AND GASTRODUODENAL ULCERS

The treatment of PUD in the setting of NSAIDs use depends upon whether or not the NSAID can be discontinued. Ideally, the patient should be changed to acetaminophen and either misoprostol or a PPI can be used. Although PPIs do decrease NSAID-related endoscopic ulcers, no studies have documented a decrease in the rate of ulcer complications. If an NSAID must be continued, ulcer healing will be entirely dependent on the agent chosen for treatment, and long-term antisecretory therapy will likely be needed.

H2RAs have been used to treat NSAID-related ulcers; however, their efficacy is likely impaired by ongoing NSAID use. Among active NSAID users, 6 to 12 weeks of treatment with H2RAs has been reported to heal approximately 75% of GUs and 87% of DUs.[52,173,174] Healing appears to be dependent on the initial size of the ulcer, as one report noted a healing rate with cimetidine of 90% for small (<5 mm) GUs, but only 25% of larger ulcers healed.[52,175] The decreased efficacy of H2RAs among patients who continue to take NSAIDs does not seem to occur with PPIs. Yeomans et al reported 79% and 80% healing rates in patients on 40 mg and 20 mg of omeprazole, respectively, versus a 63% healing rate on ranitidine.[176] Similar results were seen with lansoprazole,[177] suggesting that PPIs are more effective than H2RAs regardless of whether or not NSAIDS are continued and should therefore be used as first-line agents in NSAID-related PUD.

PROPHYLAXIS

Because a significant proportion of patients with PUD complications from NSAIDs will be asymptomatic,[52,80,93-95] high-risk patients should always be placed on some form of prophylaxis. These include patients who are elderly, have a history of PUD, are on concomitant steroid therapy, using high NSAID doses, have a short duration of therapy (less than 2 weeks), or have serious comorbid conditions. A recent American College of Rheumatology update recommended either gastroprotective therapy (mucosal protective agents or antisecretory therapy) or changing to a COX-2 selective NSAID in these situations. As discussed below, owing to recent reports regarding the risk of thrombotic events, which prompted the removal of rofecoxib from the market, the widespread use of these agents will certainly decrease.

Mucosal Protective Agents

While it had been suggested that sucralfate may be of benefit in prophylaxis of GI injury among NSAID users, a large randomized controlled trial demonstrated no benefit.[178] Only the prostaglandin E analogue misoprostol has been shown to provide mucosal protection. Misoprostol has been shown to be effective over placebo in preventing ulcers and decreasing the incidence of ulcer-related complications.[179-181] It has little effect on the dyspeptic symptoms associated with NSAIDS, however, and causes diarrhea and abdominal pain in many of those receiving higher doses.[182] While it was observed that lower doses are better tolerated,[182] the drug must be taken at least 3 times per day to be effective.

Antisecretory Therapy

H2RAs have been demonstrated to relieve the dyspeptic symptoms associated with NSAIDS,[52,183-185] but they have also been associated with a higher rate of complications, suggesting ongoing mucosal injury despite symptom relief.[95] Moreover, while they do prevent endoscopic DUs, they are not effective against the development of GUs.[52,186] For these reasons, the use of H2RAs among high-risk NSAID takers is not recommended.

Several recent studies have established PPIs as effective agents for prophylaxis of NSAID-induced endoscopic ulcers. After 6 months of treatment with either ranitidine or omeprazole among osteoarthritis patients taking NSAIDs, 16.3% of patients treated with ranitidine had GUs and 4.2% had DUs versus 5.2% and 0.5%, respectively, in those receiving omeprazole.[176] Another study showed omeprazole to be superior to misoprostol in preventing the recurrence of both DUs and GUs.[187] Although no studies have demonstrated the ability of PPIs to decrease ulcer complications, these agents are well tolerated. Moreover, despite a paucity of data to suggest benefit in this regard, they are the recommended antisecretory agent for prophylaxis among high-risk NSAID users.

COXIBs

Highly selective COX-2 inhibitors afford the same level of anti-inflammatory activity and pain relief with decreased GI toxicity.[45-49] Both celecoxib and rofecoxib appear to maintain their selectivity for COX-2 at doses substantially higher than those required to decrease inflammation.[52] Furthermore, they have been demonstrated to cause endoscopic ulcers at a rate similar to that of placebo.[188,189] While promising, several questions still remain. COX-2 might generate endogenous prostanoids that are biologically important; mice with a disrupted COX-2 gene have defects in renal function and bone resorption, and females have impaired reproductive physiology.[190] Furthermore, in September 2004, the data safety monitoring board overseeing a long-term trial evaluating the use of rofecoxib in patients at risk of developing recurrent colon polyps recommended that the study be terminated because of the recognition of an increased risk of serious thrombotic events, including myocardial infarctions and cerebrovascular accidents, some of which were fatal, among patients taking rofecoxib compared to patients receiving placebo. Once aware of these findings, Merck & Co (Whitehouse Station, NJ) the manufacturer of Vioxx, announced the voluntary withdrawal of their rofecoxib product from the market. While other selective COX-

2 inhibitors remain available, it is unlikely that the prothrombotic properties and increased risk of thromboembolic events are limited to a single agent in this class. The use of aspirin was permitted in studies evaluating celecoxib, which may have masked any potential increased risk of these adverse events with this agent. It is our opinion that patients receiving other selective COX-2 inhibitors be closely monitored for similar adverse effects.[191,192]

TREATMENT OF COMPLICATIONS

Bleeding

When a patient presents with evidence of GI bleeding from PUD, empiric therapy with an intravenous (IV) PPI should be initiated, and the patient should be referred for urgent upper endoscopy. If an ulcer is identified to be the source of bleeding at endoscopy, endoscopic hemostasis should be attempted. Hemostasis may be achieved using epinephrine injection, thermo- or electro-coagulation, or mechanical therapy (ie, hemoclips). After hemostasis has been achieved, it has been shown that rebleeding rates are markedly reduced by continuation of an IV PPI infusion for 72 hours.[193] A thorough search for *H. pylori* infection should be undertaken as well. Because bleeding can effect the results of several of the noninvasive tests for *H. pylori*,[113] a serologic test should be obtained if other tests are negative. With advances in endoscopic treatments, as well as the development of more potent antisecretory agents, the need for surgery has been significantly decreased. However, if a patient rebleeds after all endoscopic modalities have been utilized, it is reasonable to refer the patient for surgery to obtain hemostasis.

Obstruction

The initial management of a gastric outlet obstruction should be conservative with NG suction, IV hydration, antisecretory medication, and hyperalimentation if clinically indicated. It is important to establish that the obstruction is emanating from a benign cause, which can be done via endoscopy. Once it is established that the obstruction is due to an ulcer, a plan should be formulated with a gastroenterologist and a surgeon. Most cases will resolve with medical therapy alone, although recurrence is common. More definitive therapy can be achieved using endoscopic dilation or a surgical drainage procedure.

Perforation

Once the diagnosis of a perforated viscus is determined, an immediate referral should be made to a surgeon, because operative treatment is required in approximately 95% of cases. Medical therapy consists of IV antisecretory medication, IV hydration, NG suction, and antibiotics and can be considered for DUs if there is a long-standing perforation (>24 hours), evidence of a contained perforation on contrast UGI series, a lack of peritoneal signs, and the presence of comorbidities that would significantly increase the risk of surgery. Perforated GUs, however, should always be managed surgically.

TREATMENT OF HYPERSECRETORY SYNDROMES

The goal of therapy of ZES is surgical removal of the gastrinoma, which is only possible in 50% of patients with sporadic gastrinomas.[21] It is also not possible to achieve prolonged disease-free states in patients with familial forms of ZES,[194] and acid suppressive therapy thus becomes the mainstay of therapy. All patients with ZES should be treated initially with a PPI at twice the usual dose.[195] The relief of all symptoms is desired; however, the relief of pain does not reliably predict the absence of mucosal injury.[196] The goal of therapy is a basal acid output of 1 to 10 mmol/hour, which should be measured 1 hour before the next dose is to be administered.[196] If complete acid inhibition is demonstrated, the dose should be decreased by 50% and the patient reassessed. If the basal acid output is >10 mmol/hr, the dose should be increased incrementally, and for doses greater than 60 mg of omeprazole (or equivalent doses for other PPIs), the dose should be divided and given twice daily.[21] If significant acid suppression is unable to be achieved and the tumor cannot be located, which occurs only infrequently, a total gastrectomy may be considered.

References

1. *Merriam-Webster's Medical Dictionary.* Springfield, Mass: Merriam-Webster; 1997.

2. Schwarz K. Uber penetrierende magen-und jejunalgeshwure. *Beitr Klin Chirurgie.* 1910;5:96-128.

3. Marshall BJ, Warren JR. Unidentified curved bacilli in the stomach of patients with gastritis and peptic ulceration. *Lancet.* 1984;1(8390):1311-1315.

4. Talley NJ, Zinsmeister AR, Schleck CD, Melton LJ 3rd. Dyspepsia and dyspepsia subgroups: a population-based study. *Gastroenterology.* 1992;102(4 Pt1):1259-1268.

5. Sonnenberg A, Everhart JE. The prevalence of self-reported peptic ulcer in the United States. *Am J Public Health.* 1996;86(2):200-205.

6. Sonnenberg A, Everhart JE. Health impact of peptic ulcer in the United States. *Am J Gastroenterol.* 1997;92(4):614-620.

7. Sonnenberg A, Wasserman IH. Associations of peptic ulcer and gastric cancer with other diseases in US veterans. *Am J Public Health.* 1995;85(9):1252-1255.

8. Sonnenberg A. Concordant occurrence of gastric and hypertensive diseases. *Gastroenterology.* 1988;95(1):42-48.

9. Kang JY, Tinto A, Higham J, Majeed A. Peptic ulceration in general practice in England and Wales 1994-98: period prevalence and drug management. *Aliment Pharmacol Ther.* 2002;16(6):1067-1074.

10. Munnangi S, Sonnenberg A. Time trends of physician visits and treatment patterns of peptic ulcer disease in the United States. *Arch Intern Med.* 1997;157(13):1489-1494.

11. Xia HH, Phung N, Altiparmak E, Berry A, Matheson M, Talley NJ. Reduction of peptic ulcer disease and *Helicobacter pylori* infection but increase of reflux esophagitis in Western Sydney between 1990 and 1998. *Dig Dis Sci.* 2001;46(12):2716-2723.

12. Lewis JD, Bilker WB, Brensinger C, Farrar JT, Strom BL. Hospitalization and mortality rates from peptic ulcer disease and GI bleeding in the 1990s: relationship to sales of nonsteroidal anti-inflammatory drugs and acid suppression medications. *Am J Gastroenterol.* 2002;97(10):2540-2549.

13. el-Serag HB, Sonnenberg A. Opposing time trends of peptic ulcer and reflux disease. *Gut.* 1998;43(3):327-333.

14. Varanasi RV, Fantry GT, Wilson KT. Decreased prevalence of *Helicobacter pylori* infection in gastroesophageal reflux disease. *Helicobacter.* 1998;3(3):188-194.

15. Nomura AM, Perez-Perez GI, Lee J, Stemmermann G, Blaser MJ. Relation between *Helicobacter pylori* cagA status and risk of peptic ulcer disease. *Am J Epidemiol.* 2002;155(11):1054-1059.

16. Perez-Perez GI, Peek Rm, Legath AJ, et al. The role of CagA status in gastric and extragastric complications of *Helicobacter pylori*. *J Physiol Pharmacol*. 1999;50(5):833-845.

17. Wolfe MM, Soll AH. The physiology of gastric acid secretion. *N Engl J Med*. 1988;319(26):1707-1715.

18. Prinz C, Scott DR, Hurwitz D, et al. Gastrin effects on isolated rat enterochromaffin-like cells in primary culture. *Am J Physiol*. 1994;267(4 Pt 1):G663-G675.

19. Waldman HSA. The enterochromaffin-like (ECL) cells. *Acta Oncol*. 1993;32:141-147.

20. Feldman M, Richardson CT. Total 24-hour gastric acid secretion in patients with duodenal ulcer. Comparison with normal subjects and effects of cimetidine and parietal cell vagotomy. *Gastroenterology*. 1986;90(3):540-544.

21. Wolfe MM, Sachs G. Acid suppression: optimizing therapy for gastroduodenal ulcer healing, gastroesophageal reflux disease, and stress-related erosive syndrome. *Gastroenterology*. 2000;118(2 Suppl 1):S9-S31.

22. Isenberg JI, SElling JA, Elashoff JD, et al. Impaired proximal duodenal mucosal bicarbonate secretion in patients with duodenal ulcer. *N Engl J Med*. 1987;316(7):374-379.

23. Kurata JH, Nogawa AN. Meta-analysis of risk factors for peptic ulcer. Nonsteroidal antiinflammatory drugs, *Helicobacter pylori*, and smoking. *J Clin Gastroenterol*. 1997;24(1):2-17.

24. Marshall B. *Helicobacter pylori*: 20 years on. *Clin Med*. 2002;2(2):147-152.

25. Odum L, Petersen HD, Andersen IB, et al. Gastrin and somatostatin in *Helicobacter pylori* infected antral mucosa. *Gut*. 1994;35(5):615-618.

26. Moss SF, et al. Effect of *Helicobacter pylori* on gastric somatostatin in duodenal ulcer disease. *Lancet*. 1992;340(8825):930-932.

27. Graham DY, Lew GM, Lechago J. Antral G-cell and D-cell numbers in *Helicobacter pylori* infection: effect of *H. pylori* eradication. *Gastroenterology*. 1993;104(6):1655-1660.

28. Ge Z, Taylor DE. Contributions of genome sequencing to understanding the biology of *Helicobacter pylori*. *Annu Rev Microbiol*. 1999;53:353-387.

29. de Bernard M, Papini E, de Filippis V, et al. Low pH activates the vacuolating toxin of *Helicobacter pylori*, which becomes acid and pepsin resistant. *J Biol Chem*. 1995;270(41):23937-23940.

30. Atherton JC, Cao P, Peek RM Jr, et al. Mosaicism in vacuolating cytotoxin alleles of *Helicobacter pylori*. Association of specific vacA types with cytotoxin production and peptic ulceration. *J Biol Chem*. 1995;270(30):17771-17777.

31. Covacci A, Censini S, Bugnoli M, et al. Molecular characterization of the 128-kDa immunodominant antigen of *Helicobacter pylori* associated with cytotoxicity and duodenal ulcer. *Proc Natl Acad Sci U S A*. 1993;90(12):5791-5795.

32. Censini S, Lange C, Xiang Z, et al. CAG, a pathogenicity island of *Helicobacter pylori*, encodes type I-specific and disease-associated virulence factors. *Proc Natl Acad Sci U S A*. 1996;93(25):14648-14653.

33. Schoen RT, Vender RJ. Mechanisms of nonsteroidal anti-inflammatory drug-induced gastric damage. *Am J Med*. 1989;86(4):449-458.

34. Carson JL, Strom BL, Morse MI, et al. The relative gastrointestinal toxicity of the nonsteroidal anti-inflammatory drugs. *Arch Intern Med*. 1987;147(6):1054-1059.

35. Graham DY, et al. Nonsteroidal anti-inflammatory effect of sulindac sulfoxide and sulfide on gastric mucosa. *Clin Pharmacol Ther*. 1985;38(1):65-70.

36. Lanza FL, Royer Jr GL, Nelson RS. Endoscopic evaluation of the effects of aspirin, buffered aspirin, and enteric-coated aspirin on gastric and duodenal mucosa. *N Engl J Med.* 1980;303(3):136-138.

37. Henry D, Dobson A, Turner C. Variability in the risk of major gastrointestinal complications from nonaspirin nonsteroidal anti-inflammatory drugs. *Gastroenterology.* 1993;105(4):1078-1088.

38. Maliekal J, Elboim CM. Gastrointestinal complications associated with intramuscular ketorolac tromethamine therapy in the elderly. *Ann Pharmacother.* 1995;29(7-8):698-701.

39. Allen A, Hutton DA, Leonard AJ, et al. The role of mucus in the protection of the gastroduodenal mucosa. *Scand J Gastroenterol Suppl.* 1986;125:71-78.

40. Allen A, Carroll NJ. Adherent and soluble mucus in the stomach and duodenum. *Dig Dis Sci.* 1985;30(11 Suppl):55S-62S.

41. Huang JZ. Treatment of acute gastric and duodenal ulcer. In: Wolfe M, ed. *Therapy of Digestive Disorders.* Philadelphia: WB Saunders; 2000:133-143.

42. Masferrer JL, Seibert K, Zweifel B, et al. Endogenous glucocorticoids regulate an inducible cyclooxygenase enzyme. *Proc Natl Acad Sci U S A.* 1992;89(9):3917-3921.

43. Crofford LJ. COX-1 and COX-2 tissue expression: implications and predictions. *J Rheumatol Suppl.* 1997;49:15-19.

44. DeWitt DL, Smith WL. Primary structure of prostaglandin G/H synthase from sheep vesicular gland determined from the complementary DNA sequence. *Proc Natl Acad Sci U S A.* 1988;85(5):1412-1416.

45. Hla T, Neilson K. Human cyclooxygenase-2 cDNA. *Proc Natl Acad Sci U S A.* 1992;89(16):7384-7388.

46. Needleman P, Isakson PC. The discovery and function of COX-2. *J Rheumatol Suppl.* 1997;49:6-8.

47. Goldstein JL, Correa P, Zhao WW, et al. Reduced incidence of gastroduodenal ulcers with celecoxib, a novel cyclooxygenase-2 inhibitor, compared to naproxen in patients with arthritis. *Am J Gastroenterol.* 2001;96(4):1019-1027.

48. Wolfe F, Anderson J, Burke TA, et al. Gastroprotective therapy and risk of gastrointestinal ulcers: risk reduction by COX-2 therapy. *J Rheumatol.* 2002;29(3):467-473.

49. Hunt RH, Harper S, Watson DJ, et al. The gastrointestinal safety of the COX-2 selective inhibitor etoricoxib assessed by both endoscopy and analysis of upper gastrointestinal events. *Am J Gastroenterol.* 2003;98(8):1725-1733.

50. Bjarnason I, MacPherson A, Mackintosh C, et al. A randomized, double-blind, crossover comparative endoscopy study on the gastroduodenal tolerability of a highly specific cyclooxygenase-2 inhibitor, flosulide, and naproxen. *Scand J Gastroenterol.* 1997;32(2):126-130.

51. Lipsky PE, Isakson PC. Outcome of specific COX-2 inhibition in rheumatoid arthritis. *J Rheumatol Suppl.* 1997;49:9-14.

52. Wolfe MM, Lichtenstein DR, Singh G. Gastrointestinal toxicity of nonsteroidal antiinflammatory drugs. *N Engl J Med.* 1999;340(24):1888-1899.

53. Wallace JL, McKnight W, Miyasaka M, et al. Role of endothelial adhesion molecules in NSAID-induced gastric mucosal injury. *Am J Physiol.* 1993;265(5 Pt 1):G993-G998.

54. Wallace JL, Keenan CM, Granger DN. Gastric ulceration induced by nonsteroidal anti-inflammatory drugs is a neutrophil-dependent process. *Am J Physiol.* 1990;259(3 Pt 1):G462-G467.

55. Eastwood GL. Is smoking still important in the pathogenesis of peptic ulcer disease? *J Clin Gastroenterol.* 1997;25 (Suppl 1):S1-S7.

56. McCready DR, Clark L, Cohen MM. Cigarette smoking reduces human gastric luminal prostaglandin E2. *Gut.* 1985;26(11):1192-1196.

57. Quimby GF, Bonnice CA, Burstein SH, et al. Active smoking depresses prostaglandin synthesis in human gastric mucosa. *Ann Intern Med.* 1986;104(5):616-619.

58. Murthy SN, Dinoso VP, Clearfield HR, et al. Simultaneous measurement of basal pancreatic, gastric acid secretion, plasma gastrin, and secretin during smoking. *Gastroenterology.* 1977;73(4 Pt 1):758-761.

59. Murthy SN, Dinoso VP, Clearfield HR, et al. Serial pH changes in the duodenal bulb during smoking. *Gastroenterology.* 1978;75(1):1-4.

60. Ainsworth MA, Hogan DL, Koss MA, et al. Cigarette smoking inhibits acid-stimulated duodenal mucosal bicarbonate secretion. *Ann Intern Med.* 1993;119(9):882-886.

61. Bateson MC. Cigarette smoking and *Helicobacter pylori* infection. *Postgrad Med J.* 1993;69(807):41-44.

62. O'Connor HJ, Kanduru C, Bhutta AS, et al. Effect of *Helicobacter pylori* eradication on peptic ulcer healing. *Postgrad Med J.* 1995;71(832):90-93.

63. Marshall BJ, Goodwin CS, Warren JR, et al. Prospective double-blind trial of duodenal ulcer relapse after eradication of Campylobacter pylori. *Lancet.* 1988;2(8626-8627):1437-1442.

64. Borody TJ, George LL, Brandl S, et al. Smoking does not contribute to duodenal ulcer relapse after *Helicobacter pylori* eradication. *Am J Gastroenterol.* 1992;87(10):1390-1393.

65. Tomassetti P, Salomone T, Migliori M, et al. Optimal treatment of Zollinger-Ellison syndrome and related conditions in elderly patients. *Drugs Aging.* 2003;20(14):1019-1034.

66. Gibril F, Schumann M, Pace A, Jensen RT. Multiple endocrine neoplasia type 1 and Zollinger-Ellison syndrome: a prospective study of 107 cases and comparison with 1009 cases from the literature. *Medicine (Baltimore).* 2004;83(1):43-83.

67. Everhart JE, Byrd-Holt D, Sonnenberg A. Incidence and risk factors for self-reported peptic ulcer disease in the United States. *Am J Epidemiol.* 1998;147(6):529-536.

68. Hein HO, Suadicani P, Gyntelberg F. Genetic markers for peptic ulcer. A study of 3387 men aged 54 to 74 years: the Copenhagen Male Study. *Scand J Gastroenterol.* 1997;32(1):16-21.

69. Suadicani P, Hein HO, Gyntelberg F. Genetic and life-style determinants of peptic ulcer. A study of 3387 men aged 54 to 74 years: The Copenhagen Male Study. *Scand J Gastroenterol.* 1999;34(1):12-17.

70. Laine L, Cominelli F, Sloane R, et al. Interaction of NSAIDs and *Helicobacter pylori* on gastrointestinal injury and prostaglandin production: a controlled double-blind trial. *Aliment Pharmacol Ther.* 1995;9(2):127-135.

71. Thillainayagam AV, Tabaqchalli S, Warrington SJ, Farthing MJ. Interrelationships between *Helicobacter pylori* infection, nonsteroidal antiinflammatory drugs and gastroduodenal disease. A prospective study in healthy volunteers. *Dig Dis Sci.* 1994;39(5):1085-1089.

72. Kim JG, Graham DY. *Helicobacter pylori* infection and development of gastric or duodenal ulcer in arthritic patients receiving chronic NSAID therapy. The Misoprostol Study Group. *Am J Gastroenterol.* 1994;89(2):203-207.

73. Goggin PM, Collins DA, Jazrawi RP, et al. Prevalence of *Helicobacter pylori* infection and its effect on symptoms and non-steroidal anti-inflammatory drug induced gastrointestinal damage in patients with rheumatoid arthritis. *Gut.* 1993;34(12):1677-1680.

74. Friedman GD, Siegelaub AB, Seltzer CC. Cigarettes, alcohol, coffee and peptic ulcer. *N Engl J Med.* 1974;290(9):469-473.

75. Anda RF, Williamsson DF, Escobedo LG, Remington PL. Smoking and the risk of peptic ulcer disease among women in the United States. *Arch Intern Med.* 1990;150(7):1437-1441.

76. Korman MG, Hansky J, Eaves ER, Schmidt GT. Influence of cigarette smoking on healing and relapse in duodenal ulcer disease. *Gastroenterology.* 1983;85(4):871-874.

77. Kato I, Nomura AM, Stemmermann GN, Chyou PH. A prospective study of gastric and duodenal ulcer and its relation to smoking, alcohol, and diet. *Am J Epidemiol.* 1992;135(5):521-530.

78. Ippoliti A, Elashoff J, Valenzuela J, et al. Recurrent ulcer after successful treatment with cimetidine or antacid. *Gastroenterology.* 1983;85(4):875-880.

79. Lichtenstein DR, Syngal S, Wolfe M. Nonsteroidal antiinflammatory drugs and the gastrointestinal tract. The double-edged sword. *Arthritis Rheum.* 1995;38(1):5-18.

80. Singh G, Triadafilopoulos G. Epidemiology of NSAID induced gastrointestinal complications. *J Rheumatol Suppl.* 1999;56:18-24.

81. Bjorkman DJ. Nonsteroidal anti-inflammatory drug-induced gastrointestinal injury. *Am J Med.* 1996;101(1A):25S-32S.

82. Longstreth GF. Epidemiology of hospitalization for acute upper gastrointestinal hemorrhage: a population-based study. *Am J Gastroenterol.* 1995;90(2):206-210.

83. Greene JM, Winickoff RN. Cost-conscious prescribing of nonsteroidal anti-inflammatory drugs for adults with arthritis. A review and suggestions. *Arch Intern Med.* 1992;152(10):1995-2002.

84. Gabriel SE, Jaakkimainen L, Bombardier C. Risk for serious gastrointestinal complications related to use of nonsteroidal anti-inflammatory drugs. A meta-analysis. *Ann Intern Med.* 1991;115(10):787-796.

85. Griffin MR, Piper JM, Daugherty JR, et al. Nonsteroidal anti-inflammatory drug use and increased risk for peptic ulcer disease in elderly persons. *Ann Intern Med.* 1991;114(4):257-263.

86. Garcia Rodriguez LA, Jick H. Risk of upper gastrointestinal bleeding and perforation associated with individual non-steroidal anti-inflammatory drugs. *Lancet.* 1994;343(8900):769-772.

87. Hallas J, Lauritsen J, Villadsen HD, Gram LF. Nonsteroidal anti-inflammatory drugs and upper gastrointestinal bleeding, identifying high-risk groups by excess risk estimates. *Scand J Gastroenterol.* 1995;30(5):438-444.

88. Hochain P, Berkelmans I, Czernichow P, et al. Which patients taking non-aspirin non-steroidal anti-inflammatory drugs bleed? A case-control study. *Eur J Gastroenterol Hepatol.* 1995;7(5):419-426.

89. Piper JM, Ray WA, Daugherty JR, Griffin MR. Corticosteroid use and peptic ulcer disease: role of nonsteroidal anti-inflammatory drugs. *Ann Intern Med.* 1991;114(9):735-740.

90. Shorr RI, Ray WA, Daugherty JR, Griffin MR. Concurrent use of nonsteroidal anti-inflammatory drugs and oral anticoagulants places elderly persons at high risk for hemorrhagic peptic ulcer disease. *Arch Intern Med.* 1993;153(14):1665-1670.

91. Horrocks JC, De Dombal FT. Clinical presentation of patients with "dyspepsia." Detailed symptomatic study of 360 patients. *Gut.* 1978;19(1):19-26.
92. Earlam R. A computerized questionnaire analysis of duodenal ulcer symptoms. *Gastroenterology.* 1976;71(2):314-317.
93. Larkai EN, Smith JL, Lidsky MD, Graham DY. Gastroduodenal mucosa and dyspeptic symptoms in arthritic patients during chronic nonsteroidal anti-inflammatory drug use. *Am J Gastroenterol.* 1987;82(11):1153-1158.
94. Armstrong CP, Blower AL. Non-steroidal anti-inflammatory drugs and life threatening complications of peptic ulceration. *Gut.* 1987;28(5):527-532.
95. Singh G, Ramey DR, Morfeld D, et al. Gastrointestinal tract complications of nonsteroidal anti-inflammatory drug treatment in rheumatoid arthritis. A prospective observational cohort study. *Arch Intern Med.* 1996;156(14):1530-1536.
96. Gilbert DA. Epidemiology of upper gastrointestinal bleeding. *Gastrointest Endosc.* 1990;36(5 Suppl):S8-S13.
97. Silverstein FE, Gilbert DA, Tedesco FJ, et al. The national ASGE survey on upper gastrointestinal bleeding. II. Clinical prognostic factors. *Gastrointest Endosc.* 1981;27(2):80-93.
98. Laine L, Peterson WL. Bleeding peptic ulcer. *N Engl J Med.* 1994;331(11):717-727.
99. Yavorski RT, Wong RK, Maydonovitch C, et al. Analysis of 3,294 cases of upper gastrointestinal bleeding in military medical facilities. *Am J Gastroenterol.* 1995;90(4):568-573.
100. Boonpongmanee S, et al. The frequency of peptic ulcer as a cause of upper-GI bleeding is exaggerated. *Gastrointest Endosc.* 2004;59(7):788-794.
101. Canoy DS, Hart AR, Todd CJ. Epidemiology of duodenal ulcer perforation: a study on hospital admissions in Norfolk, United Kingdom. *Dig Liver Dis.* 2002;34(5):322-327.
102. Svanes C, Lie RT, Kvale G, et al. Incidence of perforated ulcer in western Norway, 1935-1990: cohort- or period-dependent time trends? *Am J Epidemiol.* 1995;141(9):836-844.
103. Pappas T, Lapp JA. Gastrointestinal emergencies. In: Taylor M, ed. *Complications of Peptic Ulcer Disease: Perforation and Obstruction.* Baltimore, Md: Williams & Wilkins; 1997:87-99.
104. Talley NJ, Axon A, Bytzer P, et al. Management of uninvestigated and functional dyspepsia: a Working Party report for the World Congresses of Gastroenterology 1998. *Aliment Pharmacol Ther.* 1999;13(9):1135-1148.
105. Westbrook JI, McIntosh JH, Duggan JM. Accuracy of provisional diagnoses of dyspepsia in patients undergoing first endoscopy. *Gastrointest Endosc.* 2001;53(3):283-288.
106. Keller R, Dinkel KC, Christl SU, et al. Interrelation between ABH blood group 0, Lewis(B) blood group antigen, *Helicobacter pylori* infection, and occurrence of peptic ulcer. *Z Gastroenterol.* 2002;40(5):273-276.
107. Perez-Trallero E, Montes M, Alcorta M, et al. Non-endoscopic method to obtain *Helicobacter pylori* for culture. *Lancet.* 1995;345(8950):622-623.
108. Meurer LN, Bower DJ. Management of *Helicobacter pylori* infection. *Am Fam Physician.* 2002;65(7):1327-1336.
109. Hahn M, Fennerty MB, Corless CL, et al. Noninvasive tests as a substitute for histology in the diagnosis of *Helicobacter pylori* infection. *Gastrointest Endosc.* 2000;52(1):20-26.

110. Klein PD, Graham DY. Minimum analysis requirements for the detection of *Helicobacter pylori* infection by the 13C-urea breath test. *Am J Gastroenterol.* 1993;88(11):1865-1869.

111. Sheu BS, Lee SC, Lin PW, et al. Carbon urea breath test is not as accurate as endoscopy to detect *Helicobacter pylori* after gastrectomy. *Gastrointest Endosc.* 2000;51(6):670-675.

112. Wu IC, Ke HL, Lo YC, et al. Evaluation of a newly developed office-based stool test for detecting *Helicobacter pylori*: an extensive pilot study. *Hepatogastroenterology.* 2003;50(54):1761-1765.

113. van Leerdam ME, van der Ende A, ten Kate FJ, et al. Lack of accuracy of the non-invasive *Helicobacter pylori* stool antigen test in patients with gastroduodenal ulcer bleeding. *Am J Gastroenterol.* 2003;98(4):798-801.

114. Wu DC, Kuo CH, Lu CY, et al. Evaluation of an office-based urine test for detecting *Helicobacter pylori*: a prospective pilot study. *Hepatogastroenterology.* 2001;48(39):614-617.

115. Armstrong D. *Helicobacter pylori* infection and dyspepsia. *Scand J Gastroenterol Suppl.* 1996;215:38-47.

116. Blum AL, Talley NJ, O'Morain C, et al. Lack of effect of treating *Helicobacter pylori* infection in patients with nonulcer dyspepsia. Omeprazole plus clarithromycin and amoxicillin effect one year after treatment (OCAY) study group. *N Engl J Med.* 1998;339(26):1875-1881.

117. McColl K, Murray L, El-Omar E, et al. Symptomatic benefit from eradicating *Helicobacter pylori* infection in patients with nonulcer dyspepsia. *N Engl J Med.* 1998;339(26):1869-1874.

118. Sharma TK, Prasad VM, Cutler AF. Quantitative noninvasive testing for *Helicobacter pylori* does not predict gastroduodenal ulcer disease. *Gastrointest Endosc.* 1996;44(6):679-682.

119. Palli D, Menegatti M, Masala G, et al. *Helicobacter pylori* infection, anti-cagA antibodies and peptic ulcer: a case-control study in Italy. *Aliment Pharmacol Ther.* 2002;16(5):1015-1020.

120. Rokkas T, Liatsos C, Karameris A, et al. Serologic detection of CagA positive *Helicobacter pylori* strains predicts the presence of peptic ulcer in young dyspeptic patients. *Gastrointest Endosc.* 1999;50(4):511-515.

121. Graham DY, Genta RM, Graham DP, et al. Serum CagA antibodies in asymptomatic subjects and patients with peptic ulcer: lack of correlation of IgG antibody in patients with peptic ulcer or asymptomatic *Helicobacter pylori* gastritis. *J Clin Pathol.* 1996;49(10):829-832.

122. Allan RN, Dykes PW, Toye DK. Diagnostic accuracy of early radiology in acute gastrointestinal haemorrhage. *Br Med J.* 1972;4(835):281-284.

123. Forrest JA, Finlayson ND, Shearman DJ. Endoscopy in gastrointestinal bleeding. *Lancet.* 1974;2(7877):394-397.

124. Katon RM, Smith FW. Panendoscopy in the early diagnosis of acute upper gastrointestinal bleeding. *Gastroenterology.* 1973;65(5):728-734.

125. Morrissey JF, Thorsen WB. Gastroscopy: a review of the English and Japanese literature. *Gastroenterology.* 1967;53:456-476.

126. Eisen GM, Dominitz JA, Faigel DO, et al. The role of endoscopy in dyspepsia. *Gastrointest Endosc.* 2001;54(6):815-817.

127. Howden CW, Hunt RH. Guidelines for the management of *Helicobacter pylori* infection. Ad hoc committee on practice parameters of the American College of Gastroenterology. *Am J Gastroenterol.* 1998;93(12):2330-2338.

128. Lai KC, Lam SK. Bleeding ulcers have high false negative rates for antral *Helicobacter pylori* when tested with urease test. *Gastroenterology.* 1996;110(A167).

129. Mignon M, Cadiot G. Diagnostic and therapeutic criteria in patients with Zollinger-Ellison syndrome and multiple endocrine neoplasia type 1. *J Intern Med.* 1998;243(6):489-494.

130. Norton JA, Jensen RT. Current surgical management of Zollinger-Ellison syndrome (ZES) in patients without multiple endocrine neoplasia-type 1 (MEN1). *Surg Oncol.* 2003;12(2):145-151.

131. Akerstrom G, Hessman O, Skogseid B. Timing and extent of surgery in symptomatic and asymptomatic neuroendocrine tumors of the pancreas in MEN 1. *Langenbecks Arch Surg.* 2002;386(8):558-569.

132. Brandi ML, Gagel RF, Angeli A, et al. Guidelines for diagnosis and therapy of MEN type 1 and type 2. *J Clin Endocrinol Metab.* 2001;86(12):5658-5671.

133. Gogel HK, Buckman MT, Cardieux D, et al. Gastric secretion and hormonal interactions in multiple endocrine neoplasia type I. *Arch Intern Med.* 1985;145(5):855-859.

134. Jensen RT. Management of the Zollinger-Ellison syndrome in patients with multiple endocrine neoplasia type 1. *J Intern Med.* 1998;243(6):477-488.

135. Salas M, Ward A, Caro J. Are proton pump inhibitors the first choice for acute treatment of gastric ulcers? A meta analysis of randomized clinical trials. *BMC Gastroenterol.* 2002;2(1):17.

136. Peterson WL, Sturdevant RA, Frankl HD, et al. Healing of duodenal ulcer with an antacid regimen. *N Engl J Med.* 1977;297(7):341-345.

137. Shields HM. Rapid fall of serum phosphorus secondary to antacid therapy. *Gastroenterology.* 1978;75(6):1137-1141.

138. Herzog P, Grendahl T, Linden JVD JR, et al. Adverse effects of high dose antacid regimens. Results of a randomized, double-blind trial. *Gastroenterology.* 1980;80:1173.

139. Hjortrup A, Svendsen LB, Beck H, et al. Two daily doses of sucralfate or cimetidine in the healing of gastric ulcer. A comparative randomized study. *Am J Med.* 1989;86(6A):113-115.

140. Black JW, Duncan WA, Durant CJ, et al. Definition and antagonism of histamine H 2 -receptors. *Nature.* 1972;236(5347):385-390.

141. Simon B, Muller P, Dammann HG, et al. Inhibition of acid secretion with substituted benzimidazole. A new principle in ulcer therapy? *Fortschr Med.* 1982;100(5):159-160.

142. Jones DB, Howden CW, Burget DW, et al. Acid suppression in duodenal ulcer: a meta-analysis to define optimal dosing with antisecretory drugs. *Gut.* 1987;28(9):1120-1127.

143. Gitlin N, McCullough AJ, Smith JL, et al. A multicenter, double-blind, randomized, placebo-controlled comparison of nocturnal and twice-a-day famotidine in the treatment of active duodenal ulcer disease. *Gastroenterology.* 1987;92(1):48-53.

144. Bank S, Greenberg RE, Magier D, et al. The efficacy and tolerability of famotidine and ranitidine on the healing of active duodenal ulcer and during six-month maintenance treatment, with special reference to NSAID/aspirin-related ulcers. *Clin Ther.* 1991;13(2):304-318.

145. Khasawneh SM, Ffarah HB. Morning versus evening dose: a comparison of three H2-receptor blockers in duodenal ulcer healing. *Am J Gastroenterol.* 1992;87(9):1180-1182.

146. Kihira K, Yoshida Y, Kasano T, et al. Effect of a proton pump inhibitor AG-1749 (lansoprazole) on intragastric pH: 24-hour intragastric pH monitoring. *Nippon Shokakibyo Gakkai Zasshi.* 1991;88(3):672-680.

147. Berlin I, Molinier P, Duchier A, et al. Dose ranging study of lansoprazole, a new proton pump inhibitor, in patients with high gastric acid secretion. *Eur J Clin Pharmacol.* 1992;43(2):117-119.

148. Holt S, Howden CW. Omeprazole. Overview and opinion. *Dig Dis Sci.* 1991;36(4):385-393.

149. Poynard T, Lemaire M, Agostini H. Meta-analysis of randomized clinical trials comparing lansoprazole with ranitidine or famotidine in the treatment of acute duodenal ulcer. *Eur J Gastroenterol Hepatol.* 1995;7(7):661-665.

150. Bader JP, Delchier JC. Clinical efficacy of pantoprazole compared with ranitidine. *Aliment Pharmacol Ther.* 1994;8 (Suppl 1):47-52.

151. Florent C. Progress with proton pump inhibitors in acid peptic disease: treatment of duodenal and gastric ulcer. *Clin Ther.* 1993;15 (Suppl B):14-21.

152. Witzel L, Gutz H, Huttermann W, et al. Pantoprazole versus omeprazole in the treatment of acute gastric ulcers. *Aliment Pharmacol Ther.* 1995;9(1):19-24.

153. Dekkers CP, Beker JA, Thjodleifsson B, et al. Comparison of rabeprazole 20 mg vs. omeprazole 20 mg in the treatment of active gastric ulcer—a European multicenter study. The European rabeprazole study group. *Aliment Pharmacol Ther.* 1998;12(8):789-795.

154. De Graef J, Woussen-Colle MC. Influence of the stimulation state of the parietal cells on the inhibitory effect of omeprazole on gastric acid secretion in dogs. *Gastroenterology.* 1986;91(2):333-337.

155. Laine L. Eradication of *Helicobacter pylori* reduces gastric and duodenal ulcer recurrence. *Gastroenterology.* 1992;103(5):1695-1696.

156. Graham DY, Lew GM, Klein PD, et al. Effect of treatment of *Helicobacter pylori* infection on the long-term recurrence of gastric or duodenal ulcer. A randomized, controlled study. *Ann Intern Med.* 1992;116(9):705-708.

157. Hentschel E, Brandstatter G, Dragosics B, et al. Effect of ranitidine and amoxicillin plus metronidazole on the eradication of *Helicobacter pylori* and the recurrence of duodenal ulcer. *N Engl J Med.* 1993;328(5):308-312.

158. Logan RP, Bardhan KD, Celestin LR, et al. Eradication of *Helicobacter pylori* and prevention of recurrence of duodenal ulcer: a randomized, double-blind, multicentre trial of omeprazole with or without clarithromycin. *Aliment Pharmacol Ther.* 1995;9(4):417-423.

159. Fujioka T, Uribe RU, Kubota T, et al. Peptic ulcer recurrence after *Helicobacter pylori* eradication: a 5-year follow-up study. *Eur J Gastroenterol Hepatol.* 1995;7 (Suppl 1): S35-S38.

160. Van der Hulst RW, Rauws EA, Koycu B, et al. Prevention of ulcer recurrence after eradication of *Helicobacter pylori*: a prospective long-term follow-up study. *Gastroenterology.* 1997;113(4):1082-1086.

161. Wong BC, Lam SK, Lai KC, et al. Triple therapy for *Helicobacter pylori* eradication is more effective than long-term maintenance antisecretory treatment in the prevention of recurrence of duodenal ulcer: a prospective long-term follow-up study. *Aliment Pharmacol Ther.* 1999;13(3):303-309.

162. Rokkas T, Karameris A, Mavrogeorgis A, et al. Eradication of *Helicobacter pylori* reduces the possibility of rebleeding in peptic ulcer disease. *Gastrointest Endosc.* 1995;41(1):1-4.

163. Jaspersen D, Koerner T, Schorr W, et al. *Helicobacter pylori* eradication reduces the rate of rebleeding in ulcer hemorrhage. *Gastrointest Endosc.* 1995;41(1):5-7.

164. Blaser MJ, Parsonnet J. Parasitism by the "slow" bacterium *Helicobacter pylori* leads to altered gastric homeostasis and neoplasia. *J Clin Invest.* 1994;94(1):4-8.

165. Laine L, Estrada R, Trujillo M, et al. Randomized comparison of differing periods of twice-a-day triple therapy for the eradication of *Helicobacter pylori*. *Aliment Pharmacol Ther.* 1996;10(6):1029-1033.

166. Fennerty B, Pruitt R, et al. 10 vs 14 day triple therapy with lansoprazole, amoxicillin, and clarithromycin in the eradicaion of *Helicobacter pylori*. *Am J Gastroenterol.* 1997;92:1653 (abstract).

167. Pilotto A, Leandro G, Franceschi M, et al. The effect of antibiotic resistance on the outcome of three 1-week triple therapies against *Helicobacter pylori*. *Aliment Pharmacol Ther.* 1999;13(5):667-673.

168. Lehmann DF, Medicis JJ, Franklin PD. Polymorphisms and the pocketbook: the cost-effectiveness of cytochrome P450 2C19 genotyping in the eradication of *Helicobacter pylori* infection associated with duodenal ulcer. *J Clin Pharmacol.* 2003;43(12):1316-1323.

169. Furuta T, Ohashi K, Kamata T, et al. Effect of genetic differences in omeprazole metabolism on cure rates for *Helicobacter pylori* infection and peptic ulcer. *Ann Intern Med.* 1998;129(12):1027-1030.

170. Furuta T, Shirai N, Xiao F, et al. Polymorphism of interleukin-1beta affects the eradication rates of *Helicobacter pylori* by triple therapy. *Clin Gastroenterol Hepatol.* 2004;2(1):22-30.

171. Hamilton-Miller JM. The role of probiotics in the treatment and prevention of *Helicobacter pylori* infection. *Int J Antimicrob Agents.* 2003;22(4):360-366.

172. Rollan A, Giancapero R, Arrese M, et al. Accuracy of invasive and noninvasive tests to diagnose *Helicobacter pylori* infection after antibiotic treatment. *Am J Gastroenterol.* 1997;92(8):1268-1274.

173. Davies J, Collins AJ, Dixon SA. The influence of cimetidine on peptic ulcer in patients with arthritis taking anti-inflammatory drugs. *Br J Rheumatol.* 1986;25(1):54-58.

174. Croker JR, Cotton PB, Boyle AC, et al. Cimetidine for peptic ulcer in patients with arthritis. *Ann Rheum Dis.* 1980;39(3):275-278.

175. O'Laughlin JC, Silvoso GK, Ivey KJ. Resistance to medical therapy of gastric ulcers in rheumatic disease patients taking aspirin. A double-blind study with cimetidine and follow-up. *Dig Dis Sci.* 1982;27(11):976-980.

176. Yeomans ND, Tulassay Z, Juhasz L, et al. A comparison of omeprazole with ranitidine for ulcers associated with nonsteroidal antiinflammatory drugs. Acid Suppression Trial: Ranitidine versus Omeprazole for NSAID-associated Ulcer Treatment (ASTRONAUT) Study Group. *N Engl J Med.* 1998;338(11):719-726.

177. Agrawal NM, Campbell DR, Safdi MA, et al. Superiority of lansoprazole vs ranitidine in healing nonsteroidal anti-inflammatory drug-associated gastric ulcers: results of a double-blind, randomized, multicenter study. NSAID-associated gastric ulcer study group. *Arch Intern Med.* 2000;160(10):1455-1461.

178. Agrawal NM, Roth S, Graham DY, et al. Misoprostol compared with sucralfate in the prevention of nonsteroidal anti-inflammatory drug-induced gastric ulcer. A randomized, controlled trial. *Ann Intern Med.* 1991;115(3):195-200.

179. Graham DY, Agrawal NM, Roth SH. Prevention of NSAID-induced gastric ulcer with misoprostol: multicenter, double-blind, placebo-controlled trial. *Lancet.* 1988;2(8623):1277-1280.

180. Graham DY, White RH, Moreland LW, et al. Duodenal and gastric ulcer prevention with misoprostol in arthritis patients taking NSAIDs. Misoprostol Study Group. *Ann Intern Med.* 1993;119(4):257-262.

181. Silverstein FE, Graham DY, Senior JR, et al. Misoprostol reduces serious gastrointestinal complications in patients with rheumatoid arthritis receiving nonsteroidal anti-inflammatory drugs. A randomized, double-blind, placebo-controlled trial. *Ann Intern Med.* 1995;123(4):241-249.

182. Raskin JB, White RH, Jackson RE, et al. Misoprostol dosage in the prevention of nonsteroidal anti-inflammatory drug-induced gastric and duodenal ulcers: a comparison of three regimens. *Ann Intern Med.* 1995;123(5):344-350.

183. Bijlsma JW. Treatment of NSAID-induced gastrointestinal lesions with cimetidine: an international multicenter collaborative study. *Aliment Pharmacol Ther.* 1988;2 (Suppl 1):85-95.

184. Lanza FL, Aspinall RL, Swabb EA, et al. Double-blind, placebo-controlled endoscopic comparison of the mucosal protective effects of misoprostol versus cimetidine on tolmetin-induced mucosal injury to the stomach and duodenum. *Gastroenterology.* 1988;95(2):289-294.

185. Saunders JH, Oliver RJ, Higson DL. Dyspepsia: incidence of a non-ulcer disease in a controlled trial of ranitidine in general practice. *Br Med J (Clin Res Ed).* 1986;292(6521):665-668.

186. Taha AS, Hudson N, Hawkey CJ, et al. Famotidine for the prevention of gastric and duodenal ulcers caused by nonsteroidal antiinflammatory drugs. *N Engl J Med.* 1996;334(22):1435-1439.

187. Hawkey CJ, Karrasch JA, Szczepaski L, et al. Omeprazole compared with misoprostol for ulcers associated with nonsteroidal antiinflammatory drugs. Omeprazole versus misoprostol for NSAID-induced Ulcer Management (OMNIUM) Study Group. *N Engl J Med.* 1998;338(11):727-734.

188. Lanza FL, Rack MF, Callison DA, et al. A pilot endoscopic study of the gastroduodenal effects of SC-58635, a novel COX-2 selecitve inhibitor. *Gastroenterology.* 1997;112 (Supplement):A194.

189. Lanza F, Simon T, Quan H, et al. Selective inhibition of cyclooxygenase-2 (cox-2) with MK-0966(250mg qd) is associated with less gastroduodenal damage then aspirin (ASA) 650mg qid, or ibuprofen 800mg tid. *Gastroenterology.* 1997;112 (Supplement): A194.

190. Wolfe MM. Future trends in the development of safer nonsteroidal anti-inflammatory drugs. *Am J Med.* 1998;105(5A):44S-52S.

191. Clark DW, Layton D, Shakir SA. Do some inhibitors of COX-2 increase the risk of thromboembolic events? Linking pharmacology with pharmacoepidemiology. *Drug Saf.* 2004;27(7):427-456.

192. McAdam BF, Catella-Lawson F, Mardini IA, et al. Systemic biosynthesis of prostacyclin by cyclooxygenase (COX)-2: the human pharmacology of a selective inhibitor of COX-2. *Proc Natl Acad Sci U S A.* 1999;96(1):272-277.

193. Lau JY, Sung JJ, Lee KK, et al. Effect of intravenous omeprazole on recurrent bleeding after endoscopic treatment of bleeding peptic ulcers. *N Engl J Med.* 2000;343(5):310-316.

194. Norton JA, Fraker DL, Alexander HR, et al. Surgery to cure the Zollinger-Ellison syndrome. *N Engl J Med.* 1999;341(9):635-644.

195. Metz DC, Strader DB, Orbuch M, et al. Use of omeprazole in Zollinger-Ellison syndrome: a prospective nine-year study of efficacy and safety. *Aliment Pharmacol Ther.* 1993;7(6):597-610.

196. Wolfe MM, Jensen RT. Zollinger-Ellison syndrome. Current concepts in diagnosis and management. *N Engl J Med.* 1987;317(19):1200-1209.

Complications of Peptic Ulcer Disease: Recognition, Management, Bleeding, Perforation, and Obstruction

Paul J. Bandini Jr, MD and Nikhil Deshpande, MD

Complications of Peptic Ulcer Disease

Despite a better understanding of the pathogenesis and etiology of PUD, complications still arise leading to significant morbidity and mortality, particularly among the elderly. Foremost are bleeding and perforation. Obstruction and penetration still occur, although much less frequently, despite our ability to heal, prevent, and remove the major causes of ulcer disease. Stress-related mucosal disease remains a serious threat to critically ill patients in an intensive care unit (ICU) setting. The following sections will address the latest principals of management of each of these potential complications.

Bleeding

UGI bleeding accounts for over 300,000 hospitalizations annually in the United States. PUD remains the single most common cause requiring hospitalization and accounts for 45% of all UGI tract bleeding. Despite the advent of ICUs, sophisticated hemodynamic monitoring, and improved endoscopic and angiographic interventions, the mortality from UGI bleeding over the past 40 years has remained approximately 10%. Lack of substantial decrease in the mortality rate may reflect the aging population. Persons older than 60 years old now account for 35% to 40% of all cases of UGI hemorrhage. Improved survival from advances in treatment has been offset by the rising number of high-risk elderly patients who comprise an increasing proportion of the 10% who die from a bleeding episode. Nearly 85% of deaths from PUD occur in persons over 65. Fortunately, 70% to 80% of patients with UGI bleed will stop within 48 hrs. However, 10% to 20% of these will experience a reoccurrence of bleeding. Analysis of patients that either continue to bleed or those that initially stop and then experience recurrent bleeding reveals that these are the patients for whom mortality is the highest; 40% to 50% of these patients will succumb during the hospitalization either from the GI bleeding or as a consequence of underlying diseases aggravated by the bleeding (Table 7-1).

Table 7-1

MORTALITY ASSOCIATED WITH UNDERLYING DISEASES AGGRAVATED BY GASTROINTESTINAL BLEEDING

Associated Medical Illnesses	Mortality (%)
Renal disease	29.4
Acute renal failure	63.6
Liver disease	24.6
Jaundice	42.4
Pulmonary disease	22.6
Respiratory failure	57.4
Cardiac disease	12.5
Congestive heart failure	28.4

MORTALITY FROM GASTROINTESTINAL BLEEDING

There are a number of clinical factors that are associated with a high risk of rebleeding, surgery, and mortality, including:

- Age >60.
- Concurrent illness.
- Hemodynamic instability.
- Coagulopathy.
- Transfusion requirement of >6 units.
- Fresh blood emesis or hematochezia.
- Onset of bleeding when in the hospital for another illness.

PREDISPOSING FACTORS

The most important pathogenic factors in the development of peptic ulcers and peptic ulcer complications are *H. pylori* infection and NSAIDs. Characteristics of patients in the United States with bleeding PUD are represented in Table 7-2.

Although each independently is associated with an increased risk, there has been controversy as to whether these 2 factors interact additively or even synergistically. A recent meta-analysis examining the role of *H. pylori* and NSAIDs suggested a synergistic relationship.[1] Irrespective of *H. pylori* status, this analysis showed that uncomplicated ulcers were 4-fold more common in those that took NSAIDs than those who did not. *H. pylori* infection alone increased the risk 3.5 fold. However, in patients who were both infected with *H. pylori* and taking NSAIDs, the risk was increased 60-fold compared to those taking NSAIDs who were not infected. A similar synergy was also seen with the complication of bleeding PUD. The presence of *H. pylori* was associated with

Table 7-2

CHARACTERISTICS OF PATIENTS IN THE UNITED STATES WITH BLEEDING PEPTIC ULCER DISEASE

	Mean Age	% H. pylori +	% NSAID/ASA use
DU	62.9	49.6	52.9
GU	65.1	45.3	57.2

a 1.79-fold increase in bleeding and NSAID use with a 4.85-fold increase. With both factors present, the risk of bleeding increased 6.13-fold. The conclusion reached by these investigators was that *H. pylori* and NSAIDs act independently both to increase the risk of uncomplicated ulcers and the complication of bleeding from ulcer disease.

The risk of bleeding from aspirin therapy has also been assessed in large randomized, controlled trials. Today, the cardiovascular benefits of aspirin have been well established. All cause mortality benefits have been clearly demonstrated for secondary prophylaxis (eg, in coronary artery disease and diabetes mellitus). In this group, there is a 2.5-fold increase in the risk of GI bleeding, but the risk is offset by the benefit.[2] However, when consideration is given for the use of aspirin in primary prevention of cardiovascular events, the indication represents a trade-off between an individual's cardiovascular risk and the probability of an adverse event such as hemorrhagic stroke or GI bleeding. In a meta-analysis of over 50,000 patients, aspirin reduced nonfatal and fatal myocardial infarction by 28%, but it also increased the risk of hemorrhagic stroke by 40% and major GI bleeding by 70%.[3]

Aspirin causes GI bleeding in a dose-related fashion[4]; however, even a dose as low as 75 mg is associated with a 2.3-fold increased risk of ulcer bleeding[5] that continues in a linear fashion over an 8- to 10-year period of time.[6] The risk is not decreased with either a buffered or enteric-coated preparation because bleeding is due to a systemic antiprostaglandin effect of aspirin. Also, the concomitant use of aspirin with a traditional NSAID increases the risk of ulcer disease to twice that of low-dose aspirin alone. Unfortunately, the use of selective COX-2 inhibitors does not provide a solution to this problem and several have now been taken off the market due to cardiovascular toxicity. Although the COX-2 inhibitors reduce the incidence of ulcer complications by 50% to 60% compared to traditional NSAIDS, this effect is negated by the concomitant use of aspirin as shown by the CLASS Study.[7] Here, 800 patients in 2 groups were receiving either celecoxib, ibuprofen, or diclofenac. No difference in GI complications was seen in these 2 groups. However, if the patients not taking aspirin were looked at separately, there was a clear reduction in GI complications in the group receiving the COX-2 inhibitor. This was a retrospective study not specifically designed to evaluate the interaction of aspirin, NSAIDs, and coxibs. In a prospective study of patients with osteoarthritis randomized to 12 weeks of enteric-coated aspirin alone, enteric-coated aspirin plus rofecoxib, ibuprofen 2400 mg daily, or placebo alone, there was no difference in the incidence of endoscopic gastroduodenal ulcers in the group taking low-dose aspirin with rofecoxib compared to ibuprofen alone.[8]

Other factors for NSAID-associated ulcer complications include a past history of complicated ulcer, multiple NSAIDs, high-dose NSAIDs, concomitant use of anticoagulants, steroids and age greater than 70 years old.

Given the importance of *H. pylori* and NSAID/aspirin use in causing bleeding PUD, it is important to test a patient with a history of UGI bleeding before leaving the hospital for *H. pylori* and assessing the ongoing need for NSAID and/or aspirin therapy. When treating *H. pylori* in patients with prior complications of PUD, urea breath or stool antigen testing should document eradication. PPI therapy should be continued for 6 to 8 weeks. If NSAIDS or aspirin need to be restarted, cotherapy with a PPI is essential to prophylax against ulcer recurrence.

CLINICAL PRESENTATION

Acute UGI bleeding usually manifests itself in several ways:

- Hematemesis (50%).
- Hematemesis and melena (20%).
- Melena alone (20%).
- Hematochezia (10%).

Hematemesis may involve the vomiting of bright red blood or dark blood that is "coffee-ground" in appearance. Melena is usually black, tarry, and foul smelling. As little as 50 to 100 mL of blood is needed to produce this color change. Hematochezia is the passage of bright red or maroon blood from the rectum and indicates more severe bleeding of at least 1000 mL and portends a worse prognosis. In the older patient, a history of unexplained syncope should heighten the suspicion of significant GI bleeding. A large volume of blood may be sequestered in the GI tract without immediate hematemesis or hematochezia. Also, antecedent symptoms of epigastric pain or dyspepsia may be absent in the elderly particularly if taking NSAIDs.

CLINICAL PROGNOSTIC FACTORS

A careful, focused history and physical examination are key to determining the nature, severity, and origin of bleeding in a patient with acute GI bleeding. Among the most widely used outcomes measures have been the number of units or blood transfused, the need for emergency surgery, and death. A number of clinical prognostic factors have been identified that determine these endpoints and are associated with a poor clinical outcome. These include factors that reflect significant comorbidity and ongoing active bleeding[9]:

- Age greater than 60 years.
- Presence of comorbid medical conditions.
- Coagulopathy.
- Onset of bleeding in the hospital.
- Hemodynamic instability on presentation.
- Severe hemorrhage.
- Red NG aspirate.
- History of hematochezia or hematemesis.
- Multiple transfusions (>5).

Table 7-3

ROCKALL SCORING SYSTEM FOR SEVERITY OF ACUTE UPPER GASTROINTESTINAL TRACT BLEEDING*

Variable	Score			
	0	1	2	3
Age	<60	61 to 79	>80	
Shock	No shock	(Tachycardia)	(Hypotension)	
	HR <100	HR >100	HR >100	
	SBP >100	SBP >100	SBP <100	
Comorbidity	Nil major		Cardiac failure (eg, IHD)	Renal failure Liver failure Disseminated malignancy
Diagnosis	M-W tear No lesion No SRH	All other diagnoses	Malignancy of the UGI tract	
Major SRH	None or dark spot		Blood in the UGI tract, adherent clot, visible or spurting vessel	

HR = heart rate; SBP = systolic blood pressure; IHD = ischemic heart disease; M-W tear = Mallory-Weiss tear; SRH = stigmata of recent hemorrhage
* A score of <3 is associated with excellent prognosis; score >8 is associated with a high risk of death.

- Need for emergency surgical intervention.
- Continued or recurrent bleeding.

A number of different clinical scoring systems have been devised to be predictive of rebleeding/death after UGI tract bleeding. These include the Baylor College scoring system, the Cedars-Sinai Medical Center predictive index, and the Rockall risk scoring system (Table 7-3). Despite differences in institution, geographic location, patient demographics, and methodology, these systems are similar in their identification of a common group of predictive variables that seem to be closely associated with adverse patient outcome. Variables include the presence of comorbidity, evidence of acute hemodynamic disturbance as a result of the bleeding episode, and the presence of high-risk endoscopic stigmata of recent hemorrhage. Central to all these systems is the pivotal role of upper endoscopy in predicting patient outcome.[10]

Risk stratification with respect to adverse outcome is a logical strategy both for triage of those at high risk to inpatient care and for identification of patients at low risk of an adverse outcome who can be safely managed on an outpatient basis.

In a comparison study,[11] Rockall's score accurately predicted rebleeding in low and intermediate-risk categories (<6) but not in high-risk patients. The rates of rebleeding were significantly higher than the ones predicted by the low-risk categories of either the Cedars-Sinai index or the Baylor score. The predicted and the observed mortality were not significantly different throughout all the categories of Rockall's score, except for a score of 4. All the scores had a better discriminative ability for mortality than for rebleeding. Unfortunately, there is a lack of clear objective evidence that risk scores are better prognostic instruments compared with clinical judgment and intuition of the physician, and this may explain in part the under utilization of these risk-stratification systems. Ultimately the use of any risk-stratification system lies in its proven ability to positively and significantly impact the cost-effective care of the patient and concomitantly improve the overall quality of care, which hopefully will reduce the incidence of recurrent bleeding and mortality rate.

ROLE OF ENDOSCOPY AND ENDOSCOPIC PROGNOSTIC FEATURES

The effectiveness of upper endoscopy in the diagnosis and treatment of bleeding PUD has been well established. Not only does endoscopy allow prompt diagnosis and provide information leading to risk stratification, but it also offers the opportunity to perform endoscopic hemostasis in high-risk patients. Its use has been associated with a reduction in blood transfusions and length of intensive care and total hospital stay when performed early on in the hospital course (within 24 hours of hospital admission). Controlled and observational studies have shown that early discharge of patients found to have low-risk stigmata for recurrent bleeding is safe and effective.

A key to an accurate diagnosis is adequate visualization of the entire UGI tract. The presence of uncleared blood and clot reduces the diagnostic and therapeutic yield and has been shown to be associated with considerable morbidity and mortality. Two randomized controlled trials have demonstrated the efficacy of IV erythromycin (250 mg or 3 mg/kg over 30 minutes) 30 to 90 minutes before upper endoscopy in promoting gastric motility and emptying of blood and clot. Such an effect improves the quality of the examination with regard to mucosal visibility and results in a reduced need for a second-look endoscopy.

A great deal of the morbidity and mortality that accompanies PUD bleeding is associated with rebleeding. Although clinical prognostic factors are important in predicting outcome, the endoscopic appearance of the ulcer may be more important in assessing the risk of rebleeding (risk stratification). In addition, endoscopy is essential for the selection of patients who will benefit from endoscopic therapy. The risk of rebleeding is 80% to 90% for an actively bleeding (Forrest IA) or oozing ulcer (Forrest IB), 50% with a non-bleeding visible vessel (Forrest IIA), 33% with an adherent clot (Forrest IIB), 10% with a flat spot, and 5% with a clean-based ulcer. Endoscopic treatment of stigmata of recent hemorrhage (actively bleeding ulcers and those with a visible vessel) has been shown to be effective in reducing the risk of rebleeding, mortality, and the need for urgent surgery.

INITIAL ASSESSMENT AND MEDICAL MANAGEMENT

First and foremost in the initial evaluation of patients with UGI bleeding is an accurate assessment of hemodynamic and cardiopulmonary status, the degree of blood loss, and prompt volume resuscitation, if necessary. This requires close monitoring of EKG, blood pressure, pulse oximetry, urine output, and postural changes. Both the extent and rate of hemorrhage and presence of comorbid medical conditions determine the clinical manifestations of bleeding. Orthostatic hypotension, defined as a greater than 10 mmHg change in systolic blood pressure, usually indicates a 20% or greater reduction in blood volume. Associated symptoms may include lightheadedness, syncope, sweating, nausea, and vomiting. Frank hypotension and tachycardia occur when there is a 25% to 40% loss of blood volume. Clinical signs may be blunted in the elderly or those on beta and calcium channel blockers. Initial hemoglobin and hematocrit may not adequately reflect the degree of blood loss since equilibration with the extravascular fluid and hemodilution often occur over 8 hours.

The role and value of NG aspiration has been controversial. Physician assessment of NG aspirate for the presence of active UGI bleeding was found to have a low sensitivity and specificity (79% and 55%, respectively) in one study.[12] The same held true for assessment of the presence of bile (sensitivity 48%, specificity 74%). The conclusion by the authors was that the visual characteristics of the NG aspirate were not accurate enough to assess either the activity or location of bleeding. Also, the assessment of the presence of bile was unreliable. Despite these limitations, a NG aspirate can provide some useful information. A survey by the American Society of Gastrointestinal Endoscopy on UGI bleeding determined that a clear gastric aspirate was associated with 8% mortality in contrast to 18% mortality when red blood was aspirated. When both stool and NG aspirate contained red blood, mortality rose to 30%.[13] Valuable information as to the location of bleeding may also be obtained when a patient presents with melena or hematochezia alone. The presence of dark blood with a "coffee-ground" appearance usually signifies a source above the ligament of Trietz. Although a negative or clear aspirate reduces the likelihood of a UGI source, it does not completely rule it out. A clear gastric aspirate has been found in approximately 15% to 20% of patients with endoscopically documented UGI source of bleeding.[12-14] Orogastric or NG aspiration also aids in facilitating upper endoscopy by removing particulate matter, blood, and clots and decreasing the risk of aspiration. There is no evidence that gastric lavage with fluid of any temperature, particularly iced saline, is effective in achieving hemostasis or preventing rebleeding and is no longer recommended.

Those patients who manifest frank shock; orthostatic hypotension; decrease in hematocrit of 6% or more or require greater than 2 units of packed red blood cells; or with ongoing bleeding manifest as hematemesis, bright red blood per NG tube, or hematochezia should be monitored in an ICU. Crystalloid fluids should be infused via 2 peripheral large bore (18 gauge) catheters or central venous catheter to maintain an adequate blood pressure. Packed red cells should be given to high-risk patients such as the elderly with comorbid medical illness and show evidence of ongoing active bleed, significant blood loss, or cardiac ischemia. Hematocrit can be maintained above 30% in these patients or greater than 20% in an otherwise healthy adult. If an underlying coagulopathy is present (ie, INR >1.5 or platelet count <50,000), fresh frozen plasma, and platelets, respectively, can be administered. Elective endotracheal intubation may be required in patients with persistent hematemesis or altered mental or respiratory status to prevent aspiration and facilitate upper endoscopy.

Several studies have examined the role of acid suppression given before or after endoscopy without endoscopic therapy. The rationale for the use of these agents comes from in vitro data showing that hemostatic mechanisms are highly pH dependent. At a pH of <6, disaggregation of platelets takes place. Platelet aggregation and plasma coagulation are nearly abolished below a pH of 5.4. Below a pH of 4, fibrin clots are dissolved by the proteolytic action of pepsin in the gastric juice. Theoretically, therefore, a profound reduction in gastric acidity to near neutrality could stabilize a clot overlying an ulcer and possibly either help diminish bleeding or its reoccurrence.

Those studies evaluating the role of H2 receptor antagonists have produced conflicting and disappointing results.[15-17] A recent meta-analysis concluded that H2 antagonists appeared to be of minimal benefit in reducing the rate of continued bleeding, the need for surgery, and the risk of death. These benefits were seen only in patients with gastric and not DUs.[18] Subsequently, a multicenter trial of 1005 patients compared an infusion of famotidine with placebo and found no difference in the rate of rebleeding between the 2 groups.[17] The reasons the H2 receptor antagonists may not be effective are incomplete acid suppression, their ability to only reduce basal acid secretion, and the development of tolerance (ie, tachyphylaxis) to their acid-suppressing effects.

In contrast, studies on the use of PPIs have been more favorable and have focused mostly on the use of IV omeprazole. In studies not allowing endotherapy, PPI administration has been shown to reduce further bleeding but not reduce mortality or need for surgery when compared to placebo or H2 receptor antagonists for oozing ulcers and for ulcers with previous bleeding. A recent comprehensive review of these studies concluded that PPI therapy was warranted in all patients with UGI bleeding severe enough to require endoscopic intervention. Moreover, PPI therapy can be recommended in patients with suspected peptic ulcer bleeding associated with hemodynamic instability, patients in whom endoscopic evaluation is delayed or unavailable, and/or those requiring blood transfusion.[19] The benefits appear to be independent of either the oral or IV route of PPI administration. However, there are no studies comparing the oral to the IV routes. In the United States, PPIs now approved for IV use include pantoprazole, lansoprazole, and esomeprazole. The suggested dose of pantoprazole is 80 mg IV bolus followed by an infusion of 8 mg/hr.

ENDOSCOPIC HEMOSTATIC THERAPY

The role of upper endoscopy and the effectiveness of endoscopic therapy in the treatment of UGI bleeding from PUD have been firmly established. Initial hemostatic rates of 80% to 95% can be achieved with endoscopic techniques. However, after the initial control, bleeding may still reoccur in 10% to 30% of patients. Numerous trials have demonstrated the benefit of endoscopic intervention when compared to medical management alone, no therapy, or sham therapy. The rebleeding rates, surgery rates, and mortality rate are all significantly benefited by endoscopic therapy in patients with high-risk lesions.[20] According to recent consensus recommendations, a finding of high-risk stigmata of ulcer bleeding such as an actively bleeding or visible vessel is an indication for immediate endoscopic hemostatic therapy. An ulcer with a clean, white base or flat red or black spot has a low risk of rebleeding and therefore requires no endoscopic intervention. If no lesion is found on upper endoscopy, further evaluation with enteroscopy and colonoscopy may be warranted.

Endoscopic therapy can be broadly divided into 3 categories: injection, thermal, and mechanical. Each of the methods has advantages and disadvantages related to the hemostatic mechanism and technical aspects of the procedure. It is not entirely clear whether one single modality consistently offers the best results. However, it is generally agreed that injection and thermal modalities are equally effective.[21,22] Also, the combination of an injection and thermal method is superior to either modality alone.

Injection Therapy

The mechanism of action of injection therapy is mainly through tamponade of the bleeding vessel although some agents also exert a pharmacologic effect. A variety of agents have been used: distilled water; hypertonic saline; diluted epinephrine; sclerosants such as absolute alcohol, ethanolamine, polidocanol, or sodium tetradecyl sulfate; thrombin; fibrin seal; and cyanoacrylate glue.

The most commonly used agent is epinephrine. It is safe, inexpensive, effective, and technically easy to instill. Very often it is the first therapeutic modality used for peptic ulcer bleeding. When diluted to 1:10,000 or 1:20,000, epinephrine causes vaso-constriction, vessel compression, and probably promotes platelet aggregation without resulting in tissue necrosis. Large volumes of epinephrine can be used with a low risk of complications because submucosal injections do not usually damage tissue or have clinically significant systemic cardiovascular effects even when plasma epinephrine levels rise 4 to 5 times above baseline immediately after injection. Injection of larger volumes (35 to 45 mL) of epinephrine has been shown to be superior to lower volumes (15 to 25 mL) when used as monotherapy to achieve sustained hemostasis in ulcers involving the gastric body. Ulcers here require a larger volume to achieve sustained mechanical compression because of the large surface area of the gastric body. Smaller volumes may dissipate widely within the submucosal layer, blunting the compressive effect of the injection. For ulcers in the duodenum, where the surface area is smaller, lesser amounts of epinephrine are required. Although initial reported rates of hemostasis with epinephrine alone range from 85% to 100%, rebleeding recurs in 15% to 35%. For this reason, injection therapy with epinephrine alone is not recommended and studies have demonstrated that epinephrine injection followed by a second modality is more effective than epinephrine alone.[23] A commonly used method is to inject 1 mL aliquots of 1:10,000 epinephrine into and adjacent to the bleeding vessel up to 45 mL. After hemostasis is achieved, thermal coaptive coagulation is then applied using either a heater probe or bipolar electrocoagulation.

Sclerosants primarily produce direct tissue injury and thrombosis of the bleeding vessel. Because epinephrine does not induce vessel thrombosis, there is at least a theoretical advantage to adding a sclerosant to epinephrine. Clinical trials have not consistently shown any advantage to adding a sclerosant agent to epinephrine. They are no more effective than epinephrine and carry a high risk of complications. Similarly, available clinical data do not show convincing superiority of either thrombin or fibrin sealant alone or together with epinephrine or sclerosing agents.

Thermal Therapy

Thermal therapy can be delivered by contact or coaptive techniques (heater probe or bipolar thermocoagulation) or noncontact techniques (Nd:YAG) laser or argon plasma coagulator (APC). With coaptive coagulation, the probe is used to physically compress and tamponade the visible vessel then seal it with thermal energy. With the heater probe, a succession of 4 pulses at 25 to 30 Joules should be delivered before changing the probe position. With the bipolar thermocoagulation probe, a relatively low power setting of 15 to 20 watts should be applied for longer duration (10 to 14 seconds) in order to ensure adequate depth of penetration. The use of larger 3.2-mm probes is also recommended. With either of these techniques, vessels up to 2 to 2.5 mm can be successfully cauterized.

Noncontact methods such as the Nd:YAG laser are not frequently used because of issues of training, cost, and portability. However, the APC is a relatively new device and may offer an advantage over contact devices. Because of its ability to bend the electrical current toward adjacent tissue, this enables the endoscopist to work in an area that would otherwise be inaccessible and where direct application of a probe would be difficult if not impossible.

No one thermal modality has demonstrated clear superiority over the other in comparative studies. In one study comparing heater probe, bipolar electrocoagulation, and the Nd:YAG laser in patients with actively bleeding ulcers, there were no significant differences among the 3 groups with respect to rebleeding rate, length of hospital stay, or need for surgery.[24] Randomized controlled trials conducted by the CURE Homeostasis Research Group compared heater probe therapy with bipolar or multipolar thermocoagulation and found a trend toward lower rates of rebleeding and emergency surgery with heater probe therapy. However, statistical significance was not achieved.[25,26]

Mechanical Therapy

Mechanical therapy also involves physical compression of the bleeding vessel. The most extensively studied device has been the hemoclip, which is essentially an endoscopic version of surgical ligation of the bleeding artery. Here, also, firm conclusions concerning the relative efficacy of hemoclips versus more traditional modalities such as injection and thermal cannot be assessed.

A study by Gevers et al randomized patients to receive hemoclips alone, injection therapy with epinephrine and polidocanol, or combination therapy.[27] No statistical difference in the rates of initial failure or early recurrence of bleeding was found between the 3 groups.[27] The 3 groups, however, differed significantly in overall failure rate with the highest rate occurring in the hemoclip group. The unsuccessful placement of the hemoclip was considered by the authors to be the reason for less effective control of bleeding. Other prospective randomized trials comparing hemoclips with heater probe have produced conflicting results. In a study by Cipolletta et al, a significantly lower rate of rebleeding, length of hospital stay, and transfusion requirement was seen with the hemoclip group compared to the heater probe group.[28] A randomized study by Lin et al found a higher rate of initial and ultimate hemostasis in the heater probe group and similar rebleeding rates in the heater probe and hemoclip groups.[29] Factors that may limit the efficacy of hemoclips include a firm, scarred ulcer base that may impair adequate tamponade and location of an ulcer high along the lesser curvature of the stomach and posterior wall of the duodenal bulb.

COMBINED ENDOSCOPIC MODALITIES

Although several published guidelines have agreed that there is no clear-cut evidence that any endoscopic technique is superior to injection of epinephrine alone for the endoscopic treatment of high-risk bleeding peptic ulcers, these guidelines have not made clear recommendations concerning epinephrine in combination with a second hemostatic technique.[30,31] Several randomized controlled trials have shown that the addition of thermal therapy or a sclerosant to epinephrine injection does further reduce bleeding rates as compared with epinephrine injection alone, especially in patients with spurting hemorrhage.[21,32,33] More evidence supporting this evidence comes from a recent meta-analysis that clearly suggests that combined therapy is the treatment of choice for high-risk bleeding peptic ulcers (ie, those with Forrest I bleeding ulcers).[23] The absolute reduction in hemostatic efficacy, although small at 5% to 10%, still represented a 30% to 50% reduction in the relative risk of a recurrent hemorrhage. Furthermore, subanalysis showed that the risk of further bleeding decreased regardless of whether thermal or injection of sclerosant as a second procedure was applied. Based on this evidence, combined therapy should be considered as standard procedure for high-risk bleeding peptic ulcers.

ACID SUPPRESSIVE THERAPY AS ADJUNCT TO ENDOSCOPIC THERAPY

Although endoscopic intervention in patients with high-risk stigmata of recent hemorrhage has improved outcomes, there still remains a 10% to 30% rebleeding rate after initial hemostatic control with endoscopic treatment. Evidence, from a number of well-designed trials, has now shown that the addition of acid-suppressive therapy with PPIs has further reduced the risk of rebleeding in patients who require endoscopic therapy. Lau et al randomized 240 patients to receive either high-dose IV omeprazole infusion or placebo following endoscopic therapy for ulcers with active bleeding, adherent clots, and visible vessels. Significant reduction in rebleeding rates from 20% seen with placebo to less than 5% with omeprazole therapy was observed.[34] Another study by the same investigators compared the effect of combined endoscopic and IV PPI therapy with PPI therapy alone in high-risk ulcer patients. IV PPI was inferior to the combination therapy of PPI and endoscopic therapy.[35] Lin et al compared the efficacy of the combination of endoscopic therapy plus either high-dose omeprazole (80 mg bolus followed by 8 mg/hr) or continuous infusion with cimetidine (300 mg IV bolus followed by 50 mg/hr by continuous infusion).[36] Combination therapy with omeprazole was found to be superior to combination therapy with cimetidine infusion in terms of reducing bleeding rates, gastric acid control, and volume of blood transfused.[36] These studies have now set the standard for adjunctive antisecretory therapy in patients with high-risk peptic ulcer bleeding. However, it must be understood that no study, including a number of meta-analyses, has yet demonstrated a positive outcome effect for this approach on mortality or the need for surgical intervention.[37]

A number of controversies still exist such as to whether PPIs are better than H2 receptor antagonists, the route and dosing of PPIs, the duration of therapy, and whether the stigmata of ulcer bleeding were important predictors of additional benefit from PPIs.

For several decades, oral and IV H2 receptor antagonists had been used as sole therapy for patients with bleeding ulcers without any supporting evidence for their efficacy in decreasing the rate of recurrent bleeding in these patients. Only one meta-analysis, conducted in 1985, of 27 available randomized trials in which more than 2500 patients were entered suggested that H2 receptor antagonists might reduce the rates of bleeding, surgery, and death by 10%, 20%, and 30%, respectively.[38] The implication of the analysis was that treatment with H2 blockers appeared to be moderately promising, but the benefit seemed to be confined to GUs and not DUs. In 2002, an updated meta-analysis of this earlier study concluded that there was no benefit of IV H2 receptor antagonists over placebo in clinically important outcomes of bleeding DU and at best only a small benefit in bleeding GU.[39] In contrast to H2 receptor antagonists alone for the treatment of bleeding peptic ulcer, PPIs when given as monotherapy without endoscopic therapy have proven to be superior to both placebo and H2 blockers in significantly reducing the odds of rebleeding. However, mortality is not reduced. Interestingly, the benefits of PPI are independent of the route and method of administration (ie, whether given orally or by IV bolus or infusion).[40]

When H2 receptor antagonists are compared to PPIs in combination with endoscopic therapy, the results are less clear. A meta-analysis by Gisbert et al in 2001 was performed to evaluate whether PPIs were more effective than H2 receptor antagonists for the treatment of bleeding peptic ulcer. The author's conclusion was that PPIs are more effective than H2 receptor antagonists in preventing persistent or recurrent bleeding from peptic ulcer, although this advantage seemed to be more evident in patients not having adjunctive endoscopic therapy.[41] The beneficial effect seemed to be similar or even more marked in patients with Forrest IA, IB, or IIA ulcers. Recently, Barkum and colleagues presented the results of a multinational study comparing IV pantoprazole (80 mg bolus followed by 8 mg/hr continuous infusion) with ranitidine (50 mg bolus followed by 13.3 mg/hr continuous infusion) for the prevention of ulcer rebleeding. In an unexpected final analysis, pantoprazole did not decrease rebleeding compared to ranitidine but did show numerical superiority. In subgroup analysis, pantoprazole showed a statistically significant rebleeding difference relative to ranitidine for arterial spurters and a strong trend toward lower rates of rebleeding with PPI in patients with a GU.[42] Finally, a more recent meta-analysis came to the conclusion that when PPIs or H2 receptor antagonists were given as adjunct to endoscopic therapy, no differences in the outcome of bleeding patients was seen between the 2 drugs, even when PPIs were given as continuous infusion or intermittent bolus.[43] What can be gleaned from these studies is that both types of antisecretory agents, PPIs and H2 receptor antagonists, are effective in reducing further bleeding when given as adjunct to endoscopic therapy. The combination of some endoscopic treatment with either PPIs or H2 receptor antagonists is definitely indicated for Forrest IIA and Forrest IIB ulcers with the intent to reduce further bleeding and need for surgery. The value of combined therapy may also extend to Forrest IA and Forrest IB ulcers, but current data are not sufficient to support the claim.

The question as to the optimal dose and route of PPI to use in bleeding PUD remains unclear. The current standard of care is to use pantoprazole as an 80-mg IV bolus followed by an infusion of 8 mg/hour for 72 hours. A recent Canadian consensus conference on the management of patients with nonvariceal UGI bleeding recommended this regimen for patients who have undergone successful endoscopic therapy.[44] For the most part, this regimen has been based on studies that extrapolated data from studies that used IV omeprazole at these doses and also dose-ranging studies with pantoprazole that found this to be the optimal dose to achieve an intragastric pH >6 to 7. Recently, the outcomes of this high-dose IV regimen were compared to lower-dose oral and IV PPIs after endoscopic hemostasis in patients with ulcer bleeding. Both oral and IV PPI, high and low dose, were associated with lower rates of rebleeding after endoscopic therapy, but the high-dose regimen was associated with greater incremental benefit for reductions in surgery and mortality.[43] Bardou et al performed a meta-analysis also comparing high-dose oral PPI therapy (at least twice the usual daily dose) with trials using the conventional high-dose PPI intravenously and concluded that both the high-dose oral and IV regimens are effective for reducing bleeding.[45] However, the oral regimen is not associated with a decrease in surgery or mortality as was observed with the high-dose IV PPI regimen.[45] It must be understood that these meta-analysis are not as clinically reliable as well conducted, randomized, controlled, double blind studies. Head to head comparisons of oral to IV PPI therapy are still needed.

WHAT TO DO WITH AN ULCER WITH ADHERENT CLOT

The optimal management of ulcers with adherent clot has been a matter of much controversy since 1989. The National Institute of Health Consensus Conference recommended against the removal of clot for fear of precipitating bleeding and suggested only gentle washing.[46] A meta-analysis by Cook et al came to the conclusion that only patients with active bleeding or nonbleeding vessels derived benefit from endoscopic therapy.[47] Rebleeding was not reduced in patients with ulcers containing flat spots or adherent clots.

Recently, the recommendation not to remove adherent clot has been challenged, and more aggressive treatment, which employs removing the clot and treating the underlying lesion, has been advocated. Much of the controversy concerning treatment of adherent clots stems from the widely variable reported prevalence of clots in patients with bleeding ulcers, ranging from 0% to 50% and bleeding rates of 8% to 36%.[48-50] Several reasons have been put forth to explain this variability in reported rates of adherent clot and bleeding. Among them are a relatively poor agreement among endoscopists in labeling stigmata of clots or visible vessels and the degree of aggressiveness in irrigating ulcers with clots. Some studies have performed very little or gentle irrigation with a syringe or no irrigation at all. Others have used vigorous measures such as application of suction with the endoscope, manipulation with a biopsy forceps or tip of the endoscope, irrigating with a large diameter heater or bipolar electrocoagulation probe, guillotining with a snare, or use of a WaterPik (WaterPik Technologies, Fort Collins, Colo). The rationale for more aggressive treatment of clot is that gentle irrigation with a syringe may fail to expose the underlying stigmata that would indicate a high risk of rebleeding. More vigorous irrigation could help stratify patients with clots into low-risk or high-risk stigmata. Laine et al reported that with vigorous irrigation of clot for up to 5 minutes with a 3.2-mm bipolar probe the clot remained adherent in 57% of patients and without endoscopic therapy, the rebleeding rate was only 8%. In the remainder of patients, the clot washed away, revealing low-risk stigmata in 13% and high-risk stigmata in 30% that then required endoscopic intervention.[51]

Recently, several randomized controlled trials were designed to evaluate endoscopic therapy for adherent clot. Bleau et al randomized 56 patients with adherent clots and no active bleeding to receive endoscopic therapy or medical therapy alone.[50] Endoscopic therapy consisted of injection of the base of the clot with 1:10,000 epinephrine in 4 quadrants, followed by vigorous attempts to remove clot by various means including suction, snare removal, and manipulation with biopsy forceps or the tip of the endoscope. The underlying lesions were then treated with heater probe coagulation. Patients who received endoscopic therapy had a significantly lower bleeding rate compared to those receiving medical therapy alone (4.8% vs. 34.3%, respectively).[50] Jensen et al also used an aggressive technique to remove clot.[49] After epinephrine injection into the 4 quadrants, a disposable snare without electrocoagulation was used to shave down the clot by cold guillotining to 3 to 4 mm above the ulcer base. The residual clot or the underlying stigmata were then treated with coaptive coagulation to achieve flattening of the residual small clot or visible vessel, a white coagulum, or no bleeding of the ulcer. This technique resulted in significantly lower rates of rebleeding and the need for further endoscopic intervention (0% for both) as compared to medically treated patients (35% and 24%, respectively).[49] Although results of these studies are promising, both have limitations. More controlled studies are needed, but for now it seems prudent to aggressively remove clot and treat high-risk stigmata in selected patients with independent predictors of rebleeding such as comorbid illness, shock, or hemoglobin less than 10. Following endoscopic therapy in this subset of patients, constant IV infusion of a PPI (80-mg bolus followed by 8 mg/hr for pantoprazole) better prevents recurrent bleeding than those treated by endoscopic therapy alone.[51]

Perforation

Today, with effective medical management with H2-receptor antagonists, PPIs, and eradication of *H. pylori*, the hospitalization rate for treatment of PUD has decreased. However, the rate of complicated ulcer disease has remained unchanged. Free perforation of a peptic ulcer is often a sudden, catastrophic, and life-threatening complication. Nearly one half of patients presenting with perforation have no history of ulcer disease and 10% to 20% have no history of ulcer symptoms. Patients tend to be elderly; chronically ill; and 40% to 70% are taking aspirin, other NSAIDs, or both. Alcohol, smoking, and crack cocaine use are other major risk factors. The association of *H. pylori* and perforated peptic ulcer remains controversial. Chowdhary et al reported on a series of 45 patients, 15 of which had a perforated peptic DU.[52] None of the 15 had evidence of *H. pylori* infection.[52] Reinbach and colleagues concluded that there was no clear-cut association between perforated DU and *H. pylori*.[53] Only 47% of the perforated DU patients were positive for *H. pylori* and this was similar to the value of 50% in controls.[53] Others[54,55] have suggested that *H. pylori* plays an important role in the etiology of non-NSAID ulcers and that eradication of infection may prevent ulcer reoccurrence after simple, surgical closure. Although the association of *H. pylori* and perforated ulcer cannot be convincingly established, most likely it is a causal factor in a subset of patients.

Classically, 3 phases of perforated peptic ulcer have been described:

1. Initially, there is the sudden onset of severe abdominal pain, primarily in the epigastrium but quickly becoming generalized. Often, this is accompanied by syncope and frank shock. This scenario develops over several hours and is the result of the leakage of acidic gastric fluid into the peritoneal cavity and release of vasoactive mediators that initiate the physiologic response. The patient is often tachycardic, clammy with cool extremities (cold shock), and may have a subnormal temperature. During this phase, which may last minutes to hours, abdominal rigidity begins to set in.

2. In the second or latent stage, the patient may actually look and feel better and be complaining of less abdominal pain. This may be the result of fluid transudating out of injured tissue, buffering and diluting the caustic gastric juice. The clinician may be lulled into believing that the patient is improving and that the situation is less critical at this point. However, pain usually remains generalized and increases with movement and the abdomen may display board-like rigidity. Dullness over the liver may be lost due to free peritoneal air, tenderness in the right lower quadrant may develop as fluid accumulates in the right paracolic gutter, and rectal exam may reveal tenderness due to the collection of inflammatory fluid in the pelvis and irritation of the pelvic peritoneum. When fluid flows into the right or left paracolic gutters, the point of maximal tenderness may localize in these areas, simulating acute appendicitis and diverticulitis, respectively.

3. In the third phase, as the peritonitis advances, there is frank peritonitis manifest as fever, abdominal distension and cardiovascular collapse. Death ensues unless therapy has been initiated well before this stage.

In the elderly, these phases and signs and symptoms may be minimal. When the clinical presentation of patients over 60 years of age with perforated peptic ulcer is examined, up to 85% have only mild abdominal pain in one series.[56] Other symptoms were dyspepsia, anorexia, nausea, and vomiting. Only 16% complained of severe abdominal pain and the duration of symptoms ranged from 4 hours to 10 days. Although most patients have abdominal tenderness, only 66% had classic signs of peritonitis and about 6% had no abdominal findings.

Plain x-rays of the abdomen with the patient in the upright position may show free air within the abdominal cavity in approximately 70%. Thus, as many as 30% may have a negative plain film of the abdomen, particularly in the elderly. A left lateral decubitus film has been shown to be most sensitive in detecting pneumoperitoneum. Placing the patient in the upright or left lateral decubitus position for 10 minutes before taking the x-ray may improve detection of free air. In equivocal cases, use of a water-soluble contrast agent (eg, gastrograffin) with an UGI tract series or computed tomography may increase the yield of revealing the site of the perforation, but even these studies will be negative if the perforation has already sealed.

DUs that perforate are usually located on the anterior wall. Perforated GUs usually involve the lesser sack. In 10% of patients, bleeding accompanies the perforation and usually occurs in the posterior wall of the duodenum opposite the one that perforated anteriorly.

Management consists of vigorous fluid resuscitation and transfusion if indicated, IV administration of broad-spectrum antibiotics, antisecretory drugs, and NG suction. Surgery is then indicated to irrigate the peritoneum and close the perforation with an omental patch. A small, highly select group of patients such as those who are not surgical candidates because of severe medical problems or deemed unable to tolerate anesthesia or who present late (24 to 36 hrs after perforation) may be managed conservatively and expectantly. Nonoperative treatment should be considered only if the patient is stable, without signs of generalized peritonitis, and the abdominal x-ray or gastrograffin study reveals no free air or leak into the peritoneal cavity respectively. Operative intervention would then be considered at the first sign of clinical deterioration.

Penetration

Penetration occurs when a peptic ulcer burrows through the wall of the stomach or duodenum without free perforation or leakage of luminal contents into the peritoneal cavity. Penetration could be found in as many as 20% of ulcers at the time of operation as reported by older surgical literature.[57]

Penetration is mostly associated with symptoms typical of PUD and thus, only a small proportion of penetrating ulcers become clinically evident.[57] Patients with penetration may report a change in the typical pattern of their ulcer symptoms, which may be gradual or sudden (eg, increase in intensity or duration of pain, radiation of pain to the back, loss of cyclicity of the pain with meals, or eating no longer relieves the discomfort). A long-standing ulcer history is common but not invariable in patients who develop penetration.[57]

Penetration occurs in descending order of frequency into the pancreas, gastrohepatic omentum, biliary tract, liver, greater omentum, mesocolon, colon, and vascular structures. Penetration can eventually lead to fistula formation or formation of perivisceral abscess.[58] Mild hyperamylasemia can develop with posterior penetration of either gastric or DU, but clinical pancreatitis is uncommon. Pyloric or prepyloric ulcers can penetrate the duodenum, eventually leading to a gastroduodenal fistula ("double" pylorus). Penetrating GUs often involve the left lobe of the liver. Penetrating DUs can result in the development of fistulas between the duodenum and the common bile duct (choledochoduodenal fistula). This can present as extrahepatic biliary obstruction, pneumobilia, or hematobilia. Fistula between the stomach and the colon (gastrocolic fistula) may result from penetrating ulcers of greater curvature of stomach, particularly marginal ulcers.[59,60] A duodenocolic fistula can also occur. The gastrocolic and duodenocolic fistulas can present with diarrhea and weight loss; feculent vomiting is infrequent. Fistula between penetrating DU and pancreatic duct has been reported.[61] Erosion into vascular structures leading to massive hemorrhage can result from aortoenteric fistula[62] or erosion into the cystic artery.

It is rare to diagnose uncomplicated penetrating PUD because it requires either imaging procedures like CT scanning or surgery, both of which are not routinely indicated in the diagnosis and management of PUD. The diagnosis of penetrating ulcer is suspected clinically when an ulcer in the proper region is found and the patient reports suggestive symptoms or when new symptoms arise as a result of fistulae formation.

Medical management of penetrating peptic ulcers should be the same as aggressive treatment of refractory PUD (robust acid suppression with proton pimp inhibitors, eradicate *H. pylori* infection, and remove precipitating or exacerbating factors such as NSAID). Surgical treatment is needed for penetrating peptic ulcers that have fistulized.

Obstruction

Peptic ulcerations of the antrum, pylorus, and duodenum can cause gastric outlet obstruction as a result of the swelling and edema that accompanies the active ulceration or as a consequence of the scarring that occurs with ulcer healing. Most cases are associated with duodenal or pyloric channel ulceration.[59]

EPIDEMIOLOGY

Gastric outlet obstruction is the least frequent complication of PUD. Until the 1970s, PUD was the most common cause of gastric outlet obstruction.[63] Obstruction has accounted for 10% to 30% of patients undergoing ulcer surgery in past surgical series, but with more effective medical and endoscopic management, this frequency appears to be decreasing as compared to bleeding and perforation. As peptic ulcer and its complications have become less frequent, malignancy has emerged as a prominent cause of obstruction, despite the lower overall rates of gastric cancer.[64-66]

PATHOPHYSIOLOGY

Acute inflammation associated with ulcer of the antrum, pyloric channel, or duodenum can cause gastric outlet obstruction due to potentially reversible elements like spasm, edema, and inflammation. Pyloric and antral dysmotility can be associated with acute ulceration, further worsening the stomach emptying. Intensive medical therapy may reverse this.

Long-standing or healed ulcers can cause fibrosis, scarring, and deformity, leading to obstruction that is difficult to reverse. Gastric atony may develop after prolonged obstruction, contributing to gastric retention.

CLINICAL PRESENTATION

Symptoms of gastric retention include early satiety, bloating, anorexia, nausea, vomiting, epigastric pain, and weight loss.[59,67] Vomiting may relieve the discomfort temporarily. High-grade outlet obstruction can cause significant dehydration, electrolyte disturbance, and weight loss. Physical examination may reveal a succussion splash (ie, an audible splash of gastric contents produced by shaking the patient's trunk) in about a third of cases. Appetite and food intake may be preserved in association with delayed, large volume vomiting of undigested food. Conversely, some patients may have minimal or intermittent obstruction, but complain of considerable pain, bloating, nausea, and vomiting. Some patients with symptomatic peptic ulcer may have visceral hyposensitization; thus, high-grade outlet obstruction may be present in these patients without significant gastric distress.

DIAGNOSIS

Aspiration of gastric contents through a NG tube often reveals substantial quantities of retained fluid in patients with gastric outlet obstruction. A gastric aspirate volume of more than 300 mL at 4 hours after a meal or more than 200 mL after an overnight fast is indicative of delayed gastric emptying.[68] Obstruction to gastric emptying can be confirmed with a saline load test in which 750 mL of saline is delivered in the stomach through a NG tube and the gastric contents are aspirated 30 minutes later.[69] Aspiration of more than 300 mL of the saline is considered evidence of delayed gastric emptying. Saline load test is now rarely used.

Mechanical obstruction of the gastric outlet can be confirmed by endoscopy or by barium contrast study. Endoscopy is generally preferred because it can make a specific diagnosis of the lesion causing the obstruction and can also provide the opportunity for biopsy and endoscopic treatment in suitable cases. If significant gastric retention is suspected, the gastric contents should be evacuated using a large-bore NG tube (like Ewald tube) prior to the endoscopic procedure, to facilitate the endoscopic examination. A careful inspection at endoscopy is imperative. Gastric biopsies should be taken to determine *H. pylori* status. Multiple jumbo biopsies should be taken from the lesion causing the obstruction. Deep needle aspiration/biopsy should be considered if the lesion appears to be submucosal or if the index of suspicion for malignancy remains high despite negative path from forceps biopsy. CT scan with oral and IV contrast may also be useful in detecting malignancy and in revealing the local anatomy.

Other causes of gastric outlet obstruction include carcinomas of the stomach, pancreas, liver, and bile ducts as well as other extrinsic intra-abdominal masses that may compress the stomach or duodenum. Gastric outlet obstruction must be distinguished from gastroparesis, in which the stomach fails to empty despite the absence of mechanical obstruction. Malignancy must be excluded in all cases of gastric outlet obstruction.[64,65] Patients with gastric outlet obstruction secondary to malignancy are usually older and mostly do not have a history of peptic ulcer or NSAID use.[64] Gastric distension and retained food results in hypergastrinemia, which should correct after the outlet obstruction is relieved. Persistent hypergastrinemia should prompt workup to rule out gastrinoma.[70]

MANAGEMENT

About 70% of cases with gastric outlet obstruction secondary to PUD can be managed medically and endoscopically. Only 30% will need an operation to bypass the outlet obstruction.[71,72] A NG tube should be placed to intermittent suction to decompress the stomach. IV fluids should be given and electrolytes should be corrected. Nutritional status should be assessed and IV hyperalimentation should be considered in malnourished patients. IV H2 blocker or, preferably, IV PPI should be used to decrease gastric secretions and expedite ulcer healing. This regimen will decrease edema, spasm, and inflammation and may yield clinical improvement in patients without significant scarring. Oral medications and liquid diet can be started in 3 to 4 days if significant improvement is noted on repeat saline load test or UGI series. NSAID use must be discontinued in cases with NSAID induced PUD.[73] Continued use is associated with high incidence of recurrence. Case reports and small series have shown that eradication of *H. pylori* infection can heal the ulcers, resolve the outlet obstruction, and even prevent recurrence of obstruction in most, but not all patients.[74-76]

ENDOSCOPIC BALLOON DILATATION

Endoscopic balloon dilatation is useful for patients who do not respond to initial medical therapy. This can be achieved by through the scope (TTS) balloon or by using a balloon placed over a guidewire positioned under fluoroscopic guidance. Proper positioning of the balloon will provide optimal results. Long duodenal strictures are the most difficult to dilate. Symptoms usually improve significantly with successful dilatation to 12 mm. There may be an advantage to postponing dilatation beyond 15 mm until after a period of medical management.[59] Stepwise dilatation for tight obstruction will probably lower the risk of perforation. Nevertheless, because of the risk of perforation, patients should be appropriately prepared for surgery before dilatation, and monitored closely after dilatation before resuming oral intake. An immediate postprocedure gastrograffin study is appropriate to detect perforation in a timely fashion. Dilation is rarely a permanent solution and recurrence is common, requiring multiple dilations or, in some cases, surgery.[67,73,77]

SURGICAL MANAGEMENT

An adequate trial of medical treatment and endoscopic dilation in suitable cases should be given before considering surgery. Surgery is indicated when the pylorus is obstructed and cannot be safely dilated, or when the obstruction persists or recurs despite adequate medical and endoscopic management.

Before endoscopic or surgical intervention, the patient should be stabilized and fluid and electrolyte balance should be restored. Surgery is generally delayed if the patient's nutritional status is compromised. Serum albumin of less than 2.8 g/dL is considered to be a predictor of poor surgical outcome. Dilation can be an effective bridge to surgery in a malnourished patient. Undertaking surgery in a patient with marked gastric dilatation is associated with increased postoperative incidence of gastric atony. This may be prevented by preoperative decompression of the dilated stomach.

Pyloric obstruction of short duration may be treated with vagotomy and pyloroplasty. For advanced cases, antrectomy and truncal vagotomy is commonly performed, but truncal vagotomy and gastrojejunostomy may be preferred in case of extensive surrounding inflammation and scarring. Both open and laparoscopic approaches are used depending on the local anatomy, nature of the procedure planned, and the surgeon's preference.

Gastric dysmotility is a well-known complication of any surgical management for gastric outlet obstruction. Rates ranging from 10% to 50% have been reported and are determined by factors like patient selection, their preoperative status, and surgical technique.[78,79]

Stress Ulcers

Severe physiologic stress is often associated with peptic injury of the UGI tract.[80] A number of terms have been used to describe stress-related peptic injury, including stress erosion, stress gastritis, stress ulcer, stress-related erosive syndrome, and stress-related mucosal disease (SRMD). Acute peptic ulcers associated with severe burns are called Curling's ulcers. Peptic ulcers associated with acute head injuries are called Cushing's ulcers.

The spectrum of stress-related peptic lesions ranges from the typical, asymptomatic gastric erosions to deep ulcerations of the stomach and duodenum that can be complicated by life-threatening hemorrhage and perforation. Typically, they occur as multiple, superficial erosions in the fundus and body of the stomach, but they sometimes develop in the antrum, duodenum, or distal esophagus. These may cause oozing of blood from superficial capillary beds and can be difficult to control because of its diffuse nature.

Stress ulcerations are the most common cause of GI bleeding in ICU patients, and the presence of GI bleeding due to these lesions is associated with a 5-fold increase in mortality compared to ICU patients without bleeding.[81,82] Mortality ranges from 50% to 70% in critically ill patients who develop bleeding during hospitalization. In addition to increased mortality, clinically important stress-related mucosal bleeding can also lead to prolonged hospital stay, thereby having an impact on hospital costs.[83] In general, the mean length of hospital stay is reportedly increased in ICU patients who bleed compared with patients who do not have this complication (30 days vs. 11 days, respectively).[84] More specifically, the excess length of ICU stay attributed to stress ulcer bleeding is estimated at 4 to 8 days.[83]

Endoscopic studies have shown the presence of acute mucosal lesions of UGI tract in at least 75% of the patients within 72 hours of major trauma or serious illness.[85] Although up to 50% of these early mucosal lesions may have endoscopic evidence of recent or ongoing bleeding, only a small percentage of these patients experience hemodynamic compromise due to acute blood loss.[86] The frequency of hemodynamically significant bleeding from stress-related mucosal lesions has declined substantially since the 1970s as a result of advances in the medical management of critically ill patients. In a prospective study of more than 2000 patients admitted to ICUs, only 1.5% developed clinically significant bleeding.[87]

The stress-related mucosal damage in the GI tract is thought to result from derangements in the balance between gastric acid production and mucosal protective mechanisms. Multiple factors may be responsible.

ISCHEMIA

Shock, sepsis, and trauma can lead to impaired perfusion of the gut, which can in turn lead to gastric mucosal ischemia and diminished secretion of protective mucus and bicarbonate.[82,88]

HYPERSECRETION OF ACID

Cushing's ulcers (associated with head trauma) are associated with hypergastrinemia and hypersecretion of gastric acid, which is not the case in other stress-related peptic injuries.[89-92] Acid secretion tends to be normal or subnormal in most other patients, in whom stress ulcerations result from a breakdown of mechanisms normally protecting the gastric mucosa.

DEFECTS IN PROTECTIVE GASTRIC MUCOUS LAYER

The stomach mucosa is normally protected by a glycoprotein mucous layer, which forms a physical barrier to the gastric acid and also neutralizes the gastric acid in the area adjacent to the stomach wall. In critically ill patients, increased concentrations of refluxed bile salts or the presence of uremic toxins can denude the glycoprotein mucous barrier, thereby allowing gastric mucosal injury.[83,84]

H. PYLORI

The influence of *H. pylori* infection on the development of stress ulcers in critically ill patients has not been well studied but does not appear to be an important factor.[93] While *H. pylori* seropositivity may be present in more than 50% of ICU patients, there is little evidence to date that it plays a substantial role in the pathogenesis of stress-induced bleeding or that it is an independent risk factor for clinically important bleeding.[94]

RISK FACTORS

The two major risk factors associated with clinically significant bleeding due to stress ulcers are mechanical ventilation for more than 48 hours and coagulopathy.[81] Additional risk factors for stress ulcerations are[86,95-98] shock, sepsis, hepatic failure, acute renal failure, multiorgan failure, multiple trauma, burns over 35% of total body surface area, organ transplant, head or spinal trauma, prior history UGI bleeding, or PUD.[99,100]

PROPHYLACTIC MEASURES

Acid suppression has become the mainstay of stress ulcer prophylaxis. Various degrees of acid suppression produce different outcomes. For example, pepsin begins to be inactivated at a pH of 4.5, but raising the pH to 5.0 completely inactivates this enzyme and neutralizes 99.9% of gastric acid. Although a higher pH may be desirable, an intragastric pH of 4 or greater is considered appropriate to prevent mucosal bleeding.[101] A meta-analysis of 42 trials investigating the efficacy of antacids and H2Rs for stress ulcer prophylaxis found that most trials maintained the intragastric pH at 3.5 or higher and that the degree of acid suppression was associated with a decreased risk of clinically important bleeding.[25] An argument can be made that a pH of 6.5 or greater is more effective because it keeps pepsin inactivated and maintains normal blood coagulation.[82] However, evidence from a randomized controlled trial suggests that achieving a pH of 3.5 seems sufficient.[61]

The majority of studies evaluating PPIs in critically ill adult patients reported significant increases in pH following drug administration, although the effects were dependent on dose, time, and probably route. Assuming that acid suppression is the predominant mechanism for the reduced bleeding associated with antisecretory therapies, the PPIs would be expected to be at least as effective as H2 receptor antagonists with repetitive administration. Regardless of the antisecretory agent used for stress ulcer prophylaxis, maintenance of a gastric pH equal to or greater than 4 does not guarantee the prevention of clinically important bleeding.

ANTACIDS

Antacids decrease gastric acidity by direct neutralization of stomach acid. Studies assessing their efficacy as compared to H2 blockers have shown conflicting results.[81,86] Although their cost is low, antacids need to be administered orally or via NG tube at frequent intervals, which makes their use less practical. Side effects can include hypermagnesemia, hypophosphatemia, diarrhea, constipation, NG tube obstruction, and (possibly) increased risk of nosocomial pneumonia secondary to overflow aspiration.

H2 BLOCKERS

H2 blockers raise gastric pH by blocking the stimulatory effects of histamine on parietal cell acid secretion. Their effectiveness in preventing stress ulceration has been documented in most but not all trials.[86,102] H2 blockers are effective when given orally, via NG tube, or via IV route.[103] Administration by continuous infusion provides better control of gastric pH than bolus infusion, but this has not been shown to translate into increased efficacy in preventing clinically significant bleeding.[104,105] Following initiation of H2 blocker therapy, pH is rapidly elevated, but within 24 to 48 hours of treatment, tolerance develops, pH falls, and higher doses of H2Rs are required to maintain a sustained response.[106] H2 blockers are generally well tolerated, but rarely can be responsible for interstitial nephritis, confusion, or thrombocytopenia. Development of thrombocytopenia in critically ill patients is likely multifactorial; the likelihood that H2 receptor antagonists cause thrombocytopenia is relatively small.

Cimetidine (but not other H2 blockers) may affect pharmacokinetics of theophylline and warfarin. The costs of H2 blockers can be substantial.

PROTON PUMP INHIBITORS

Omeprazole oral suspension is more effective than IV H2 blocker in preventing stress-related GI bleeding. Oral PPIs are more effective at maintaining gastric pH above 4.0 as compared to IV H2 blockers. In addition, oral PPI therapy is more cost-effective in limiting the morbidity and mortality of stress ulcers. Therefore, oral PPIs, rather than IV H2 blockers, should be used as first line prophylaxis against stress-related mucosal damage. For patients who cannot tolerate oral or NG feeds, IV H2 blockers should be the first choice for prophylaxis against stress-related GI bleeding. While IV PPIs may be slightly more efficacious than IV H2 blockers, IV PPIs are far more expensive, with little available cost-effectiveness data to justify more widespread use.[107-112]

PPIs inhibit acid secretion by irreversibly binding to the hydrogen-potassium ATP-ase pump that resides on the luminal surface of the parietal cell. Thus, PPIs block the final common pathway to acid secretion by the 3 chemical stimuli: acetylcholine, histamine, and gastrin. Because of this mechanism of action, PPIs cause significant acid suppression, and tolerance does not develop as opposed to the H2 blockers. Theoretically, therefore, PPIs would provide an advantage over H2 blockers, sucralfate, and antacids in preventing stress ulceration. Recently, several liquid preparations have been developed in order to obviate administration problems in patients not able to take them orally either because of swallowing difficulties, altered mental status, or prolonged mechanical ventilation. Although attempts have been made to deliver these preparations to critically ill patients, there is no firm evidence that they are effective. A major issue that needs to be addressed with these preparations is the bioavailability that may be affected by impaired absorption or GI dysmotility in this clinical setting.

Currently available data concerning the use of PPIs in stress ulcer prophylaxis have been encouraging. However, more studies are needed particularly comparison studies with sucralfate and H2 blockers. Until bioavailability issues with the newer, extemporaneously formulated liquid preparations are settled, it is not unreasonable to use IV H2 blockers as the first choice for prophylaxis against stress-related GI bleeding in patients who cannot tolerate oral or NG feeds. While IV PPIs may be more efficacious than IV H2 blockers as far as overall acid suppression is concerned, they are far more expensive with little available cost-effectiveness data to justify more widespread use. In patients able to take orally, a PPI is a better choice than an H2 blocker because of better acid control and lack of tachyphylaxis.

SUCRALFATE

Sucralfate can be administered orally or via a NG tube. It has little effect on gastric pH and volume but coats the mucosa of the UGI tract, creating a mechanical barrier between the acid and mucosa. Concerns about its potential for causing elevations of plasma aluminum concentration appear theoretical and have not been observed in critically ill patients receiving 6 g/day of sucralfate for 14 days, even in the presence of renal insufficiency.[99] Sucralfate is less expensive than parenteral H2 blockers,[113] but its use can be inconvenient for busy ICU nurses.

PROSTAGLANDIN ANALOGS

Prostaglandin analogs like misoprostol have both antisecretory as well as cytoprotective effects, possibly resulting from capillary bed vasodilation, thereby preventing local ischemia.[114,115] Misoprostol may be as effective as antacids or H2 blockers in preventing stress ulceration, but its use is associated with significant diarrhea, which has limited its usefulness.[85,96]

NUTRITION

Several studies have reported that enteral nutrition may reduce the risk of bleeding due to stress ulcerations.[116,117] The effect of enteral nutrition is not mediated by an increase in gastric pH.[118] Nutrition may prevent exhaustion of gastric epithelial energy stores and thereby prevent necrosis and ulcer formation; this mechanism may explain the protective effect against stress ulceration that has been reported with total parenteral nutrition (TPN).[116]

RISK OF NOSOCOMIAL PNEUMONIA

It has been suggested that by raising the gastric pH, antacids and antisecretory agents (H2-blockers and presumably PPIs) predispose to the growth of gram-negative bacteria in the stomach, which in turn accounts for the increased rates of nosocomial pneumonia in patients treated with these agents. Because sucralfate does not affect the gastric pH, lower rates of nosocomial pneumonia are observed in patients treated with it.[119] This hypothesis has not been tested in well-designed vigorous clinical trials.

References

1. Huang JQ, Sridhar S, Hunt RH. Role of *Helicobacter pylori* infection and NSAIDs in peptic ulcer disease: a meta-analysis. *Lancet.* 2005;359(9300):14.
2. Weisman SM, Graham DY. Evaluation of the risks and benefits of low-dose aspirin in the secondary prevention of cardiovascular and cerebrovascular events. *Arch Intern Med.* 2002;162(19):2197-2202.
3. Hayden M, Pignone M, Phillips C, et al. Aspirin for the primary prevention of cardiovascular events: a summary of the evidence for the U.S. Preventive Services Task Force. *Ann Int Med.* 2002;136(2):161-172.
4. Shorrock CJ, Langman MJS, Warlow C. Risks of upper GI bleeding during TIA prophylaxis with aspirin. *Gastroenterology.* 1992;102 (Suppl):A165.
5. Weil J, Colin-Jones D, Langman M, et al. Prophylactic aspirin and risk of peptic ulcer bleeding. *BMJ.* 1995;310:827-830.

6. Serrano P, Lanas A, Arroyo MT, Ferriera IJ. Risk of upper gastrointestinal bleeding in patients taking low-dose aspirin for the prevention of cardiovascular diseases. *Aliment Pharmacol Ther.* 2002;16:1945-1953.

7. Silverstein FE, Faich G, Goldstein J, et al. Gastrointestinal toxicity with celecoxib vs. nonsteroidal anti-inflammatory drugs for osteoarthritis and rheumatoid arthritis: The CLASS Study. A randomized controlled trial. Celecoxib Long-Term Arthritis Safety Study. *JAMA.* 2000;284:1247-1255.

8. Lanie L, Maller ES, Quan H, Simon T. Ulcer formation with low-dose enteric coated aspirin and the effect of COX-2 selective inhibition: a double blind trial. Unpublished observations. 2003

9. Huang CS, Lichtenstein DR, Nonvariceal UGI bleeding. *Gastroenterology Clinics.* 2003;32(4):1053-1078.

10. Das A, Wong RCK. Prediction of outcomes of acute GI hemorrhage: a review of risk scores and predictive models. *Gastrointest Endosc.* 2004;60(1):85-93.

11. Camellini L, Merighi A, Pagnini C, et al. Comparison of three different risk-scoring systems in non-variceal upper gastrointestinal bleeding. *Dig Liver Dis.* 2004;36(4):248-250.

12. Cuellar R, Gavaler J, Alexander J, et al. Gastrointestinal tract hemorrhage. The value of a nasogastric aspirate. *Arch Intern Med.* 1990;150:1381-1384.

13. Silverstein FE, Gilbert DA, Tedesco FJ, Buenger NK, Persing J. The National ASGE Survey on upper gastrointestinal bleeding II. Clinical prognostic factors. *Gastrointest Endosc.* 1981;27:80-93.

14. Silverstein FE, Gilbert DA, Tedesco FJ, Buenger NK, Persing J. The National ASGE Survey on upper gastrointestinal bleeding I. Study design and baseline data. *Gastrointest Endosc.* 1981;27:73-79.

15. Lin HJ, Lo WC, Lee FY, et al. A prospective, randomized comparative trial showing that omeprazole prevents rebleeding in patients with bleeding peptic ulcer after successful endoscopic therapy. *Arch Intern Med.* 1998;158:54.

16. Collins R, Langman M. Treatment with histamine H2 antagonists in acute upper gastrointestinal hemorrhage: implications of randomized trials. *N Engl J Med.* 1985;313:660.

17. Walt RP, Cottrell J, Mann SG, et al. Continuous IV famotidine for hemorrhage from peptic ulcer. *Lancet.* 1992;340:1058.

18. Lavine JE, Leontiades GI, Sharma UK, Howden CW. Meta-analysis: The efficacy of intravenous H2-receptor antagonists in bleeding peptic ulcer. *Aliment Pharmacol Ther.* 2002;16:137.

19. Ersad BL. Proton-pump inhibitors for acute peptic ulcer bleeding. *Aliment Pharmacol Ther.* 2001;35:730-740.

20. Cook DJ, Guyatt GH, Salena BJ, Laine LA. Endoscopic therapy for acute non-variceal upper gastrointestinal hemorrhage: a meta-analysis. *Gastroenterology.* 1992;102:139-142.

21. Lin HJ, Yseng GY, Perng EL, Lee FY, Chang FY, Lee SD. Comparison of adrenaline injection and bipolar electrocoagulation for the arrest of peptic ulcer bleeding. *Gut.* 1999;44:715-719.

22. Chung SC, Leung JW, Sung JY, Lo KK, Li AK. Injection or heater probe for bleeding ulcer. *Gastroenterology.* 1991;100:33-37.

23. Calvert X, Vergara M, Brullet E, Javier P, Gisbert JP, Carpo R. Addition of a second endoscopic treatment following epinephrine injection improves outcome in high-risk bleeding ulcers. *Gastroenterology.* 2004;126:441-450.

24. Hui WM, Ng MM, Lok AS, Lai CL, Lau YN, Lam SK. A randomized comparative study of laser photocoagulation, heater probe, and bipolar electrocoagulation in the treatment of actively bleeding ulcers. *Gastrointest Endosc.* 1991;37:299-304.

25. Jensen DM. Heat probes for homeostasis of bleeding peptic ulcers: technique and results of randomized controlled trials. *Gastrointest Endosc.* 1990;36:S42-S49.

26. Gralnick IM, Jensen DM, Gornbein J, et al. Clinical and economic outcomes of individuals with severe peptic ulcer hemorrhage and non-bleeding visible vessels: an analysis of two prospective clinical trials. *Am J Gastroenterol.* 1998;93:2047-2056.

27. Gevers AM, DeGoede E, Simoens M, Hiele M, Rutgeerts P. A randomized trial comparing injection therapy with hemoclip and with injection combined with hemoclip for bleeding ulcers. *Gastrointest Endosc.* 2002;55:466-469.

28. Cipolletta L, Bianco MA, Marmo R, et al. Endoclips versus heater probe in preventing early rebleeding from peptic ulcer. A prospective and randomized trial. *Gastrointest Endosc.* 2001;53:147-151.

29. Lin HJ, Hsieh YH, Tseng GY, Perng CL, Chang FY, Lee SD. A prospective randomized trial of endoscopic hemoclip versus heater probe thermocoagulation for peptic ulcer bleeding. *Am J Gastroenterol.* 2002;97:2250-2254.

30. British Society of Gastrointest Endosc Committee. Non-variceal upper gastrointestinal hemorrhage: guidelines. *Gut.* 2002;51(suppl 4):iv 1-iv 6.

31. Feu F, Brullet E, Calvert X, et al. Guidelines for the diagnosis and treatment of acute non-variceal upper gastrointestinal bleeding. *Gastroenterol Hepatol.* 2003;26:70-85.

32. Lin HJ, Perng CL, Lee SD. Is sclerosant injection mandatory after an epinephrine injection for arrest of peptic ulcer hemorrhage? A prospective randomized, comparative study. *Gut.* 1993;34:1182-1185.

33. Chung SS, Lau JY, Sung JJ, et al. Randomized comparison between adrenaline injection alone and adrenaline injection plus heat probe treatment for actively bleeding ulcers. *BMJ.* 1997;314:1307-1311.

34. Lau JY, Sung JJ, Lee KK, et al. Effect of intravenous omeprazole on recurrent bleeding after endoscopic treatment of bleeding peptic ulcers. *N Engl J Me*d. 2000;343:310-316.

35. Sung JJ, Chan FK, Lau JY, et al. The effect of endoscopic therapy in patients receiving omeprazole for bleeding ulcers with nonbleeding visible vessels or adherent clots: a randomized comparison. *Ann Intern Med.* 2003;139:237-243.

36. Lin HJ, Lo WC, Lee FY, Perng CL, Tseng GY. A prospective randomized comparative trial showing that omeprazole prevents rebleeding in patients with bleeding peptic ulcer after successful endoscopic therapy. *Arch Intern Med.* 1998;158:54-58.

37. Leontiadis GI, McIntyre L, Sharma BK, et al. Proton pump inhibitor treatment for acute peptic ulcer bleeding. *Cochrane Database Syst Rev.* 2004;(3):CD002094.

38. Collins R, Langman M. Treatment with histamine H2 antagonists in acute upper gastrointestinal hemorrhage. Implications of randomized trials. *N Engl J Med.* 1985;313(11):660-666.

39. Levine JE, Leontiades GI, Sharma VK, Howden C. Meta-analysis. The efficacy of H2-receptor antagonists in bleeding peptic ulcer. *Aliment Pharmacol Ther.* 2002;16:1137-1142.

40. Andruilli A, Annesa V, Carusso N, et al. Proton-pump inhibitors and outcomes of endoscopic hemostasis in bleeding peptic ulcers: a series of meta-analysis. *Am J Gastroenterol.* 2005;100:207-219.

41. Gisbert JP, Gonzalez L, Calvert X, Rogue M, Gabriel R, Pajares JM. Proton pump inhibitors vs. H2-antagonists: a meta-analysis of their efficacy in treating bleeding peptic ulcer. *Aliment Pharmacol Ther.* 2001;15:912-926.

42. Barkum AN, Racz I, VanRensburg C, et al. Prevention of peptic ulcer bleeding using continuous infusion of pantoprazole vs. ranitidine: a multi-center, multinational, randomized double-blind parallel-group comparison. *Gastroenterology.* 2004;126(suppl 2):A-78.

43. Leontiadis GI, McIntire L, Sharma BK, et al The influence of PPI dose on treatment efficacy for ulcer bleeding following endoscopic hemostatic therapy (EHT): a sub-group analysis from the Cochrane Collaboration (CC) Systematic review. *Gastroenterology.* 2004;126(suppl 2):A-602.

44. Barkum AN, Mardou M, Marshall JK for the Nonvariceal Upper GI Bleeding Consensus Conference Group. Consensus recommendations for managing patients with non-variceal upper gastrointestinal bleeding. *Ann Intern Med.* 2003;139:843-857.

45. Bardou M, Toubouti Y, Martel M, Rahme E, et al. High dose oral proton pump inhibition decrease re-bleeding in high-risk patients with acute peptic ulcer bleeding: A meta-analysis. *Gastroenterology.* 2004;126(suppl 2):A-602.

46. Consensus Conference. Therapeutic endoscopy and bleeding ulcers. *JAMA.* 1989;262:1369-1372.

47. Laine L, Peterson WL. Bleeding peptic ulcer. *N Engl J M*ed. 1994;331:717.

48. Laine L, Stein C, Sharma V. A prospective outcome of patients with clot in an ulcer and the effect of irrigation. *Gastrointest Endosc.* 1996;43:107-110.

49. Jensen DM, Kovacs TOG, Jutabha R, et al. Randomized trial of medical or endoscopic therapy to prevent recurrent ulcer hemorrhage in patients with adherent clots. *Gastroenterology.* 2002;123:407-413.

50. Bleau BL, Gostout CJ, Shaw MJ, et al. Final results: rebleeding from peptic ulcers associated with adherent clots: a prospective randomized controlled study comparing endoscopic therapy with medical therapy (abst). *Gastrointest Endosc.* 1997;45:AB87.

51. Laine L, Freeman M, Cohen H. Lack of uniformity in diagnosis of endoscopic features of bleeding ulcers. *Gastrointest Endosc.* 1994;40:411-417.

52. Chowdhary SK, Bhasin DK, Panigrahi D, et al. *Helicobacter pylori* infection in patients with perforated duodenal ulcer. *Trop Gastroenterol.* 1998;19(1):19.

53. Reinbach DH, Cruickshank G, McColl KE. Acute perforated duodenal ulcer is not associated with *Helicobacter pylori* infection. *Gut.* 1993;34(10):1344.

54. Kate V, Ananthakrishnan N, Badrinath S. Effect of *Helicobacter pylori* eradication on the ulcer recurrence rate after simple closure of perforated duodenal ulcer: retrospective and prospective controlled studies. *Br J Sur*g. 2001;88(8):1054-1058.

55. Ng EK, Lam YH, Sung JJ, et al. Eradication of *Helicobacter pylori* prevents recurrence of ulcer after simple closure of duodenal ulcer perforation: randomized controlled trial. *Ann Surg.* 2000;231(2):153-158.

56. Kane E. Perforated peptic ulcer in the elderly. *J Am Geriatr Soc.* 1981;29(5):224.

57. Norris JR, Haubrich WS. The incidence and clinical features of penetration in peptic ulceration. *JAMA.* 1961;178:386.

58. Ranschaert E, Rigauts H. Confined gastric perforation: ultrasound and computed tomographic diagnosis. *Abdom Imaging.* 1993;18:318.

59. Graham DY. Ulcer complications and their nonoperative treatment. In: Sleisenger M, Fordtran J. eds. *Gastrointestinal Disease.* 5th ed. Philadelphia: WB Saunders; 1993:698.

60. Soybel DI, Kestenberg A, Brunt EM, Becker JM. Gastrocolic fistula as a complication of benign GU: report of four cases and update of the literature. *Br J Surg.* 1989;76:1298.

61. Martin LF, Booth FV, Karlstadt RG, et al. Continuous intravenous cimetidine decreased stress-related upper gastrointestinal hemorrhage without promoting pneumonia. *Crit Care Med.* 1993;21:19-30.

62. Odze RD, Begin LR. Peptic-ulcer-induced aortoenteric fistula. Report of a case and review of the literature. *J Clin Gastroenterol.* 1991;13:682.

63. Ellis H. The diagnosis of benign and malignant pyloric obstruction. *Clin Oncol.* 1976;2:11-15.

64. Shone DN, Nikoomanesh P, Smith-Meek MM, et al. Malignancy is the most common cause of gastric outlet obstruction in the era of H2 blockers. *Am J Gastroenterol.* 1995;90:1769.

65. Johnson CD, Ellis H. Gastric outlet obstruction now predicts malignancy. *Br J Surg.* 1990;77:1023.

66. Quigley RL, Pruitt SK, Pappas TN, Akwari O. Primary hypertrophic pyloric stenosis in the adult. *Arch Surg.* 1990;125:1219-1221.

67. DiSario JA, Fennerty MB, Tietze CC, et al. Endoscopic balloon dilation for ulcer-induced gastric outlet obstruction. *Am J Gastroenterol.* 1994;89:868.

68. Walker CO. Complications of peptic ulcer disease and indications for surgery. In: Sleisenger MH, Fordtran JS, eds. *Gastrointestinal Disease. Pathophysiology, Diagnosis, Management.* 2nd ed. Philadelphia: WB Saunders; 1978:914-932.

69. Goldstein H, Boyle JD. The saline load test—a bedside evaluation of gastric retention. *Gastroenterology.* 1965;49:375-380.

70. Hangen D, Maltz GS, Anderson JE, et al. Marked hypergastrinemia in gastric outlet obstruction. *J Clin Gastroenterol.* 1989;11:442.

71. Zittel TT, Jehle EC, Becker HD. Surgical management of peptic ulcer disease today—indication, technique, and outcome. *Langenbecks Arch Surg.* 2000;385:84-96.

72. Khullar SK, DiSario JA. Gastric outlet obstruction. *Gastrointest Endosc Clin North Am.* 1996;6:585-603.

73. Boylan JJ, Gradzka MI. Long-term results of endoscopic balloon dilatation for gastric outlet obstruction. *Dig Dis Sci.* 1999;44:1883.

74. Taskin V, Gurer I, Ozyilkan E, et al. Effect of *Helicobacter pylori* eradication on peptic ulcer disease complicated with outlet obstruction. *Helicobacter.* 2000;5:38.

75. Annibale B, Marignani M, Luzzi I, et al. Peptic ulcer and duodenal stenosis: role of *Helicobacter pylori* infection. *Ital J Gastroenterol.* 1995;27:26.

76. de Boer WA, Driessen WM. Resolution of gastric outlet obstruction after eradication of *Helicobacter pylori. J Clin Gastroenterol.* 1995;21:329.

77. Solt J, Bajor J, Szabo M, Horvath OP. Long-term results of balloon catheter dilation for benign gastric outlet stenosis. *Endoscopy.* 2003;35:490.

78. McCallum RW, Polepalle SC, Schirmer B. Completion gastrectomy for refractory gastroparesis following surgery for peptic ulcer disease. Long-term follow-up with subjective and objective parameters. *Dig Dis Sci.* 1991;36:1556.

79. Hom S, Sarr MG, Kelly KA, et al. Postoperative gastric atony after vagotomy for obstructing peptic ulcer. *Am J Surg.* 1989;157:282.

80. Haglund U. Stress ulcers. *Scand J Gastroenterol.* 1990;25(Suppl 175):27-33.

81. Cook DJ, Fuller HD, Guyatt GH, et al. Risk factors for gastrointestinal bleeding in critically ill patients. Canadian Critical Care Trials Group. *N Engl J Med.* 1994;330:377-381.

82. Navab F, Steingrub J. Stress ulcer: is routine prophylaxis necessary? *Am J Gastroenterol.* 1995;90:708.

83. Ritchie W. Role of bile acid reflux in acute hemorrhagic gastritis. *World J Surg.* 1981;5:189.

84. Schindlbeck NE, Lippert M, Heinrich C, Muller-Lissner SA. Intragastric bile acid concentrations in critically ill, artificially ventilated patients. *Am J Gastroenterol.* 1989;84:624.

85. DePriest JL. Stress ulcer prophylaxis: do critically ill patients need it? *Postgrad Med.* 1995;98:159.

86. Shuman RB, Schuster DP, Zuckerman GR. Prophylactic therapy for stress ulcer bleeding: a reappraisal. *Ann Intern Med.* 1987;106:562.

87. Beejay U, Wolfe MM. Acute gastrointestinal bleeding in the intensive care unit. *Gastroenterol Clin North Am.* 2000;29:309-336.

88. Geus WP, Lamers CBHW. Prevention of stress ulcer bleeding: a review. *Scand J Gastroenterol.* 1990;25 (Suppl 178):32.

89. Norton L, Greer J, Eiseman B. Gastric secretory response to head injury. *Arch Surg.* 1970;101:200-204.

90. Bowen JC, Fleming WH, Thompson JC. Increased gastrin release following penetrating central nervous system injury. *Surgery.* 1974;75:720-724.

91. Stremple JF, Molot MA, McNamara JJ, et al. Posttraumatic gastric bleeding. *Arch Surg.* 1972;105:177.

92. Watts CC, Clark K. Gastric acidity in the comatose patient. *J Neurosurg.* 1969;30:107.

93. Robertson MS, Cade JF, Clancy RL. *Helicobacter pylori* infection in intensive care: increased prevalence and a new nosocomial infection. *Crit Care Med.* 1999;27:1276.

94. Allen ME, Kopp BJ, Erstad BL. Stress ulcer prophylaxis in the postoperative period. *Am J Health-Syst Pharm.* 2004;61(6):588-596.

95. Cook DJ. Stress ulcer prophylaxis: gastrointestinal bleeding and nosocomial pneumonia. Best evidence synthesis. *Scand J Gastroenterol Suppl.* 1995;210:48.

96. Martin LF, Booth FVM, Reines D, et al. Stress ulcers and organ failure in intubated patients in surgical intensive care units. *Ann Surg.* 1992;215:332.

97. Hatton J, Lu WY, Rhoney DH, et al. A step-wise protocol for stress ulcer prophylaxis in the neurosurgical intensive care unit. *Surg Neurol.* 1996;46:493.

98. McBride DQ, Rodts GE. Intensive care of patients with spinal trauma. *Neurosurg Clin N Am.* 1994;5:755.

99. Tryba M, Cook D. Current guidelines on stress ulcer prophylaxis. *Drugs.* 1997;54:581-596.

100. Soderstrom CA, Ducker TB. Increased susceptibility of patients with cervical cord lesions to peptic gastrointestinal complications. *J Trauma.* 1985;25:1030-1038.

101. VoderBruegge WF, Peura DA. Stress-related mucosal damage: review of drug therapy. *J Clin Gastroenterol.* 1990;12(Suppl 2):S35-S40.

102. Messori A, Trippoli S, Vaiani M, et al. Bleeding and pneumonia in intensive care patients given ranitidine and sucralfate for prevention of stress ulcer: meta-analysis of randomised controlled trials. *BMJ.* 2000;321:1103.

103. Pemberton LB, Schaefer N, Goehring L, et al. Oral ranitidine as prophylaxis for gastric stress ulcers in intensive care unit patients: Serum concentrations and cost comparisons. *Crit Care Med.* 1992;21:339.

104. Baghaie AA, Mojtahedzadeh M, Levine RL, et al. Comparison of the effect of intermittent administration and continuous infusion of famotidine on gastric pH in critically ill patients: Results of a prospective randomized, crossover study. *Crit Care Med.* 1995;23:687.

105. Ballesteros MA, Hogan DL, Koss MA, Isenberg JI. Bolus or intravenous infusion of ranitidine: Effects on gastric pH and acid secretion. *Ann Intern Med.* 1990;112:334.

106. Merki HS, Wilder-Smith CH. Do continuous infusions of omeprazole and ranitidine retain their effect with prolonged dosing? *Gastroenterology.* 1994;106:60-64.

107. Maton PN. Omeprazole. *N Engl J Med.* 1991;324:965-975.

108. Levy MJ, Seelig CB, Robinson, NJ, et al. Comparison of omeprazole and ranitidine for stress ulcer prophylaxis. *Dig Dis Sci.* 1997;42:1255.

109. Azevedo JR, Soares MG, Silva G, Palacio G. Prevention of stress ulcer bleeding in high-risk patients: comparison of three drugs. *Crit Care Med.* 1999;27:41.

110. Phillips JO, Metzler MH, Palmieri MT, et al. A prospective study of simplified omeprazole suspension for the prophylaxis of stress-related mucosal damage. *Crit Care Med.* 1996;24:1793.

111. Lasky MR, Metzler MH, Phillips JO. A prospective study of omeprazole suspension to prevent clinically significant gastrointestinal bleeding from stress ulcers in mechanically ventilated trauma patients. *J Trauma.* 1998;44:527.

112. Schupp KN, Schrand LM, Mutnick AH. A cost-effectiveness analysis of stress ulcer prophylaxis. *Ann Pharmacother.* 2003;37:631.

113. Cook DJ, Witt LA, Cook RJ, Guyatt GH. Stress ulcer prophylaxis in the critically ill: a meta-analysis. *Am J Med.* 1991;91:519.

114. Wilson DE. Antisecretory and mucosal protective actions of misoprostol. *Am J Med.* 1987;83:2.

115. Dajani EZ. Overview of the mucosal protective effects of misoprostol in man. *Prostaglandins.* 1987;33(Suppl):117.

116. Pingleton SK, Hadizma S. Enteral alimentation and gastrointestinal bleeding in mechanically ventilated patients. *Crit Care Med.* 1983;11:13.

117. Raff T, Germann G, Hartmann B. The value of early enteral nutrition in the prophylaxis of stress ulceration in the severely burned patient. *Burns.* 1997;23:313.

118. Nakagawa K, Okada A, Kawashima Y. Acute gastric mucosal lesions: A new experimental model and effect of parenteral nutrition. *J Parenter Enteral Nutr.* 1985;9:571.

119. du Moulin GC, Paterson DG, Hedley-Whyte J, Lisbon A. Aspiration of gastric bacteria in antacid-treated patients: a frequent cause of postoperative colonisation of the airway. *Lancet.* 1982;1:242-245.

Section II

Motility Disorders Including Selected Functional Bowel Disorders

Oropharyngeal Dysphagia: Causes, Evaluation, and Treatment

Radu Tutuian, MD and Donald O. Castell, MD

Introduction

Dysphagia is a Greek word derived from "phagia" (to eat) and "dys" (with difficulty) and clinically is separated into oropharyngeal and esophageal dysphagia. A careful history is very helpful in differentiating these 2 types of dysphagia, and the separation is very important because the diagnostic work-up and therapeutic interventions differ for these conditions. Most commonly, oropharyngeal dysphagia arises from neurologic or myogenic diseases. Oropharyngeal dysphagia occurs in about one third of stroke patients,[1] in patients with head injuries, Parkinson's disease, and Alzheimer's disease, increasing the risks of malnutrition, aspiration, choking, and death. In the neurologic patient population, oropharyngeal dysphagia carries a high morbidity, mortality, and cost.

Frequently, a multidisciplinary team in which gastroenterologists work closely with radiologists, neurologists, speech-language pathologists, otolaryngologists, and sometimes geriatricians and palliative care physicians is required to care for patients with oropharyngeal dysphagia (Figure 8-1).

Normal oropharyngeal swallowing is the result of a complex coordination of muscular activity controlled by the medullary swallow center via the cranial nerves. The medullary swallowing center has important interactions with the respiratory centers, which translates into apnea during oropharyngeal deglutition. Boluses are transferred from the oral cavity into the esophagus by a rapid sequence of propulsions carefully timed with the opening and closing of sphincters and valves. The contraction of the tongue against the palate propels the bolus into the pharynx. Once the bolus passes the tonsillary arches, the pharyngeal phase of deglutition is initiated and this part includes the velopharyngeal closure, hypolaryngeal elevation with laryngeal closure and relaxation and opening of the upper esophageal sphincter (UES).[2,3] Tongue propulsion combined with pharyngeal contractions propels the bolus through the UES into the esophagus and pharyngeal contraction clears pharyngeal residuals. Once the bolus is in the esophagus, the tongue and pharyngeal musculature relax,

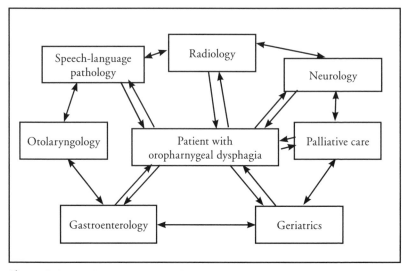

Figure 8-1. Multidisciplinary approach to patients with oropharyngeal dysphagia.

leading to velopharyngeal opening, descent of the hypopharyngeal structures with laryngeal opening, and closure of the UES. The UES together with the glossopalatal and velopharyngeal closing mechanisms prevents retrograde flow from the esophagus, penetration of the larynx, and nasopharyngeal regurgitation during and between swallows.

Causes of Oropharyngeal Dysphagia

The physiologic process of nutrients passing from the mouth into the esophagus requires coordinated contraction of the oropharyngeal musculature and a patent tract. Causes of oropharyngeal dysphagia can be grouped into structural, neurologic (both central and peripheral), and myogenic disorders (Table 8-1).

STRUCTURAL CAUSES OF OROPHARYNGEAL DYSPHAGIA

Oropharyngeal Tumors, Head and Neck Surgery, and Radiotherapy

Benign or malignant tumors of the tongue, soft and hard palate, pharynx, tonsils, and glottis can present initially with dysphagia. Occasionally extrinsic tumors (ie, thyroid tumors) can cause compression if they reach a substantial size. Pain or painful swallowing (ie, odynophagia) may accompany dysphagia in these patients. These diagnoses are typically established by endoscopy with biopsy while imaging studies (x-ray, CT scan, MRI scans) are helpful in evaluating the local and regional extension.

While tumors can cause dysphagia, the treatment of head and neck malignancies can also lead to difficulty swallowing depending on the extent of surgical resection, postsurgical reconstruction, and whether or not collateral damage to neural innerva-

Table 8-1

CAUSES OF OROPHARYNGEAL DYSPHAGIA

Structural Disorders	Neurologic Disorders	Myogenic Disorders
Oropharyngeal tumors	**CNS**	Myasthenia gravis
Head and neck surgery	Cerebrovascular accidents	Botulism
Radiotherapy	CNS tumors	Dermatomyositis
Cervical osteophytes	Multiple sclerosis	Mixed connective tissue disease
Cricopharyngeal stenosis	Cerebral palsy	
Cricopharyngeal bar	Amyotrophic lateral	Sarcoidosis
Pharyngeal diverticulum	sclerosis (ALS)	Thyrotoxic myopathy
(Zenker's diverticulum)	Extrapyramidal syndromes (Parkinson's, Huntington's, Wilson's)	Paraneoplastic syndromes
	Head trauma	Myotonic dystrophy
	Alzheimer's disease	Oculopharyngeal muscular dystrophy
	Drugs (phenothiazines, benzodiazepines)	Drugs (amiodarone, alcohol, statins)
	Peripheral nervous system	
	Spinal muscular dystrophy	
	Guillain-Barré syndrome	
	Poliomyelitis, postpolio	
	Diphtheria	
	Drugs (botulinum toxin, procainamide)	

tions occurs.[4] The extent of tongue base and oral tongue resection is very important in determining the severity of dysphagia because the tongue plays an important role in the generation of oropharyngeal propulsive forces.[5,6] Resection of the larynx (ie, laryngectomy) can cause dysphagia by a combination of anatomic derangements and pharyngeal muscle dysfunction.[7] During postlaryngectomy reconstruction, altering the muscle insertions can lead to impaired UES opening and outflow obstruction; decreased pharyngeal pump function; and development of cervical pseudodiverticuli, which may delay pharyngeal clearance.[8]

Radiotherapy alone or in conjunction with ENT surgery is a recognized cause of oropharyngeal dysphagia. Radiation can damage both muscular and neural structures in the head and neck region, leading to pharyngeal dysmotility, muscular weakness, and incoordination of the pharyngeal-UES function. Radiotherapy can also affect the salivary glands, which can lead to xerostomia, an important contributor to swallow dysfunction. Radiotherapy-induced injuries can occur any time after treatment, and it is not uncommon for these problems to manifest clinically 10 or more years after the administration of radiation therapy.

Postcricoid Web, Stenosis, and Cricopharyngeal Bar

A postcricoid web consists of a thin layer of mucosal and submucosal tissue and appears radiographically or endoscopically as a thin, usually anteriorly located constriction in the proximal esophagus within centimeters of the UES. When clinically manifested, it presents as dysphagia for solids but due to its proximal location can occasionally lead to deglutitive aspiration. A large series of videofluoroscopic examinations reported cricopharyngeal webs in 7.5% of patients evaluated for dysphagia.[9] Postcricoid webs have been associated with iron-deficiency anemia (Plummer-Vinson syndrome), although in recent years the incidence of this syndrome has declined and webs can be found independent of iron deficiency.

A cricopharyngeal bar is a common incidental radiologic finding of unclear clinical significance. Cricopharyngeal bars have been reported in 5% to 20% of patients undergoing videofluoroscopy as a posterior indentation,[10,11] but dysphagia is not more common in patients with cricopharyngeal bars compared to those without bars.[12] Furthermore, in a series of 124 patients, a second esophageal lesion was found in 23 out of 24 patients with cricopharyngeal bars and was considered to be due to the esophageal lesion in at least one third of these patients dysphagia.[13] Careful manometric examination of patients with cricopharyngeal bars usually finds normal UES resting pressure and complete deglutitive UES relaxation.[14] While some authors report inflammatory myopathic changes confined to the cricopharyngeal muscle observed on histopathologic examinations of muscle specimens from patients with cricopharyngeal bars,[15] other studies report an increased prevalence of cricopharyngeal bars in patients with polymyositis or dermatomyositis.[16,17] These observations suggest that focal or generalized myopathic changes may play a role in the genesis of cricopharyngeal bars and stenoses.

Cricopharyngeal bars should be considered of functional significance causing dysphagia if (1) the constriction is circumferential (ie, cricopharyngeal stenosis, seen on 2 perpendicular radiologic views) and additional pharyngeal or esophageal abnormalities have been excluded by radiographic, manometric, and endoscopic examinations; (2) the cricopharyngeal bar is associated with hypopharyngeal diverticula; and/or (3) coexisting pharyngeal neuromuscular dysfunction is identified.

Pharyngeal Diverticula

Pharyngeal diverticula are broadly classified according to their anatomic location into lateral and posterior. Lateral pharyngeal diverticula occur in the area of relative weakness through the thyrohyoid membrane inferior to the hyoid bone, an area with incomplete overlap between the thyrohyoid and inferior constrictor muscle. Lateral pharyngeal diverticula can be congenital or acquired and are common incidental findings on barium swallows. In contrast to the posterior diverticula (Zenker's diverticulum), lateral pharyngeal diverticula are not typically associated with altered UES dynamics, and there are only sporadic case reports of clinical improvement of dysphagia after surgical resection or removal of the diverticula.[18]

Posterior hypopharyngeal diverticula (Figure 8-2) are also know as Zenker's diverticula, bearing the name of the first physician hypothesizing that the herniation of the hypopharyngeal pouch was due to increased hypopharyngeal pressures.[19] Zenker's diverticula occur more frequently in elderly patients, the median age of clinical presentation being in the eighth decade. Over the years, UES incoordination,[20] failed UES relaxations,[21] or UES spasm[22] were postulated to be implicated in the pathogenesis

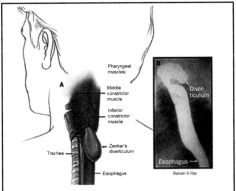

Figure 8-2. Anatomic location and radiographic view of a Zenker's diverticulum.

of the Zenker's diverticulum, but recent manometric studies have reported normal UES resting and residual pressures.[23] More recently, combined videofluoroscopy and manometry studies confirmed normal UES resting, residual UES pressures, and UES-pharyngeal coordination but identified inadequate UES opening as the cause of increased pharyngeal pressure that ultimately leads to the protrusion of pharyngeal structures through the Killian's dehiscence.[24] This is shown on manometric testing by increased hypopharyngeal intrabolus pressure. Causes of inadequate UES opening are thought to be muscle fiber degeneration of the cricopharyngeal muscle and replacement with fibroadipose tissue.

Cervical Osteophytes

Cervical osteophytes are a common incidental finding identified in 6% to 30% of elderly patients,[25] but it appears that less than 1% of patients with cervical osteophytes complain of dysphagia.[26] These anterior protrusions of the bony structures cause dysphagia by mechanical compression of the posterior pharyngeal wall and periesophageal inflammation caused by the movement of the esophagus over the cervical exostosis.[27] Still, given the high prevalence of this finding and the relative low percentage of patients with incidental cervical osteophytes complaining of dysphagia, other causes of dysphagia should be carefully excluded. If the osteophytes are the true cause of dysphagia, surgical excision alleviates dysphagia but the surgical intervention carries an increased risk of iatrogenic muscle and nerve injury.[28]

NEUROGENIC CAUSES OF OROPHARYNGEAL DYSPHAGIA

Cerebrovascular Accidents (Stroke)

Ischemic or hemorrhagic cerebrovascular accidents are an important cause of mortality and morbidity. Oropharyngeal dysphagia occurs in approximately one third of stroke patients.[29] In patients who suffered a brainstem cerebrovascular accident, dysphagia is more common and more severe than in patients with unilateral hemispheric stroke in which dysphagia may resolve after the acute phase of the stroke.[30,31] In brainstem strokes, the lesion involves the lower motor neuron innervating the cervical musculature, while in unilateral hemispheric strokes the upper, cortical motor neuron is affected. The severity of dysphagia in hemispheric strokes depends on the cortical representation of the swallowing musculature (typically located in the motor and premotor cortex) and the plasticity of the undamaged cortex to take control of swallowing function during recovery.

Dysphagia in stroke patients leading to aspiration pneumonia is one of the main causes for death after stroke. One half to two thirds of stroke patients with dysphagia die within 6 months of the stroke due to nutritional and pulmonary complications of dysphagia.[32]

Parkinson's Disease

Parkinson's disease is the result of the loss of dopaminergic central neurons, including those that coordinate the fine motions of the oropharyngeal musculature. Up to half of patients with Parkinson's disease have dysphagia. In patients with Parkinson's disease, the onset of dysphagia is a poor prognostic indicator, with studies suggesting that the median survival of Parkinson's patients from the onset of dysphagia ranges between 15 to 24 months.[33] Still there appears to be no relationship between dysphagia and the severity or duration of Parkinson's disease.[34] Virtually all phases of oropharyngeal deglutition are affected in Parkinson's disease, including impaired lingual movements and mastication, piecemeal swallows, increased oral residue, preswallow spill, swallow hesitancy, postswallow retention of liquids on the pharyngeal wall, piriform and valecular pooling, abnormal pharyngeal wall movements, and impaired UES swallowing.[35-37] Intra- and postswallow aspiration occurs in approximately one third of Parkinson's patients complaining of dysphagia.

Motor Neuron Disease—Amyotrophic Lateral Sclerosis

Given the complex muscular system that facilitates oropharyngeal bolus passage, dysphagia is a common feature of the motor neuron diseases. ALS is the most common variant of the motor neuron diseases and involves the degeneration of motor neurons in the cortex, brainstem, and spinal cord, leading to both upper and lower motor neuron weakness. The onset of ALS is insidious but the sequence of involvement of the bulbar musculature is relatively predictable. The tongue is generally involved first followed by pharyngeal muscle weakness. By the time of dysphagia, lingual dysfunction is present, and typical pharyngeal abnormalities include delayed pharyngeal swallowing response, impaired bolus clearance from the pharynx, and intra- and/or postswallow aspiration.[38]

MYOGENIC CAUSES OF OROPHARYNGEAL DYSPHAGIA

Myasthenia Gravis

Myasthenia gravis is an autoimmune disease in which the antibodies against the postsynaptic acetylcholine receptor (AChR antibodies) are produced. Patients with myasthenia gravis start complaining of ocular, facial, laryngeal, pharyngeal, respiratory, and later on limb muscle weakness. Approximately 20% of patients with myasthenia gravis complain of dysphagia at the time of diagnosis, and over the course of the disease, up to 60% of patients with myasthenia gravis will complain of dysphagia.[39,40] Patients with myasthenia gravis will present with incomplete oral clearance, premature bolus spill, deglutitive velopharyngeal incompetence, and abnormal pharyngeal wall motion with valecular and piriform sinus pooling leading to aspiration.

Inflammatory Myopathies

Inflammatory myopathies include polymyositis, dermatomyositis, and inclusion body myositis. Dysphagia occurs in 30% to 60% of patients with inflammatory myopathies and may sometimes be the only manifestation of the disease.[41] Although the clinical manifestations of inflammatory myopathies typically include subacute, progressive, symmetrical proximal muscle weakness, about 30% to 40% of patients presenting only with dysphagia do not have clinically significant proximal muscular weakness.[15] Almost all patients with dysphagia due to inflammatory myopathies will have pharyngeal dysfunction that will be associated with aspiration in 60% of them.[42] These manifestations are due to both weakness of the pharyngeal muscle as well as a decreased distensibility of the UES during deglutition. Histologic examinations of the pharyngeal and cricopharyngeal muscles in these patients will demonstrate necrosis, focal or diffuse inflammation, and fibrosis.[43,44]

Thyrotoxic Myopathies

Myopathies in patients with hyperthyroidism are thought to be secondary to mitochondrial dysfunction, and muscular weakness can occur in up to 80% of thyrotoxic patients.[45] Pharyngeal muscle weakness may be the only presentation of the thyrotoxicosis and should be remembered in the differential diagnosis of causes of dysphagia, especially in elderly patients in whom dysphagia may be the only clinical manifestation of the disease.

Oculopharyngeal Muscular Dystrophy

Oculopharyngeal muscular dystrophy is a rare autosomal dominant myopathy that affects almost exclusively the pharyngeal and ocular musculature. There is a high prevalence of the disease in the French-speaking part of Canada, although the disease has been described in groups of patients from Europe, Australia, and Japan.[46-48] Patients initially will present in their 40s to 70s with bilateral ocular ptosis followed some years later by dysphagia. Patients with oculopharyngeal muscle dystrophy will have pharyngeal weakness with impaired bolus clearance, incomplete UES opening with variable aspiration, and postnasal regurgitation.

MEDICATIONS CAUSING OROPHARYNGEAL DYSPHAGIA

Several medications can interfere with the oropharyngeal deglutitive process by influencing central or peripheral neurogenic control, impair neuromuscular transmission or muscle function, or alter salivary secretion. A list of medications that can cause oropharyngeal dysphagia is summarized in Table 8-2.

Central-acting dopamine antagonists (phenothiazines and metoclopramide) can cause extrapyramidal movement disorders very similar to the clinical picture of Parkinson's disease.[49] The extrapyramidal side effects can interfere with tongue movement and impair pharyngeal propulsive and clearing mechanisms. While most of these effects typically reverse after cessation of the medication, central-acting dopamine antagonists can also lead to tardive dyskinesia that may be irreversible.[50,51] Central-acting benzodiazepines have been documented to cause oropharyngeal dysphagia.[52,53]

Table 8-2

MEDICATIONS KNOWN TO CAUSE OROPHARYNGEAL DYSPHAGIA

Medications Influencing Central Nervous System Control
- Phenothiazines
- Metoclopramide
- Benzodiazepines (nitrazepam, clonazepam)
- Antihistamines

Medications Impairing Neuromuscular Transmission
- Botulinum toxin
- Procainamide
- Penicillamine
- Erythromycin
- Aminoglycosides

Medications Toxic to the Muscle
- Amiodarone
- Alcohol
- Cholesterol-lowering medications (lovastatin, simvastatin)
- Cyclosporine
- Steroids (prednisone)
- Chloroquine
- Colchicine

Medications With Neuromyopathic Effect
- Digoxin
- Trichloroethylene
- Vincristine

Medications Inhibiting Salivation
- Anticholinergics
- Antidepressants
- Antihistamines
- Antipsychotics
- Antiparkinsonian medications
- Antihypertensives
- Diuretics

Medications Increasing Salivation
- Anticholinesterase
- Psychotropic medication (nitrazepam, clonazepam, clozapine)

These medications probably cause oropharyngeal dysphagia through a combination of impaired pharyngeal clearing and excessive salivation.

Several medications can cause dysphagia by impairing neuromuscular transmission. Examples include botulinum toxin, used to treat spastic cervical muscle disorder (ie, torticollis), which can spread during local injection to adjacent muscles causing impaired pharyngeal propulsion and clearing[54]; penicillamine[55]; large doses of aminoglycosides[56]; and procainamide (occasionally even being able to induce anti-AchR antibodies).[57]

Other mechanisms by which medications can induce oropharyngeal dysphagia are inflammatory or toxic myopathic side effects. Penicillamine and zidovudine can cause muscular inflammation similar to that seen in polymyositis.[58,59] Amiodarone can have toxic myopathic effects as part of the amiodarone-induced thyroid dysfunction,[60] while cholesterol-lowering agents (lovastatin, simvastatin) are know to have direct toxic effects on striated muscles.[61]

Evaluation of Oropharyngeal Dysphagia

HISTORY AND PHYSICAL EXAMINATION

A carefully taken history is an extremely important initial step in evaluating patients complaining of oropharyngeal dysphagia. Location of the discomfort by the patient to the cervical region is not sufficient to classify the dysphagia as oropharyngeal because many patients with esophageal dysphagia may perceive the difficulty of swallowing to occur at the bottom of the neck. More important is the timing of the swallowing difficulty relative to the phases of deglutition. Patients with esophageal dysphagia will have no problem transferring the food from the mouth into the upper esophagus and will typically perceive the discomfort after the oral bolus has moved into the esophagus. In contrast, patients with oropharyngeal dysphagia typically complain of difficulty transferring boluses from the mouth into the esophagus (ie, "initiating" the swallow).

Another important initial distinction in patients with "throat discomforts" is separating globus sensation from oropharyngeal dysphagia. Globus is a common, nonpainful sensation of a lump, fullness, or tightness in the throat without impaired deglutitive function.[62] Oropharyngeal dysphagia occurs during swallowing, primarily during food ingestion as opposed to the globus sensation, which is a constant discomfort occurring between meals and typically alleviated by food ingestion.

Patients with oropharyngeal dysphagia may also present with symptoms indicating oral dysfunction, pharyngeal dysfunction, aspiration, or structural lesions (Table 8-3). Information on the type of onset, duration, and progression of dysphagia is helpful. Patients with malignancies frequently report a relatively short history of progressive dysphagia, associated with weight loss. A sudden onset of dysphagia often associated with other neurologic signs and symptoms (eg, dysarthria, diplopia, limb weakness) usually indicates an acute cerebrovascular insult. Patients with inflammatory myopathies, myasthenia, or ALS more frequently report a more insidious, subacute onset of symptoms. Parkinson's disease should be considered in patients reporting tremor, ataxia, or unsteadiness.

Physical examination of patients complaining of oropharyngeal dysphagia is oriented toward identifying features of underlying disease (ie, systemic disease, neurolog-

Table 8-3

TYPICAL SYMPTOMS ASSOCIATED WITH OROPHARYNGEAL DYSPHAGIA

Symptoms Indicating Oral Dysfunction

- Drooling from the mouth
- Food spillage
- Difficulty to initiate swallow
- Piecemeal swallow
- Dysarthria
- Sialorrhea or xerostomia

Symptoms Indicating Pharyngeal Dysfunction

- Bolus hold-up localized in the neck
- Postnasal regurgitation
- Need for repetitive swallow
- Dysphonia

Symptoms Suggesting Aspiration

- Choking during meals
- Cough during meals
- Pneumonia/aspiration pneumonia

Symptoms Suggestive of Structural Lesions (Malignancy, Strictures, Diverticuli)

- Pain on swallowing
- Persistent sore throat
- Dysphagia only for solids
- Delayed regurgitation of old food

ic diseases) and to detect consequences of oropharyngeal dysphagia such as impaired nutrition or pulmonary complications. While associated neurologic or systemic signs (eg, cranial nerve dysfunction, cerebellar signs, hemiparesis, movement disorders, or muscular signs) are helpful when present, oropharyngeal dysphagia and pharyngeal neuromuscular dysfunction may be the only sign of the neurologic or systemic disease. It is also important to remember that isolated clinical signs may be present in normal individuals. As an example, the gag reflex is absent in 20% to 40% of healthy adults and is neither indicative of the severity of pharyngeal dysfunction or the ability to protect airway.[63]

During the local ENT exam, particular attention should be focused on palpation of the neck region. The presence of masses or of enlarged cervical lymph nodes or thyroid may be important pieces of the diagnostic puzzle. Occasionally, a pharyngeal pouch may be identified during clinical examination because its compression may produce an audible "gurgle" as the result of regurgitating small amounts of residuals from the pouch into the pharynx.

Bilateral ptosis may suggest myasthenia while unilateral ptosis with or without additional features of Horner's syndrome may be indicative of neurologic causes located in the medullary region or malignancies compromising sympathic neural transmission.

Laryngeal ascent can be evaluated clinically by assessing the axial movements of the laryngeal and hyoid cartilages by palpating these structures during a liquid swallow. Aspiration of pharyngeal content in the airways is suggested by coughing or choking during swallowing but the clinical diagnosis of aspiration is challenging. Studies by Splaingard et al[64] and Longemann et al[65] indicate that almost half of videofluoroscopic documented aspiration episodes are missed by clinical assessment alone.

VIDEOFLUOROSCOPY

A series of brief recordings of fluoroscopic exams of the cervical region during barium swallows has become a vital test in evaluating patients with oropharyngeal dysphagia. Structural lesions (eg, diverticula, webs/bars, stenosis, tumors, osteophytes) can be identified on static images; however, dynamic recordings are important in evaluating pharyngeal function, timing, and severity of aspiration. During videofluoroscopic barium swallows (also referred to as modified barium swallow), lateral and anterior-posterior views of the oral and pharyngeal phases of swallows are recorded and reviewed in slow motion to assess the sequence of processes during oropharyngeal deglutition. This technique provides information on the presence/absence or delay of the pharyngeal swallow response, timing of aspiration (if present), velopharyngeal competence (and pharyngonasal regurgitation, if present), and competency of pharyngeal clearance.[66]

While modified barium swallow provides important information on the bolus movement in the oropharyngeal region, it does not permit quantification of pharyngeal contractile forces, intrabolus pressures, and UES relaxations.[67]

ENDOSCOPY

Flexible endoscopy is currently the best method to directly visualize and biopsy mucosal or endoluminal structures, making it indispensable when malignancies are suspected. While both gastroenterologists and ENT specialists can perform these procedures, the gastroenterological exam is usually limited to the laryngopharynx and the UES, providing limited information about glottic and pharyngeal lesions. Nasal endoscopy performed by ENT specialists can be done with topical anesthesia or under general anesthesia when more intense instrumentation is anticipated. Flexible endoscopy cannot surpass videofluoroscopy for assessment of swallow dynamics and potential aspirations.[68]

OROPHARYNGEAL MANOMETRY

Oropharyngeal manometry provides quantitative information on pharyngeal contraction, UES resting and residual pressures, and UES-pharyngeal coordination.[69]

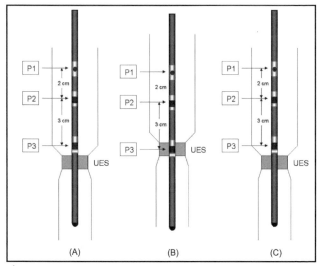

Figure 8-3. Manometry catheter position during oropharyngeal deglutition. The catheter (A) is positioned with the distal (P3) sensor approximately 1 cm above the proximal border of the UES. During deglutition, the UES ascends onto the pressure transducer (B), opens, and following the bolus passage, closes and returns to the initial position (C).

Due to the rapid sequence during oropharyngeal deglutition and radial asymmetry of the pharynx and UES, circumferential solid-state pressure transducers are preferred because of the rapid response time of the transducers and the capability to evaluate radial forces over the entire 360 degrees.[70] Because the UES ascends approximately 1 cm during deglutition, we prefer placing the UES pressure transducer about 1 cm above the sphincter. During deglutition, the sphincter will initially rise on the transducer, then open, let the bolus move through, close, and then descend into the initial position (Figure 8-3). It is our opinion that this approach allows a more accurate determination of UES dynamics. When the distal sensor is placed above the UES, a typical "M" pattern is identified manometrically in the distal channel (Figure 8-4). Initially, the pressure rises as the UES ascends on the transducer followed by the UES relaxation. The pressure will then rise again once the UES closes and return to the pharyngeal baseline when the UES descends back in the initial position. If the distal pressure transducer is placed in the UES, it will "drop" into the esophagus during deglutition, leading to an overestimation of the UES relaxation duration (because it also includes the ascent and descent of the UES) and a misinterpretation of the UES residual pressure because the transducer actually measures the esophageal baseline pressure.

In patients without structural abnormalities identified during barium swallow and/or endoscopy, oropharyngeal manometry can assist evaluating patients with dysphagia. An increased UES residual pressure is frequently found in patients with Parkinson's disease. A high intrabolus pressure suggestive of poor UES compliance is found in

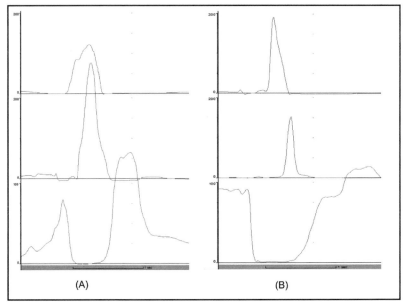

Figure 8-4. Oropharyngeal manometry tracings recorded with the distal transducer above the UES (A) and in the UES (B). When the distal sensor is placed above the UES, a typical "M" pattern is identified in the distal channel. Initially, the pressure rises as the UES ascends on the transducer followed by the UES relaxation. The pressure will then rise again once the UES closes and return to the pharyngeal baseline when the UES descends back in the initial position. If the distal pressure transducer is placed in the UES, it will "drop" in the esophagus during deglutition, leading to an overestimation of the UES relaxation duration (because it also includes the ascent and descent of the UES) and a misinterpretation of the UES residual pressure as the transducer measures the esophageal baseline pressure.

patients with Zenker's diverticulum. Decreased pharyngeal contraction amplitudes can be found in stroke patients or patients with myogenic causes of dysphagia. Patients with otherwise unexplained dysphagia may exhibit hypertensive UES, poorly relaxing UES, or short UES relaxation duration during manometry. While some authors argue that oropharyngeal manometry makes little impact on patients' management,[71] other investigators have shown that treatment of oropharyngeal motility abnormalities leads to improvement in patient symptoms.[72]

Treatment of Oropharyngeal Dysphagia

The management of patients with oropharyngeal dysphagia can be difficult and usually requires a close collaboration between different specialties (see Figure 8-1). Identifying the cause of oropharyngeal dysphagia is very important in delineating treatment strategies. Identifying treatable systemic diseases causing dysphagia (ie, thyrotoxicosis, myasthenia gravis, Parkinson's disease, inflammatory myopathies) should be sought first. Structural lesions causing oropharyngeal dysphagia (ie, tumors, diverticula, webs/bars) may be identified during videofluoroscopy and/or endoscopy and surgical interventions should be considered in these patients. A next step in the management of patients with oropharyngeal dysphagia is evaluating the risk of aspiration and the ability to have an adequate oral caloric intake. This evaluation is important in patients with high risk of aspiration, and gastrostomy feeding tubes should be considered in those not able to meet their caloric needs. In patients in whom structural lesions and treatable systemic diseases have been excluded who are not at risk of aspiration during swallowing, "local" therapies such as dietary modifications, swallow therapy, and/or surgery may be considered.

Surgical interventions are the primary option in patients with ENT tumors. Still, it is important to recognize that surgical procedures by themselves can cause oropharyngeal dysphagia by the anatomic alteration in the cervical region. When curative resection of tumors is not an option, the goals of the surgical interventions are to reduce or eliminate aspiration and restore the abilities for oral intake. Depending on the location and extension of tumors, more conservative intervention (ie, preserving the voice [ie, laryngeal suspension, epiglottoplasty, and vocal fold augmentation or medialization]) may be possible as alternatives to more destructive procedures that deprive the patient of the ability to phonate (ie, glottic closure, tracheoesophageal diversion, laryngotracheal separation, and total laryngectomy).

In patients with Zenker's diverticulum, it is important to remember that the primary cause of the formation of the diverticulum is a poorly compliant UES. Removing the diverticulum without improving the compliance of the UES (typically achieved by myotomy) frequently leads to persistent dysphagia and recurrence of the diverticulum.[73] Myotomy alone can indeed lead to symptomatic improvement and even regression of the pharyngeal pouch.[74-76] Depending on the size and location of the pouch, current treatment for Zenker's diverticulum involves myotomy alone or in combination with pouch suspension or resection.[77]

Dietary modifications include alterations of the consistency of food, manipulating the swallowing posture, and/or adjustment of the swallowing technique. The goals of the swallow therapy interventions are to improve pharyngeal bolus flow and minimize the risk of aspiration. Speech-language pathologists usually evaluate patients during videofluoroscopy in order to assess the ability of these interventions to improve bolus flow and minimize aspiration. These interventions have been primarily focused on patients with neurological, poststroke dysphagia. Dietary modifications in patients with poststroke dysphagia aim at the ability of individual patients to find ways to compensate for the lost neurologic control of the cervical musculature. Even though some authors regard these interventions as having limited efficacy,[78] these techniques should be definitely considered given their biologic plausibility, relatively low costs, low risks, and in many instances the lack of better alternatives.

Oropharyngeal dysphagia unfortunately leads to an increased risk of aspiration and inability to meet caloric needs through oral intake in many patients. In these cases, the option of enteral feeding tubes should be discussed with patients and their family members. A percutaneous endoscopic gastrostomy (PEG) tube can be placed safely and offer the ability to maintain adequate fluid and caloric balance. PEG tubes are superior to NG feeding tubes in their reliability to deliver the recommended calories[79,80] but do not reduce the risk of aspiration pneumonia.[81]

Summary

Oropharyngeal dysphagia can be caused by a wide variety of systemic and local conditions. A careful clinical history and physical exam can help distinguish oropharyngeal from esophageal dysphagia, while videofluoroscopy is probably the most important test to evaluate patients with oropharyngeal dysphagia. Treatable systemic, local, or iatrogenic (ie, medication) causes of oropharyngeal dysphagia should always be considered, and clinical diagnostics should be conducted along these lines. The goals of managing patients with oropharyngeal dysphagia should be treatment of underlying diseases, reduction or elimination of the risk of aspiration (ie, obtaining a "safe swallow"), and ensuring adequate nutritional intake.

References

1. Young EC, Durant-Jones L. Developing a dysphagia program in an acute care hospital: a needs assessment. *Dysphagia.* 1990;5(3):159-165.

2. Kahrilas PJ, Dodds WJ, Dent J, Logemann JA, Shaker R. Upper esophageal sphincter function during deglutition. *Gastroenterology.* 1988;95(1):52-62.

3. Cook IJ, Dodds WJ, Dantas RO, et al. Opening mechanisms of the human upper esophageal sphincter. *Am J Physiol.* 1989;257(5 Pt 1):G748-G759.

4. Walther EK. Dysphagia after pharyngolaryngeal cancer surgery. Part I: Pathophysiology of postsurgical deglutition. *Dysphagia.* 1995;10(4):275-278.

5. Logemann JA, Pauloski BR, Rademaker AW, et al. Speech and swallow function after tonsil/base of tongue resection with primary closure. *J Speech Hear Res.* 1993;36(5):918-926.

6. McConnel FM, Logemann JA, Rademaker AW, et al. Surgical variables affecting postoperative swallowing efficiency in oral cancer patients: a pilot study. *Laryngoscope.* 1994;104(1 Pt 1):87-90.

7. Logemann JA, Gibbons P, Rademaker AW, et al. Mechanisms of recovery of swallow after supraglottic laryngectomy. *J Speech Hear Res.* 1994;37(5):965-974.

8. Muller-Miny H, Eisele DW, Jones B. Dynamic radiographic imaging following total laryngectomy. *Head Neck.* 1993;15(4):342-347.

9. Ekberg O, Malmquist J, Lindgren S. Pharyngo-oesophageal webs in dysphageal patients. A radiologic and clinical investigation in 1134 patients. *ROFO Fortschr Geb Rontgenstr Nuklearmed.* 1986;145(1):75-80.

10. Clements JL Jr, Cox GW, Torres WE, Weens HS. Cervical esophageal webs—a roentgenanatomic correlation. Observations on the pharyngoesophagus. *Am J Roentgenol Radium Ther Nucl Med.* 1974;121(2):221-231.

11. Ekberg O, Nylander G. Dysfunction of the cricopharyngeal muscle. A cineradiographic study of patients with dysphagia. *Radiology.* 1982;143(2):481-486.

12. Curtis DJ, Cruess DF, Berg T. The cricopharyngeal muscle: a videorecording review. *Am J Roentgenol.* 1984;142(3):497-500.

13. Jones B, Ravich WJ, Donner MW, Kramer SS, Hendrix TR. Pharyngoesophageal interrelationships: observations and working concepts. *Gastrointest Radiol.* 1985;10(3):225-233.

14. Dantas RO, Cook IJ, Dodds WJ, Kern MK, Lang IM, Brasseur JG. Biomechanics of cricopharyngeal bars. *Gastroenterology.* 1990;99(5):1269-1274.

15. Shapiro J, Martin S, DeGirolami U, Goyal R. Inflammatory myopathy causing pharyngeal dysphagia: a new entity. *Ann Otol Rhinol Laryngol.* 1996;105(5):331-335.

16. Georgalas C, Baer ST. Pharyngeal pouch and polymyositis: association and implications for etiology of Zenker's diverticulum. *J Laryngol Otol.* 2000;114(10):805-807.

17. Williams RB, Grehan MJ, Hersch M, Andre J, Cook IJ. Biomechanics, diagnosis, and treatment outcome in inflammatory myopathy presenting as oropharyngeal dysphagia. *Gut.* 2003;52(4):471-478.

18. Pace-Balzan A, Habashi SM, Nassar WY. View from within: radiology in focus lateral pharyngeal diverticulum. *J Laryngol Otol.* 1991;105(9):793-795.

19. Zenker FA, von Ziemssen H. Dilatations of the esophagus. In: von Ziemssen H, ed. *Cyclopedia of the practice of medicine.* London: Low, Marston, Searle and Rivingston; 1878:46-68.

20. Ardran GM, Kemp FH, Lund WS. The etiology of the posterior pharyngeal diverticulum: a cineradiographic study. *J Laryngol Otol.* 1964;78:333-349.

21. Hurwitz AL, Nelson JA, Haddad JK. Oropharyngeal dysphagia: manometric and cine esophagraphic findings. *Am J Dig Dis.* 1975;20(4):313-324.

22. Hunt PS, Connell AM, Smiley TB. The cricopharyngeal sphincter in gastric reflux. *Gut.* 1970;11(4):303-306.

23. Knuff TE, Benjamin SB, Castell DO. Pharyngoesophageal (Zenker's) diverticulum: a reappraisal. *Gastroenterology.* 1982;82(4):734-736.

24. Cook IJ, Gabb M, Panagopoulos V, et al. Pharyngeal (Zenker's) diverticulum is a disorder of upper esophageal sphincter opening. *Gastroenterology.* 1992;103(4):1229-1235.

25. Bone RC, Nahum AM, Harris AS. Evaluation and correction of dysphagia-producing cervical osteophytosis. *Laryngoscope.* 1974;84(11):2045-2050.

26. Stuart D. Dysphagia due to cervical osteophytes. A description of five patients and a review of the literature. *Int Orthop.* 1989;13(2):95-99.

27. Papadopoulos SM, Chen JC, Feldenzer JA, Bucci MN, McGillicuddy JE. Anterior cervical osteophytes as a cause of progressive dysphagia. *Acta Neurochir.* 1989;101(1-2):63-65.

28. Welsh LW, Welsh JJ, Chinnici JC. Dysphagia due to cervical spine surgery. *Ann Otol Rhinol Laryngol.* 1987;96(1 Pt 1):112-115.

29. Horner J, Massey EW, Riski JE, Lathrop DL, Chase KN. Aspiration following stroke: clinical correlates and outcome. *Neurology.* 1988;38(9):1359-1362.

30. Horner J, Buoyer FG, Alberts MJ, Helms MJ. Dysphagia following brain-stem stroke. Clinical correlates and outcome. *Arch Neurol.* 1991;48(11):1170-1173.

31. Veis SL, Logemann JA. Swallowing disorders in persons with cerebrovascular accident. *Arch Phys Med Rehabil.* 1985;66(6):372-375.

32. Schmidt J, Holas M, Halvorson K, Reding M. Videofluoroscopic evidence of aspiration predicts pneumonia and death but not dehydration following stroke. *Dysphagia.* 1994;9(1):7-11.

33. Muller J, Wenning GK, Verny M, et al. Progression of dysarthria and dysphagia in postmortem-confirmed parkinsonian disorders. *Arch Neurol.* 2001;58(2):259-264.

34. Robbins JA, Logemann JA, Kirshner HS. Swallowing and speech production in Parkinson's disease. *Ann Neurol.* 1986;19(3):283-287.

35. Leopold NA, Kagel MC. Prepharyngeal dysphagia in Parkinson's disease. *Dysphagia.* 1996;11(1):14-22.

36. Johnston BT, Li Q, Castell JA, Castell DO. Swallowing and esophageal function in Parkinson's disease. *Am J Gastroenterol.* 1995;90(10):1741-1746.

37. Ali GN, Wallace KL, Schwartz R, DeCarle DJ, Zagami AS, Cook IJ. Mechanisms of oral-pharyngeal dysphagia in patients with Parkinson's disease. *Gastroenterology.* 1996;110(2):383-392.

38. Bosma JF, Brodie DR. Disabilities of the pharynx in amyotrophic lateral sclerosis as demonstrated by cineradiography. *Radiology.* 1969;92(1):97-103.

39. Osserman KE, Genkins G. Studies in myasthenia gravis: review of a twenty-year experience in over 1200 patients. *Mt Sinai J Med.* 1971;38(6):497-537.

40. Viets HR. Diagnosis of myasthenia gravis in patients with dysphagia. *JAMA.* 1947;134(12):987-992.

41. Dalakas MC. Polymyositis, dermatomyositis and inclusion-body myositis. *N Engl J Med.* 1991;325(21):1487-1498.

42. Johnson ER, McKenzie SW. Kinematic pharyngeal transit times in myopathy: evaluation for dysphagia. *Dysphagia.* 1993;8(1):35-40.

43. Porubsky ES, Murray JP, Pratt LL. Cricopharyngeal achalasia in dermatomyositis. *Arch Otolaryngol.* 1973;98(6):428-429.

44. Verma A, Bradley WG, Adesina AM, Sofferman R, Pendlebury WW. Inclusion body myositis with cricopharyngeus muscle involvement and severe dysphagia. *Muscle Nerve.* 1991;14(5):470-473.

45. Sweatman MC, Chambers L. Disordered esophageal motility in thyrotoxic myopathy. *Postgrad Med J.* 1985;61(717):619-620.

46. Johnson CC, Kuwabara T. Oculopharyngeal muscular dystrophy. *Am J Ophthalmol.* 1974;77(6):872-879.

47. Blumbergs PC, Chin D, Burrow D, Burns RJ, Rice JP. Oculopharyngeal dystrophy: clinicopathological study of an Australian family. *Clin Exp Neurol.* 1983;19:102-109.

48. Dobrowski JM, Zajtchuk JT, LaPiana FG, Hensley SD Jr. Oculopharyngeal muscular dystrophy: clinical and histopathologic correlations. *Otolaryngol Head Neck Surg.* 1986;95(2):131-142.

49. Bashford G, Bradd P. Drug-induced Parkinsonism associated with dysphagia and aspiration: a brief report. *J Geriatr Psychiatry Neurol.* 1996;9(3):133-135.

50. Miller LG, Jankovic J. Metoclopramide-induced movement disorders. Clinical findings with a review of the literature. *Arch Intern Med.* 1989;149(11):2486-2492.

51. Hayashi T, Nishikawa T, Koga I, Uchida Y, Yamawaki S. Life-threatening dysphagia following prolonged neuroleptic therapy. *Clin Neuropharmacol.* 1997;20(1):77-81.

52. Lim HC, Nigro MA, Beierwaltes P, Tolia V, Wishnow R. Nitrazepam-induced cricopharyngeal dysphagia, abnormal esophageal peristalsis and associated bronchospasm: probable cause of nitrazepam-related sudden death. *Brain Dev.* 1992;14(5):309-314.

53. Wyllie E, Wyllie R, Cruse RP, Rothner AD, Erenberg G. The mechanism of nitrazepam-induced drooling and aspiration. *N Engl J Med.* 1986;314(1):35-38.

54. Borodic GE, Joseph M, Fay L, Cozzolino D, Ferrante RJ. Botulinum A toxin for the treatment of spasmodic torticollis: dysphagia and regional toxin spread. *Head Neck.* 1990;12(5):392-399.

55. Masters CL, Dawkins RL, Zilko PJ, Simpson JA, Leedman RJ. Penicillamine-associated myasthenia gravis, antiacetylcholine receptor and antistriational antibodies. *Am J Med.* 1977;63(5):689-694.

56. Kaeser HE. Drug-induced myasthenic syndromes. *Acta Neurol Scand Suppl.* 1984;100:39-47.

57. Miller CD, Oleshansky MA, Gibson KF, Cantilena LR. Procainamide-induced myasthenia-like weakness and dysphagia. *Ther Drug Monit.* 1993;15(3):251-254.

58. Doyle DR, McCurley TL, Sergent JS. Fatal polymyositis in D-penicillamine-treated rheumatoid arthritis. *Ann Intern Med.* 1983;98(3):327-330.

59. Dalakas MC, Illa I, Pezeshkpour GH, Laukaitis JP, Cohen B, Griffin JL. Mitochondrial myopathy caused by long-term zidovudine therapy. *N Engl J Med.* 1990;322(16):1098-1105.

60. Berbegal J, Lluch V, Morera J, de Gracia MC. Dysphagia as the presentation of amiodarone-induced hyperthyroidism. *Med Clin.* 1993;100(11):437-438.

61. London SF, Gross KF, Ringel SP. Cholesterol-lowering agent myopathy (CLAM). *Neurology.* 1991;41(7):1159-1160.

62. Cook IJ, Dent J, Collins SM. Upper esophageal sphincter tone and reactivity to stress in patients with a history of globus sensation. *Dig Dis Sci.* 1989;34(5):672-676.

63. Davies AE, Kidd D, Stone SP, MacMahon J. Pharyngeal sensation and gag reflex in healthy subjects. *Lancet.* 1995;345(8948):487-488.

64. Splaingard ML, Hutchins B, Sulton LD, Chaudhuri G. Aspiration in rehabilitation patients: videofluoroscopy vs bedside clinical assessment. *Arch Phys Med Rehabil.* 1988;69(8):637-640.

65. Logemann JA, Roa Pauloski B, Rademaker A, et al. Impact of the diagnostic procedure on outcome measures of swallowing rehabilitation in head and neck cancer patients. *Dysphagia.* 1992;7(4):179-186.

66. Logemann JA. Role of the modified barium swallow in management of patients with dysphagia. *Otolaryngol Head Neck Surg.* 1997;116(3):335-338.

67. Williams RB, Wallace KL, Ali GN, Cook IJ. Biomechanics of failed deglutitive upper esophageal sphincter relaxation in neurogenic dysphagia. *Am J Physiol Gastrointest Liver Physiol.* 2002;283(1):G16-G26.

68. Langmore SE, Schatz K, Olsen N. Fiberoptic endoscopic examination of swallowing safety: a new procedure. *Dysphagia.* 1988;2(4):216-219.

69. Castell JA, Dalton CB, Castell DO. Pharyngeal and upper esophageal sphincter manometry in humans. *Am J Physiol.* 1990;258(2 Pt 1):G173-G178.

70. Olsson R, Castell JA, Castell DO, Ekberg O. Solid-state computerized manometry improves diagnostic yield in pharyngeal dysphagia: simultaneous videoradiography and manometry in dysphagia patients with normal barium swallows. *Abdom Imaging.* 1995;20(3):230-235.

71. Malhi-Chowla N, Achem SR, Stark ME, DeVault KR. Manometry of the upper esophageal sphincter and pharynx is not useful in unselected patients referred for esophageal testing. *Am J Gastroenterol.* 2000;95(6):1417-1421.

72. Hatlebakk JG, Castell JA, Spiegel J, Paoletti V, Katz PO, Castell DO. Dilatation therapy for dysphagia in patients with upper esophageal sphincter dysfunction—manometric and symptomatic response. *Dis Esophagus.* 1998;11(4):254-259.

73. Ellis FH Jr, Schlegel JF, Lynch VP, Payne WS. Cricopharyngeal myotomy for pharyngo-esophageal diverticulum. *Ann Surg.* 1969;170(3):340-349.

74. Konowitz PM, Biller HF. Diverticulopexy and cricopharyngeal myotomy: treatment for the high-risk patient with a pharyngoesophageal (Zenker's) diverticulum. *Otolaryngol Head Neck Surg.* 1989;100(2):146-153.

75. Ellis FH Jr, Gibb SP, Williamson WA. Current status of cricopharyngeal myotomy for cervical esophageal dysphagia. *Eur J Cardiothorac Surg.* 1996;10(12):1033-1038.

76. Ekberg O, Lindgren S. Effect of cricopharyngeal myotomy on pharyngoesophageal function: pre- and postoperative cineradiographic findings. *Gastrointest Radiol.* 1987;12(1):1-6.

77. Jamieson GG, Duranceau AC, Payne WS. Pharyngo-esophageal diverticulum. In: Jamieson GG, ed. *Surgery of the Esophagus.* Edinburgh: Churchill Livingstone Press; 1988:435-443.

78. DePippo KL, Holas MA, Reding MJ, Mandel FS, Lesser ML. Dysphagia therapy following stroke: a controlled trial. *Neurology.* 1994;44(9):1655-1660.

79. Baeten C, Hoefnagels J. Feeding via nasogastric tube or percutaneous endoscopic gastrostomy. A comparison. *Scand J Gastroenterol Suppl.* 1992;194:95-98.

80. Park RH, Allison MC, Lang J, et al. Randomised comparison of percutaneous endoscopic gastrostomy and nasogastric tube feeding in patients with persisting neurological dysphagia. *BMJ.* 1992;304(6839):1406-1409.

81. Cole MJ, Smith JT, Molnar C, Shaffer EA. Aspiration after percutaneous gastrostomy. Assessment by Tc-99m labeling of the enteral feed. *J Clin Gastroenterol.* 1987;9(1):90-95.

chapter **9**

Motility Disorders of the Esophagus

John G. Lieb II, MD and David A. Katzka, MD

Esophageal motility disorders remain an interesting but enigmatic group of problems. Part of the challenge of these diseases rests in the fact their diagnosis is often made by a motility tracing as opposed to a pathology or blood specimen. As a result, the diagnosis is often open to variable interpretation. Furthermore, it is often difficult to know whether these abnormal motility findings represent a clear diagnosis or merely an epiphenomenon of another or perhaps several diseases. In this chapter, discussion will focus on dysmotility of the esophageal body and LES, with a brief overview of normal physiology. An attempt will be made to clarify and classify these challenging disorders.

Normal Physiology of Swallowing

The esophageal motility function is dependent upon intact function by the muscular layers of the esophageal wall and an intact local and CNS stimulation and regulation. The muscle of the esophagus consists mostly of a muscularis propria, the thickest and strongest contractile element of the esophageal wall. In the proximal esophagus, this muscle is striated whereas in the distal two thirds of the esophagus, this component consists of longitudinal and circular smooth muscle layers. The function of these layers is mostly under local control by the enteric nervous system, consisting of a network of neural plexus throughout the gut wall that regulate wall movement through the activation of local reflexes. Peristalsis is accomplished through the activation of muscular contraction proximal and muscular relaxation distal to a swallowed bolus. With continued movement of the bolus down the esophagus, this wave of ascending contraction and descending relaxation moves caudad so that it eventually reaches a point just above the LES. Specifically, lumen-occluding contractions of esophageal circular muscle produce a pressure wave cephalad to the bolus (53 mmHg in the upper to 35 mmHg in the middle to 69 mmHg in the lower third of the esophagus) traveling toward the stomach.[1] The junction of striated and smooth muscle in the middle third of the esophagus may account for the lower amplitude of the peristaltic wave.

The contractile pressure wave is mediated predominantly by cholinergic innervation and travels 3 cm/s, 5 cm/s, and 2.5 cm/s, respectively down the upper, mid, and lower esophagus. The pressures are lower when measured in the upright position[2] and with dry or air swallows.[3] Nitric oxide- and vasoactive intestinal peptide-mediated relaxation of circular muscle caudad to the bolus and marked contractile rebound from such relaxation cephalad to the bolus also contribute to the peristaltic wave[4-8] and forward progress of the bolus. The longitudinal muscles contract to shorten the length of the esophagus. Collectively, this action of moving a bolus introduced to the esophagus by the oropharynx and propelled to the distal esophagus is termed primary peristalsis. In contrast, secondary peristalsis can be induced when a pressure stimulus is applied to the esophagus such as from residual food left from an unsuccessful primary peristalsis or from refluxed gastric contents[9] such that further peristaltic action is required to clear the bolus into the stomach past the LES.

The LES is defined manometrically as a 2 to 4 cm zone of high resting pressure at the GEJ. This high resting pressure is contributed to by an extrinsic component of the surrounding crural diaphragm and an intrinsic smooth muscle component. The smooth muscle of the LES is distinct from the body of the esophagus in that it is tonically contracted. This tonicity is believed to be due to higher intracellular calcium, more actin, fewer gap junctions, and perhaps higher vagal Ach tone than in the body of the esophagus.[10] Motilin and intra-abdominal pressure also cause LES contraction, which is abolished by atropine.[10] Relaxation of the LES occurs under several circumstances. The first is a result of primary peristalsis secondary to esophageal distention just proximal to the LES. With primary peristalsis and relaxation of the LES, a bolus is propelled into the stomach within 8 to 10 seconds.[11] A second type of relaxation is transient LES relaxation. This occurs in eructation and vomiting and is activated through partly local and brainstem mechanisms. It may be elicited by pharyngeal stimulation, proximal gastric distention, and introduction of fat into the duodenum.

Manometry

A brief summary of manometry is useful before discussing the disorders of motility. The manometer is a flexible tube with solid state transducers covering 360 degrees at multiple locations. With the patient within no more than 30 degrees of supine—a necessary standard because of the effect of gravity on pressure—measurement of pressures can began with the manometer inserted into the gastric fundus. Measurement of esophageal pressures occurs by monitoring the pressure of non-compliant containers of castor oil inside the manometer. A sharp rise with deep inspiration in the distal transducers confirms placement into the stomach. The manometer is then zeroed and pulled caudally until the proximal transducer (scout) reads an increase in baseline pressure, marking the distal border of the LES. Pulling more caudad reaches the highest LES pressure zone, and the difference between the midrespiratory pressure at this point and the intragastric pressure is the maximal LES pressure. At the point of respiratory reversal, the pressure with inspiration becomes negative, indicating the location of the diaphragm and entrance into the thoracic half of the LES (assuming no hiatal hernia). The LES is then observed during test swallows of several milliliters of liquid to ascertain the LES relaxation pressure, which is defined as the difference between the lowest pressure achieved during LES relaxation and the gastric baseline pressure. Normal tracings of LES relaxation pressures and esophageal body contractions are shown in the figures including a basal LES pressure of 10 to 45 mmHg, relaxation of the LES with swallows to <8 mm above gastric pressure, and peristaltic velocity of 2 to 8 cm/s.[10] With the above background, a discussion of abnormal esophageal motility can begin.

Achalasia

INTRODUCTION

Classic or "idiopathic" achalasia, as its Greek root for "lack of relaxation" implies, is a foregut disease defined by poor relaxation of the LES and aperistalsis of the esophageal body. It is a rare disorder occurring in 1 in 10,000[12]—common enough for most gastroenterologists to have seen a few cases, but uncommon enough to make its characterization difficult and arguably incomplete. It is not uncommon that achalasia is recognized or diagnosed years after the development of symptoms. Many questions regarding the causes, diagnosis, and treatment of achalasia remain, and we will try to address those here.

ETIOLOGY

Several steps have been hypothesized to contribute to the pathogenesis of achalasia. The first is the occurrence of viral exposure in a genetically susceptible individual. This viral exposure is suggested firstly by histologic evidence: the mucosa of affected esophagi display papillomatosis and hyperplasticity, perhaps from stasis or squamous-tropic viral infection, like HPV.[13] In addition, VZV has been detected in cardiomyotomy specimens,[14] but PCR studies of VZV and other neurotrophic viruses like CMV and HSV have not borne out.[15] wallerian degeneration in vagal axons resembles axons distal to a vagotomy.[16] The vagal nuclei in the medulla themselves have been shown to be pathologic on autopsy.[17] As regards genetic susceptibility, HLA-DQB1 and DRB1 has been found more commonly in patients with achalasia.[18]

The next step in pathogenesis is the development of an autoimmune reaction characterized by antibodies presumably against the myenteric plexus of the LES and esophagus. Specific examples of antibodies that may be found in achalasia include antimyenteric, antimuscarinic, and antineuronal antibodies. This autoimmune reaction results in an inflammatory response in the myenteric plexus of the LES where lymphocytic inflammation is observed in histology specimens. This inflammatory neuritis leads to a depletion of inhibitory neuropeptides NO and VIP that consequently promotes smooth muscle contraction.[19] As a result, there is a net stimulatory effect on LES contraction accounting for the hypertension and incomplete relaxation commonly seen. With continued inflammation, collagen deposition and greater ganglial depletion result, leading to more end-stage achalasia.

Familial achalasia constitutes 1% of all cases as part of the triple-A syndrome of alacrima, achalasia, autoimmune neuropathy, deafness, vitiligo, microcephaly, and short stature.[20] However, 20% of patients with achalasia have some dry eye symptoms, pointing to a possible polygenic component to classic achalasia. Although no conclusive universal mechanism has been found to cause classic achalasia, the most widely accepted hypothesis combines the above mechanisms.

Table 9-1

SYMPTOMS OF ACHALASIA

Major Symptoms
- Dysphagia
- Chest pain
- Regurgitation
- Weight loss

Minor Symptoms
- Slow eating
- Stereotypical maneuvers during eating
- Halitosis
- Heartburn
- Accumulation of oral debris at night
- Staining of the pillow during sleep
- Nocturnal coughing or choking
- Acute airway obstruction
- Inability to belch
- Postprandial syncope
- Dental caries
- Asthma
- Pneumonia

CLINICAL PRESENTATION

The presentation of achalasia is diverse (Table 9-1). However, dysphagia is nearly universal (95%), classically for liquids as well as solids, but dysphagia for solids can predominate early in the disease. Patients may describe the dysphagia as fullness in the chest or a sticking feeling. Regurgitation occurs in 75% and is usually nonacidic but can be somewhat sour if fermentation is active in food remnants in the distal esophagus, with pHs as low as 4 having been described. Patients with achalasia may complain of thick, white phlegm in the morning from swallowed saliva overnight, which may be mistaken for chronic bronchitis, allergic rhinitis, or sinusitis. Morning regurgitation of the previous evening meal and nocturnal cough is not uncommon. Patients and families of patients note prolonged eating time, including several maneuvers to raise intraesophageal pressure such as drinking large volumes of carbonated beverages,[21] abducting the shoulders, tilting the neck, and the Valsalva's maneuver. Patients may attempt alcohol, warm liquids, or marijuana in an attempt to open the LES,[22] or even induce vomiting, which may be mistaken for bulimia. Weight loss occurs in about 58%, in some cases up to 100 lbs.[23] Chest pain can be dull, intermittent, or constant;

Table 9-2

DIAGNOSTIC CRITERIA FOR ACHALASIA

Esophageal Manometry
- Aperistalsis of the esophageal body
- Hypertensive LES
- Incomplete relaxation of LES
- Elevated esophageal body pressure

Radiography
- Bird-beak narrowing of GEJ
- Dilated aperistaltic esophagus
- Food and fluid retention
- Sigmoidization
- Epiphrenic diverticulum

Endoscopy
- Food and/or fluid retention
- Dilated esophagus
- Tight GEJ that "pops" open
- Candida esophagitis

can worsen postprandially; and is easily confused with cardiac chest pain. Pain occurs in 17% to 95% and is more prominent earlier in the course of the disease before the distal esophagus dilates and in younger patients.[24] Some patients may present with extraesophageal manifestations such as aspiration pneumonia, lung abscess, or even esophageal-pericardial fistula.

Given the diversity of presenting symptom, it is not surprising that the average time from initial complaint to diagnosis can be as long as 4.6 years with a high of 67 years.[25]

The demographics of the patient is an important consideration since achalasia is more likely in Caucasian cohorts especially in Northwestern Europe, North America, and New Zealand. The mean age at diagnosis is between 30 and 60 with an increased incidence with age over 50. The incidence, which lacks gender predominance, is on the order of 0.5 per 100,000 and has not changed significantly in 50 years.

DIAGNOSIS

Radiographic, endoscopic, and manometric studies can confirm the diagnosis of achalasia (Table 9-2). Chest x-ray may show a wide mediastinum or an air fluid level in the esophagus especially on lateral view. Esophagogram classically shows a dilated distal esophagus with a narrow stream of barium in an elongated LES (bird's beak sign) (Figure 9-1). Most patients have residual barium in the esophagus after 5 min-

Figure 9-1. Manometric tracing of esophageal body in achalasia.

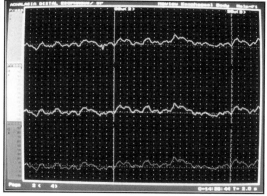

Figure 9-2. Esophagogram of early achalasia.

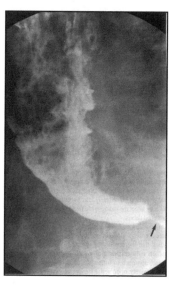

utes, and some show retained debris. In nondilated cases, fluoroscopy will still demonstrate failure of the primary peristaltic wave to clear the barium and simultaneous uncoordinated contractions. Epiphrenic (pulsion) diverticula may be seen. In extreme cases, the esophagus may attain an appearance not unlike that of the sigmoid colon, the so-called sigmoid esophagus (Figure 9-2).

Endoscopy is recommended but is often performed only at the time of intervention because it may miss early cases as a primary diagnostic tool. The distal esophageal mucosa may be red and friable. Food debris may be present, and the mucosa may appear hyperplastic and friable. Standard insufflation may not sufficiently open the LES, and a "pop" may occur as the scope is passed to the stomach.

Although not a "gold standard" meant to supersede clinical and radiographic findings, manometry is one of the best tests for achalasia and is essential prior to surgery

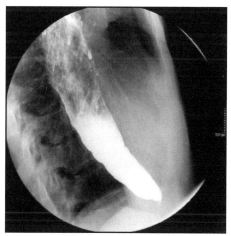

Figure 9-3. Esophagogram of advanced achalasia.

or dilation. Manometry may be difficult in very dilated cases and can sometimes be skipped if the clinical, radiographic, or endoscopic findings are classic and no intervention is planned. In achalasia, the esophageal body is aperistaltic on manometry with nonlumen occluding, low amplitude, isobaric waves, often less than 40 mmHg (Figure 9-3). Occasionally, repetitive, prolonged waves are seen.[26] However, once the distal esophagus dilates as in later stages of the disease, manometric measurements become more difficult because they require the wall of the esophagus to press against the narrow manometer. In fact, a guidewire inserted in the stomach may be required in large esophagi prior to placement of the manometer.[10] The amplitude achieved by striated esophageal contraction is reduced although peristalsis there as a whole is preserved.[27] Manometric anomalies of the LES are the physiologic sine qua non of achalasia. Although resting LES pressure can be normal (10 to 45 mmHg) in 40% of achalasia patients,[28] the finding of low LES resting pressure should raise the possibility of an alternative diagnosis.[10] LES relaxation residual pressure is usually abnormally high.[29] Complete relaxation of the LES can occasionally be seen, especially in early stage disease, but the duration of the relaxation is universally short.[30]

Vigorous achalasia can be differentiated from classic cases based on the presence of high amplitude, nonperistaltic esophageal body contractions. This may be an earlier stage of classic achalasia based on pathologic studies.[19] Clinical studies have not reported a progression, however.[31]

TREATMENT

Several caveats must be considered prior to instituting therapy for achalasia. First, there is poor correlation between symptoms and radiographic appearance both before and after treatment. Although this may be due in part to institutional variation in radiographic technique, which some have proposed standardizing,[32] other factors contribute as well. In addition, reliance upon symptomatic improvement after therapy for achalasia may not be an accurate means of evaluating these patients. As a result, a standardized "timed" barium esophagogram assessing the emptying of 100 to 200 mL of low-density barium at 1, 2, and 5 minutes has been proposed as a monitoring tool for objective response to achalasia treatment.[33] Second, older patients >45 to >60 (depending on the study) tend to have better symptomatic outcomes.[34,35] Whether this is because their physiology is more amenable to treatment or their esophagus is less sensitive and thus less likely to be symptomatic is unclear. Third, because of small numbers of patients, most studies do not stratify patients on the basis of severity and much of the methodology used in these studies is heterogeneous, even with "similar" techniques.

Until recently, pneumatic dilation of the LES has been a mainstay of therapy for primary achalasia for many decades. Current practice usually employs a 30-mm rigiflex balloon that is noncompliant at maximal inflation and is visible by fluoroscopy. The rigiflex is preceded by endoscopy to ensure proper guidewire placement, to remove food debris, and to look for carcinoma. The duration of dilation does not seem to correlate with clinical outcomes, and 6 seconds has even been reported as sufficient.[36] At 2 to 3 PSI, a "waist" can be seen indicating partial LES dilation on fluoroscopy. The balloon is then inflated to 10 PSI until obliteration of the waist (ie, opening of the LES) occurs. The patient undergoes a gastrograffin swallow as a gross assessment followed by barium cinemetric studies to rule out microperforation. Assuming there is no perforation, the patient is observed and then discharged within 4 hours if chest pain, fever, and inability to tolerate liquids are not present.

If present, perforation confined to the esophageal wall and not extending to the pleural or pericardial spaces can be managed conservatively with antibiotics and nothing by mouth.[10] Overall, perforation complicates about 2% of dilations.[37] For frank perforations, emergency laparotomy is required but most of these patients may have surgical completion of the myotomy with excellent outcomes; in some series, no different than elective Heller myotomy. The caveat, however, is getting them to surgery within hours of the perforation because waiting leads to marked mediastinal inflammation and a technically challenging operation. Risk factors for perforation include first dilation, vigorous achalasia, epiphrenic diverticulum, and malnutrition.[38-40] Chest pain is a less threatening but more common complication of dilation.

Initial symptom relief is reported in 82% of nearly 600 patients in multiple studies with a median follow up of 17 months. But at 5 years, single dilation is only 30% to 50% effective[35,41-43] and may be repeated up to 2 to 3 times, typically with a larger balloon. Use of 40-mm dilators is not routinely recommended because of high perforation rates. Less incremental benefit is gained by each successive dilation,[44] and early relapse (at 2 months) is a poor long-term predictive factor.[45] Reassessment by radiography and/or manometry may have a role especially after several dilations.[32] Older patients, heterogeneously defined as >45 or >60, may have a more favorable and lasting outcome with dilation; however, as many as 30% of patients may require eventual myotomy.[46]

Injection of botulinum toxin into the LES is an alternative to dilation, initially proposed in the mid 1990s.[47] The toxin blocks tonic contraction signals from vagal cholinergic neurons. Twenty units are injected at each quadrant of the LES and an additional 20 units either prograde or retrograde from the gastric cardia using a sclerotherapy needle. Straddling the endoscope repeatedly between stomach and esophagus and en face positioning of the scope 90 degrees perpendicular to the esophageal wall during injection ensures proper positioning (Figure 9-4).

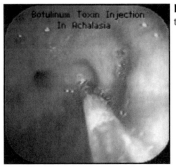

Figure 9-4. Botulinum toxin injection adjacent to pinpoint LES.

Overall, botulinum toxin provides symptom relief in 70% of patients at 18 months with lower LES pressure (43%) and decreased esophageal diameter in 17%. However, 40% at 18 months[48] and in another series 50% at 6 months required reinjection.[49] A minority of patients (up to 20%) who do not respond to the first injection may respond to a second endoscopy with injection. Factors predicting favorable botulinum toxin outcome include age greater than 60 and the presence of vigorous achalasia.[10] Some researchers have proposed that botulinum toxin may be also affecting sensory neurons because symptom improvement outpaces manometric or radiographic improvement.[50]

Botulinum toxin has several drawbacks. It is contraindicated in egg-allergic patients, in those taking aminoglycosides, and must be kept at 2° to 8°C. Agitation of the solution may precipitate and inactivate the toxin. Moreover, botulinum toxin is expensive.

Medications have been used with mixed success for patients with achalasia, including postprandial sublingual nifedipine, nitrates, sildenafil, beta-agonists, and peripheral opioid antagonists (loperamide). Isosorbide dinitrate (5 mg) has been shown to be superior to 20 mg SL nifedipine,[51] which has been superior to the non-dihydropyridine calcium channel antagonists diltiazem and verapamil.[52,53] All these agents suffer from tachyphylaxis, partial relief of symptoms, and side effects such as headache, orthostasis, myocardial ischemia (SL nifedipine), and tachy- (beta agonist and anticholinergics) and bradyarrhythmias. Even among patients with a known manometric and symptomatologic response to SL nifedipine, only 33% were still compliant at 4 years.[54] As a result, medications are rarely used for achalasia.

With the ability to perform Heller myotomy laparoscopically, surgical treatment has become a first-line therapy for many patients with achalasia. The myotomy is usually combined with a partial fundoplication (Dor or Toupe) to prevent postoperative reflux. The incision transects the LES and is usually extended down the gastric cardia. The laparoscopic approach is now becoming the standard of care.[10] Several series now demonstrate up to 95% response rates 5 years after surgery. One prospective randomized controlled trial performed by surgeons on 81 patients showed a significant benefit of surgical vs dilation therapy (95% versus 65% at 5 years). It is not surprising that some centers have altogether abandoned pneumatic dilation in favor of laparoscopic

Table 9-3

TREATMENT OPTIONS FOR ACHALASIA

Therapy	Advantages	Disadvantages
Botulinum toxin	Easy to perform	Short duration
	Generally effective	
	Safe	
	Repeatable	
	? Diagnostic utility	
Balloon dilatation	Avoids anesthesia	? Surgery better
(outpatient)	Expert	
	Generally safe	Perforation risk
Surgical myotomy	Effective	Inpatient stay
combined with		Surgery
antireflux surgery	Not 100%	

myotomy. Some surgeons report technical challenges in patients previously injected with botulinum toxin or dilation, so it is best to leave the LES alone if possible in patients with achalasia heading for surgery. A summary of treatment options is given in Table 9-3.

ACHALASIA AND CANCER

Although squamous cell carcinoma occurs 8- to 140-fold more often in patients with achalasia (in about 3% of cases), it occurs an average of 17 to 20 years after diagnosis of achalasia.[55-57] Therefore, some have questioned the value of endoscopic surveillance. At present, it is usually reserved for patients with long standing, advanced disease, which theoretically might prevent symptoms of cancer and lead to later stage diagnosis. The mechanism of this carcinogenesis is unknown but probably relates to inflammation from stasis.

PSEUDOACHALASIA

In 3% of all cases of achalasia, a secondary cause may be found that is more likely to be cancer (Table 9-4). Cancer causes achalasia by 2 mechanisms. The most common mechanism is secondary to malignant infiltration of the LES by the cancer. In addition to extrinsically compressing the GEJ, pathologic analysis demonstrates infiltration of the LES neural elements by the tumor. Carcinoma of the gastric cardia, esophagus, breast, and lung are the most common causes of achalasia by this mechanism. The second means of malignancy-induced achalasia is paraneoplastic by tumor secretion of an antineuronal antibody (anti-Hu) that injures LES neurons. Small cell lung cancer and much less commonly lymphoma can cause this type of achalasia.

Table 9-4

CAUSES OF SECONDARY ACHALASIA

Benign Causes
- Chagas' disease
- Postfundoplication
- Neurofibromatosis
- Amyloidosis
- Pancreatic pseudocyst
  Mediastinal fibrosis

Direct Infiltration of LES by Tumor
- Gastric cardia
- Esophageal
- Lung
- Breast
- Prostate
- Lymphoma
- Hepatocellular
- Pancreatic

Paraneoplastic Syndrome (anti-Hu)
- Small cell lung
- Lymphoma

Clinical predictors of secondary achalasia include old age (over age 60, 9% of cases have a secondary cause); rapid weight loss; and an elongated, narrow LES segment that is even more difficult to pass on EGD than usual for achalasia.[58]

Other less common diseases responsible for secondary achalasia include amyloid, sarcoid; medullary stroke or mass; and Chagas' disease, which is caused by trypanosome protozoa prevalent in South America and can cause megacolon and megaesophagus due to inflammation in the myenteric plexus.

Ruling out pseudoachalasia can be challenging. Because barium studies may miss 72% of GEJ tumors in patients with secondary achalasia,[59] all patients with achalasia should undergo endoscopy, which itself is imperfect because mucosal biopsies can miss 25% of malignant pseudoachalasia cases.[60] Therefore, if clinical features are suggestive, endoscopic ultrasound should accompany standard endoscopy and is more sensitive and specific than CT.[61]

Figure 9-5. Manometric tracing of esophageal body in DES.

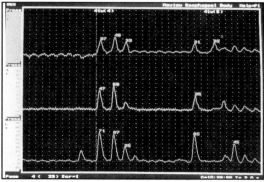

Other Motility Disorders

DIFFUSE ESOPHAGEAL SPASM

Introduction

Diffuse esophageal spasm (DES) is generally considered an abnormality of uncoordinated esophageal contraction. In this entity, peristalsis is haphazard, with multiple, sometimes spontaneous, and nearly simultaneous high-amplitude contractions (Figure 9-5) The distal, smooth muscle portion of the esophagus is predominantly involved.

Etiology

Histologic study reveals patchy esophageal neural process degeneration. Nitric oxide sequestration and donation have been shown to induce and inhibit, respectively, the contractions seen in DES,[62,63] pointing to disorganized, nitric-oxide dependent esophageal body relaxation in this disorder. This disordered contraction is either primary or may be secondary to GERD as evidenced by the disproportionate prevalence of GERD in patients with DES. In addition, some patients are hyper-responsive to the procontractile effects of cholinergic stimuli during edrophonium testing.[64]

Clinical Presentation

Chest pain is considered the cardinal feature of DES. This can be difficult to distinguish from angina pectoris especially because the majority of patients are over age 50. Pain may be provoked by swallowing, emotional distress, cholinergic stimuli, or rarely exercise, and lasts seconds to minutes but sometimes hours.[64]

Diagnosis

Spasm may be present on barium radiographs showing unprovoked multiple, non-lumen-occluding contractions that may propel the barium both caudad and cephalad. Another term used is the corkscrew esophagus.

However, manometry is considered the gold standard for diagnosis (Table 9-5). Although much debate surrounds the definition of DES, most authorities believe the following manometric criteria would rule in the diagnosis: simultaneous, poorly

Table 9-5

DIFFUSE ESOPHAGEAL SPASM: MANOMETRIC CRITERIA

- Nonpropulsive contractions
- High-amplitude contractions
- Triple peaked contractions
- Hypertensive LES
- Provocation with edrophonium

coordinated contractions with at least 10% of test swallows; contraction amplitude>30 mmHg; and repetitive and peaked contractions.[10] Additionally, only a few of the criteria may be present and still point to the diagnosis. Several provocative maneuvers during the manometry study may be useful: cold swallows may produce pain but not motor abnormalities, whereas solid boluses or edrophonium may provoke both. Because of the episodic nature of the disorder, a single normal manometry exam may not rule out DES. Additionally, one may find manometric abnormalities without symptoms or provocation of symptoms without manometric abnormalities.[65] Because diagnosis is based upon the combination of these 2, often supportive but not definitive evidence of DES is obtained.

Treatment

Because some patients have DES secondary to GER, some physicians have advocated a course of empiric reflux therapy first. Trials using twice-daily PPIs for patients with chest pain may demonstrate close to 90% efficacy with a comparable diagnostic accuracy to ambulatory pH monitoring. Whether these patients have true reflux-induced DES or chest pain as a heartburn equivalent is unclear. As a result, failure of reflux therapy might be an indication for ambulatory pH monitoring to definitively exclude acid reflux. If a diagnosis of primary DES is established, antispasmodics such as sublingual nitroglycerine,[66] nifedipine, and anticholinergics may be used but are inconsistent at relieving pain.[67,68] Some patients respond to attempts at decreasing visceral pain sensation with antidepressants such as trazodone 100 to 150 mg[69] or low dose tricyclic antidepressants.[70]

Some studies have suggested the DES may overlap or be a variant of achalasia. Accordingly, patients with DES may present with dysphagia and demonstrate manometric features of achalasia such as hypertensive LES and/or incomplete LES relaxation. Similarly, these patients may show incomplete LES opening radiographically. As a result, achalasia-type treatment such as injection of botulinum toxin and pneumatic dilation may be effective.[71] A summary of treatment options is given in Table 9-6.

Table 9-6

ALGORITHM FOR DIAGNOSIS AND TREATMENT OF DIFFUSE ESOPHAGEAL SPASM

/
DES suspected

/   /
Chest Pain   Dysphagia
/   /
Empiric course of PPI   Barium Swallow
/   /   /   /
No Response   Response   Abnormal   Normal
/   /
Incomplete opening LES   Esophageal Manometry
Other achalasia-like
features

/   /
Hypertensive LES   Normal
Incomplete relaxation

Ambulatory pH study

/   /
Normal   Abnormal   Botox   TCAs
/   Look for other
More Aggressive GERD RX   causes

/
Esophageal Manometry
/   /
Abnormal   Normal
/   /
Anticholinergics   Low-dose TCAs
(eg, hyoscyamine)
Calcium Channel Antagonists
Nitrates

NUTCRACKER ESOPHAGUS

Introduction

Nutcracker esophagus is defined by high amplitude normal peristaltic contractions. Dr. Castell and colleagues first proposed this term in 1979. By definition, the amplitude of contractions is greater than 2 standard deviations above normal, though it may not be consistently high in all swallows. It has typically been considered a variant of DES as suggested by the fact that it is the most common motility disorder of the esophagus in patients with noncardiac chest pain, accounting for 48% of cases.

Etiology

The underlying mechanism causing nutcracker esophagus is not known. However, cholinergic drugs are known to increase the amplitude of primary peristalsis. There is also some evidence that these patients may have alteration of nitric oxide metabolism similar to DES and achalasia. Endoscopic ultrasound studies demonstrate thickened muscle layers in the esophageal wall but the cause of this finding is unknown.[65] Some investigators have postulated that these forceful high amplitude contractions produce a localized esophageal ischemia and hence chest pain. As in DES, visceral hypersensitivity may exacerbate the sensation in some affected individuals.

Much criticism has been focused on nutcracker esophagus because of its non-specific nature. For example, although it is classically considered a spastic-type disorder, it may be found incidentally and is found commonly in patients with GER. As a result, it is unclear if nutcracker esophagus has several potential etiologies or merely represents an epiphenomenon or in some cases a normal variant.

Clinical Presentation

Chest pain is the predominant symptom in nutcracker esophagus that may occur spontaneously or be associated with swallowing. However, dysphagia is uncommon.

Diagnosis

Manometry is the principal method of diagnosing the nutcracker esophagus. In studies of healthy volunteers, the mean pressure of esophageal primary is 99 mmHg $\pm$ 40 mmHg to be the mean, making 180 mmHg the minimum pressure required to establish the diagnosis.[72] As a result, nutcracker esophagus is defined as greater than 80% peristaltic contractions greater than 180 mmHg. These high amplitude contractions should be confirmed at several sites along the length of the manometer, customarily at 3 and 8 cm from the LES. Contraction duration may also be longer than 6 seconds whereas in controls it is 3.9 s+0.9 s,[1] but prolonged contraction is not necessary to make the diagnosis.

Treatment

Because of the controversial clinical significance of nutcracker esophagus, the direction and efficacy of treatment is questionable. Similar to DES, first-line therapy should be for GER using twice daily PPIs. Ambulatory pH monitoring may also be helpful to either document the presence of acid reflux or further evaluate patients with lack of response to PPIs. Endoscopic evaluation of the esophagus is usually normal in these patients. If acid reflux is felt not to be a cause, therapy is also similar to DES

Table 9-7

INEFFECTIVE ESOPHAGEAL MOTILITY

- 8 to 10/10 peristaltic contractions: normal
- 6 to 7/10 peristaltic contractions: mild IEM
- 3 to 5/10 peristaltic contractions: moderate IEM
- 0 to 2/10 peristaltic contractions: severe IEM

with an emphasis on reassurance and symptomatic treatment of chest pain. Although pharmacologic agents such as calcium channel antagonists and anticholinergics can reduce amplitude of contractions to the "normal" range, this reduction has not been shown to be consistent in relieving pain, again underscoring the unclear relation between manometric findings and symptoms.[73] Some uncontrolled data in a small number of patients support the use of sildenafil in the nutcracker esophagus by promoting the action of nitric oxide although the data are limited.[74]

HYPERTENSIVE LOWER ESOPHAGEAL SPHINCTER

Patients may have high resting pressures within the LES but normal relaxation, the so-called hypertensive LES. Mean pressures by definition are greater than 45 mm.

Symptoms can be remarkably similar to disorders of LES relaxation such as achalasia including dysphagia to solids and liquids, regurgitation of undigested materials, and difficulty with belching. These patients may respond to achalasia-like treatment, including injection of botulinum toxin and pneumatic dilation. On the other hand, the finding of hypertensive LES alone is not a specific diagnosis. For example, in one report, hypertensive LES is not uncommonly seen in patients with documented GER by ambulatory pH monitoring. Thus, treatments for hypertensive LES, if necessary, will be dictated by the specific symptoms and supportive studies such as barium esophagography attending this manometric finding.

DISORDERS OF HYPOMOTILITY

Introduction, Etiology, and Definition

The disorders of esophageal motility are defined by LES hypotonicity and weak esophageal motility (Table 9-7). A hypotonic LES is defined by a manometric pressure <10 mmHg. This finding may also be suggested radiographically by a "patulous" GEJ. Many studies over decades have typically associated these findings with GER, commonly in association with a sliding hiatal hernia. Weak esophageal body motility has more recently been termed ineffective esophageal motility (IEM). Numerous investigators have referred to this concept over the years such as weakened esophageal peristalsis or failed primary peristalsis, but the term IEM was coined by Dr. Castell and colleagues in the 1990s. Manometrically, it has been described as having >2 swallows out of 10 associated with esophageal body contraction amplitudes <30 mmHg.

This is based on classic studies by Kahrilas et al,[11,60] which showed a failure of the esophageal body to propel a barium bolus when the contraction pressure is <30 mmHg. The putative cause of IEM is GER. This has been suggested from several sets of data, which include:

1. The finding and severity of gross reflux esophagitis correlates with the degree of IEM.

2. Increased acid exposure on ambulatory pH monitoring is significantly more common in IEM.

3. Improvement of IEM with surgical fundoplication for GER.

Although ostensibly convincing data, some reanalysis of the validity of IEM has occurred in recent years. This is as a result of 2 types of studies:

1. Studies showing poor correlation between the presence of IEM and the degree of acid reflux exposure on pH monitoring.

2. Studies that question the significance of IEM criteria as shown by the inaccuracy of IEM as a marker of poor esophageal motility when compared to more reliable emerging techniques for measuring esophageal function such as esophageal impedance measurements.

As a result, many investigators feel that the concept of IEM is overrated and should be redefined by a greater number of ineffective or even not normal contractions. It may also be that impedance measurements of the esophagus may altogether replace esophageal manometry as the standard test of esophageal motility.

Treatment

Treatment for IEM has focused on prevention of further injury from GERD and symptoms attributable to the dysmotility. Treatment of GER with PPIs is commonly used but there are no data showing that any treatment alters the course of IEM. Similarly, there are no studies that demonstrate that PPIs improve IEM, although there are some studies demonstrating manometric improvement with fundoplication. As a result, treatment is generally aimed at the severity of GERD as judged by other parameters (symptoms, presence of erosive esophagitis) rather than IEM alone. Some patients with IEM may complain of dysphagia secondary to slow transit through the esophagus. Again, medical therapy for GERD has not been shown to be helpful in these patients, although some patients with IEM may have some improvement of their dysphagia after fundoplication. Some investigators have tried promotility drugs effective elsewhere in the GI tract such as metoclopramide and more recently tegaserod. Unfortunately, no one has shown a clear-cut clinical benefit from these agents as of yet.

Ineffective esophageal motility may also be secondary to a systemic disease due to systemic injury to esophageal smooth muscle, the myenteric plexus, or both. The prototype disease in this situation is scleroderma. Several hypotheses have been proposed as mechanisms in the esophageal manifestations of scleroderma: collagen deposition in lamina propria and muscular layers, neuronal degeneration, spasm and vasculitis of the vaso nervorum (capillaries around nerve bodies), periaxonal collagen deposition, and even antimyenteric plexus antibodies. All of these may eventually end in atrophy and fibrosis of smooth muscle in the esophagus. Manometric hallmarks of scleroderma involving the esophagus include low LES pressure and low amplitude or absent peristalsis in the distal two thirds. Manometry is arguably more sensitive and is abnormal

Table 9-8

SECONDARY CAUSES OF INEFFECTIVE ESOPHAGEAL MOTILITY

- Scleroderma
- Hypothyroidism
- Amyloidosis
- Intestinal pseudo-obstruction
- Diabetes mellitus

in 85% to 90% of patients with scleroderma.[75] However, 40% with manometric findings are asymptomatic.[76] Radiographically, one may see a dilated atonic esophagus with a patulous LES. These patients typically have severe reflux disease resulting in erosive esophagitis, stricture formation and even Barrett's esophagus. The stasis of the severe IEM may also lead to Candida esophagitis. Treatment is aimed at controlling the acid reflux. No medical treatment aimed at the reflux, the poor motility, or the scleroderma itself has been shown to improve esophageal motility. Fundoplication is risky in these patients due to the high incidence of postoperative dysphagia.

Other systemic disorders may also cause IEM and aperistalsis of the esophageal body (Table 9-8). These include hypothyroidism, mixed connective tissue disease, rheumatoid arthritis, Raynaud's phenomenon, intestinal pseudo-obstruction, amyloidosis, diabetes mellitus and multiple sclerosis, and systemic lupus erythematosus. Treatment is aimed at the systemic disease.

References

1. Richter JE, Wu WC, Johns DN, et al. Esophageal manometry in 95 healthy volunteers. Variability of pressures with age and frequency of abnormal contractions. *Dig Dis Sci.* 1987;32:583-592.

2. Sears VW Jr, Castell JA, Castell DO. Comparison of the effects of upright versus supine body position and liquid versus solid bolus on esophageal pressures in normal humans. *Dig Dis Sci.* 1990;35:857-864.

3. Hollis JB, Castell DO. Effect of dry swallows and wet swallows of different volumes on esophageal peristalsis. *J Appl Physiol.* 1975;38:1161-1164.

4. Weisbrodt NW, Christianson J. Gradients of contractions in the opossum esophagus. *Gastroenterology.* 1972;62:1159-1166.

5. Yamato S, Saha JK, Goyal RK. Role of nitric oxide in lower esophageal sphincter relaxation to swallowing. *Life Sci.* 1992;50:1263-1272.

6. Diamant NE, El Sharkawy TY. Neural control of esophageal peristalsis. A conceptual analysis. *Gastroenterology.* 1977;72:546-556.

7. Dodds WJ, Christianson J, Dent J, et al. Pharmacologic investigation of primary peristalsis in smooth muscle portion of opossum esophagus. *Am J Physiol.* 1979;237: E561-E566.

8. Gidda JS, Boyinski JP. Swallow evoked peristalsis in opossum esophagus: role of cholinergic mechanisms. *Am J Physiol.* 1986;251:G779-G781.

9. Paterson WG, Rattan S, Goyal RK. Esophageal responses to transient and sustained esophageal distension. *Am J Physiol.* 1988;255:G587-G595.

10. Castell DO, Richter JE. *The Esophagus.* 3rd ed. Philadelphia: Lippencott, Williams, and Wilkens; 1999.

11. Kahrilas PJ, Dodds WJ, Dent J, et al. Upper esophageal sphincter function during delutition. *Gastroenterology.* 1988;95:52-62.

12. Mayberry JF. Epidemiology and demographics of achalasia. *Gastr Endosc Clin N Am.* 2001;11:235-247.

13. Lehman MB, Clark SB, Ormsby AH, Rice TW, Richter JW, Goldblum JR. Squamous mucosal alterations in esophagectomy specimens from patients with end-stage achalasia. *Am J Surg Pathol.* 2001;25:1413-1418.

14. Robertson CS, Martin BAB, Atkinson M. Varicella-zoster virus DNA in the esophageal myenteric plexus in achalasia. *Gut.* 1993;34:299-302.

15. Niwamoto H, Okamoto E, Fujimoto J, Takeuchi M, Furuyama J, Yamamoto Y. Are human herpes viruses or measles virus associated with esophageal achalasia? *Dig Dis Sci.* 1995;40(4):859-864.

16. Cassella RR, Ellis FH Jr, Brown AL Jr. Fine structure changes in achalasia of the esophagus. I. vagus nerves. *Am J Pathol.* 1965;279:46-54.

17. Casella RR, Brown AL Jr, Sayre GP, Ellis FH Jr. Achalasia of the esophagus: pathologic and etiologic considerations. *Ann Surg.* 1964;160:474-480.

18. Verne GN, Hahn AB, Pineau BC, et al. Association of LSA-DR and -DQ alleles with idiopathic achalasia. *Gastroenterology.* 1999;117:26-31.

19. Goldblum JR, Rice TW, Richter JE. Histopathologic features in esophagomyotomy specimens from patients with achalasia. *Gastroenterology.* 1996;111:648-654.

20. Erlich E, et al. Familial achalasia associated with adrenocortical insufficiency, alacrima, and neurologic dysfunction. *Am J Med Genet.* 1987;26:637-644.

21. Yang P, et al. The effect of carbonated beverages on esophageal clearance in achalasia. *Gastroenterology.* 1982;82:1215A.

22. Wong RKH, et al. Achalasia. In: Castell DO. *The Esophagus.* 3rd ed. Philadelphia: Lippincott, Williams and Wilkins; 1999:185-404.

23. Tucker HJ, Snape WJ Jr, Cohen S. Achalasia secondary to carcinoma: manometric and clinical features. *Ann Intern Med.* 1978;89:315-318.

24. Eckhart VF, Stauf B, Bernhard G. Chest pain in achalasia: patient characteristics and clinical course. *Gastroenterology.* 1999;116:1300-1304.

25. Eckhart VF. Clinical presentation and complications of achalasia. *Gastroint Endosc N Am.* 2001;11:281-292.

26. Hirano I, Tatum RP, Shi G, et al. Manometric heterogeneity in patients with idiopathic achalasia. *Gastroenterology.* 2001;120:789-798.

27. Ali GN, Hunt DR, Jorgensen JE, et al. Esophageal achalasia and coexistent upper esophageal sphincter relaxation disorder presenting with airway obstruction. *Gastroenterology.* 1995;109:1328-1332.

28. Sifirm D, Janssen J, Vantrappen G. Failing deglutitive inhibition in primary esophageal motility disorders. *Gastroenterology.* 1994;106:875-882.

29. Cohen S, Lipschutz W. Lower esophageal sphincter dysfunction in patients with achalasia. *Gastroenterology.* 1971;61:814-820.

30. Katz PO, Richter JE, Cowan R, et al. Apparent complete lower esophageal sphincter relaxation in achalasia. *Gastroenterology.* 1986;90:978-983.

31. Goldenberg SP, Burrell M, Fette GG, Vos C, Traube M. Classic and vigorous achalasia: a comparison of manometric, radiographic, and clinical findings. *Gastroenterology.* 1991;101:743-748.

32. Kostic SV, Rice TW, Baker ME, et al. Timed barium esophagogram: a simple physiologic assessment for achalasia. *J Thorac Cardiovasc Surg.* 2000;120:935-946.

33. DeOliviera JMA, Brigisson S, Doinoff C, et al. Timed barium swallow: a simple technique for evaluating esophageal emptying in patients with achalasia. *Am J Roentgenol.* 1997;169:473-479.

34. Neubrand M, Scheurlen C, Schepki M, Sauerbruch T. Long-term results and prognostic factors in the treatment of achalasia with botulinum toxin. *Endoscopy.* 2002;34:519-523.

35. Robertson CS, Fellows IW, Mayberry JF, Atkinson M. Choice of therapy for achalasia in relation to age. *Digestion.* 1988;40:244-250.

36. Khan AA, Shah SWH, Alam A, et al. Pneumatic balloon dilation in achalasia: a prospective comparison of balloon distention time. *Am J Gastroenterol.* 1998;93:1064-1067.

37. Vela MF, Richter JE. Management of achalasia at a tertiary center—a complicated disease. *Gastroenterology.* 2003;124:S1635.

38. Eckardt VF, Kanzler G, Westermeier T. Complications and their impact after pneumatic dilation for achalasia: prospective long-term follow-up study. *Gastrointest Endosc.* 1997;45:349-353.

39. Borotto E, Gaudric M, Danel B, et al. Risk factors of esophageal perforation during pneumatic dilatation for achalasia. *Gut.* 1996;39:9-12.

40. Fennerty B. Esophageal perforation during pneumatic dilatation for achalasia: a possible association with malnutrition. *Dysphagia.* 1990;5:227-228.

41. West RL, Hirsch DP, Bartelsman JFWM, et al. Long-term results of pneumatic dilation in achalasia followed for more than 5 years. *Am J Gastroenterol.* 2002;97(6):1346-1351.

42. Parkman HP, Reynolds JC, Ouyang A, et al. Pneumatic dilatation or esophagomyotomy treatment for idiopathic achalasia: clinical outcomes and cost analysis. *Dig Dis Sci.* 1993;38:75-85.

43. Penagini R, Cantu P, Mangano M, Colombo P, Bianchi PA. Long-term effects of pneumatic dilatation on symptoms and lower esophageal sphincter pressure in achalasia. *Scand J Gastroenterol.* 2002;37:380-384.

44. Eckardt VF, Aignherr C, Bernhard G. Predictors of outcome in patients with achalasia treated by pneumatic dilation. *Gastroenterology.* 1992;103:1732-1738.

45. Eckardt VF, Kanzler G, Westermeier T. Complications and their impact after pneumatic dilation for achalasia: prospective long-term follow-up study. *Gastrointest Endosc.* 1997;45:349-353.

46. Csendes A, Braghetto I, Henriques A, et al. Late results of a prospective randomized trial comparing forceful dilation and esophagomyomectomy in patients with achalasia. *Gut.* 1989;30:299-305.

47. Parischa PJ, Ravich WJ, Hendrix TR, et al. Treatment of achalasia with intrasphincteric injection of botulinum toxin. A pilot trial. *Ann Intern Med.* 1994;121:590-591.

48. Paricha PJ, Rai R, Ravich WJ. Botulinum toxin for achalasia: long-term outcome and predictor of response. *Gastroenterology.* 1996;110:1410-1415.

49. Tsai JKC. Botulinum toxin as a therapeutic agent. *Pharmacol Ther.* 1996;72:13-24.

50. Vaezi MJ, Richter JE, Wilcox CM. Botulinum toxin versus balloon dilation in the treatment of achalasia: a randomized trial. *Gut.* 1999;44:231-239.

51. Gelfand M, Rozen P, Gilat T, et al. Isosorbid dinitrate and nifedipine treatment of achalasia: a clinical, manometric, and radionuclide evaluation. *Gastroenterology.* 1982;83:963-969.

52. Becker BS, Burakoff R. The effect of verapamil on the lower esophageal sphincter in normal subjects and in achalasia. *Am J Gastroenterol.* 1983;78:773-776.

53. Triadafilopoulos G, Aaronson M, Sackel S, et al. Medical treatment of esophageal achalasia: double blind crossover study with oral nifedipine, verapamil, and placebo. *Dig Dis Sci.* 1991;36:260-267.

54. Bortolloti M. Medical therapy for achalasia. A benefit reserved for few. *Digestion.* 1999;60:11-16.

55. Brossard E, Ollyo JB, Fontolliet C, et al. Achalasia and squamous cell carcinoma of the esophagus: is an endoscopic surveillance justified? *Gastroenterology.* 1992;102: A4.

56. Meijssen MAC, Tilanus HW, van Blankenstein M, Hop SCJ, Ong GL. Achalasia complicated by esophageal squamous cell carcinoma: a prospective study of 195 patients. *Gut.* 1992;33:155-158.

57. Just-Viera JO, Haight C. Achalasia and carcinoma of the esophagus. *Surg Gynecol Obstet.* 1969;128:1081-1095.

58. Kahrilas PJ, Kishk SM, Helm JF, et al. Comparison of pseudoachalasia and achalasia. *Am J Med.* 1987;82:439-446.

59. Tracey JP, Truabe M. Difficulties in the diagnosis of pseudoachalasia. *Am J Gastroenterol.* 1994;89:2014-2018.

60. Rozman RW, Achkar E. Features distinguishing secondary achalasia from primary achalasia. *Am J Gastroenterol.* 1990;85:1327-1330.

61. Deviere J. Dunham F, Rickaert F, et al. Endoscopic ultrasonography in achalasia. *Gastroenterology.* 1989;96:1210-1213.

62. Murray JA, Ledlow A, Launspach J, et al. The effects of recombinant human hemoglobin on esophageal motor function in humans. *Gastroenterology.* 1995;109:1241-1248.

63. Konturek JW, Gillessen A, Domschke W. Diffuse esophageal spasm: a malfunction that involves nitric oxide? *Scand J Gastroenterol.* 1995;30:1041-1045.

64. Richter JE, Hackshaw BT, Wu WC et al. Edrophonium: a useful provocative test for esophageal chest pain. *Ann Intern Med.* 1985;103:14-21.

65. Goyal R. In: Wilson and Bruanwald, eds. *Harrison's Principals of Internal Medicine.* 14th ed. New York: Mcgraw Hill and Co; 1999:1592.

66. Orlando RC, Bozymski EM. Clinical and manometric effects of nitroglycerin in diffuse esophageal spasm. *N Engl J Med.* 1973;289:23-25.

67. Hongo M, Traube M, McCallum RW. Comparison of effects of nifedipine, propantheline bromide, and the combination on esophageal motor function in normal volunteers. *Dig Dis Sci.* 1984;29:300-304.

68. Davies HA, Lewis MJ, Rhoads J, et al. Trial of nifedipine for prevention of esophageal spasm. *Digestion.* 1987;36:81-83.

69. Clouse RE, Lustman PJ, Eckert TC, et al. Low dose trazodone for symptomatic patients with esophageal contraction abnormalities. a double blind, placebo controlled trial. *Gastroenterology.* 1987;92:1027-1036.

70. Cannon RO 3rd, Quyyumi AA, Mincemoyer R, et al. Imipramine in patients with chest pain despite normal coronary angiograms. *N Engl J Med.* 1994;330:1411-1417.

71. Ebert EC, Ouyang A, Wright SH, et al. Pneumatic dilation in patients with symptomatic diffuse esophageal spasm and lower esophageal sphincter dysfunction. *Dig Dis Sci.* 1983;28:481-485.

72. Achem SR, Benjamin SB. Esophageal dysmotility. In: Castell DO, ed. *The Esophagus.* 2nd ed. Boston, Mass: Little, Brown; 1995:247-268.

73. Richter JE, Dalton C, Bradley L, et al. Oral nifedipine in the treatment of noncardiac chest pain in patients with the nutcracker esophagus. *Gastroenterology.* 1987;93:21-28.

74. Eherer AJ, Schwetz I, Hammer HF, et al. Effect of sildenafil on esophageal motor function in healthy subjects and in patients with esophageal motility disorders. *Gut.* 2002;50:758-764.

75. Weihrauch TR, Korting GW. Manometric assessment of esophageal involvement in progressive systemic sclerosis, morphea, and Raynaud's disease. *Br J Dermatol.* 1982;107:325.

76. Cohen S, Lauffer I, Snape WJ, et al. The gastrointestinal manifestations of scleroderma: pathogenesis and management. *Gastroenterology.* 1980;79:155.

Unexplained (Noncardiac) Chest Pain

Ronnie Fass, MD, FACP, FACG and Ram Dickman, MD

Introduction

Unexplained chest pain (UCP) is very common in the general population. However, epidemiological studies describing the demographics, ethnic, gender, or age predilections and distribution of potential risk factors are still scarce in UCP. Furthermore, it has yet to be determined if most patients diagnosed with UCP are treated by a cardiologist, primary care physician, or gastroenterologist for further work-up. Regardless, UCP has attracted much attention in the past 2 decades due to the complexity of the underlying mechanisms for patients' symptoms and the recognition that GERD is an important contributing factor for esophageal-related UCP.

Other terms have been used to describe UCP, including irritable esophagus, functional chest pain, and chest pain of undetermined origin. The Rome II Committee for functional esophageal disorders made a distinction between UCP due to GERD and/or esophageal dysmotility and UCP without clearly identified esophageal abnormality.[1] The latter group has been termed functional chest pain of presumed esophageal origin. Abnormalities in sensory perception, centrally or peripherally, have been documented in this challenging group of patients. While PPIs have revolutionized the diagnostic and therapeutic approach to UCP, medical therapy in a significant minority has focused primarily on pain modulators.

History and Clinical Presentation

UCP patients may report squeezing or burning substernal chest pain, which may radiate to the back, neck, arms, and jaws and is indistinguishable from cardiac-related chest pain. This is compounded by the fact that patients with a history of coronary artery disease may also experience UCP. Consequently, UCP patients should first be evaluated by a cardiologist to exclude cardiac angina.[2,3]

When taking a medical history, retrosternal chest discomfort; pressure or heaviness that lasts several minutes; pain induced by exertion, emotion, exposure to cold, or a large meal; and pain that is relieved by rest or nitroglycerin usually signify typical cardiac angina. Any two of these clinical characteristics are suggestive of atypical cardiac angina, and only one or none of these characteristics is indicative of UCP.

Only 15% to 34% of ambulatory patients who present with chest pain are ultimately diagnosed with coronary artery disease.[4] In contrast, only 26% of the patients thought to have chest pain due to coronary artery disease have a normal coronary angiogram.[5] Additionally, up to 25% of the patients defined as having "atypical chest pain" were found to have an abnormal angiogram.[5] Therefore, all patients who present with chest pain, regardless of its character, should undergo a proper cardiac evaluation before being referred to a gastroenterologist for further work-up.

Heartburn and acid regurgitation, which are classic symptoms of GERD, may be encountered in 10% to 70% of the patients with GERD-related UCP.[6] These patients often report chest pain provoked by recumbency or meals and relieved by antireflux treatment.[7] The wide range in the prevalence of GERD-related symptoms represents different patient populations evaluated. However, many studies reported that most patients presenting with GERD-related UCP lacked classic symptoms of GERD.

Studies that endoscopically evaluated patients with UCP revealed a very low incidence of esophageal mucosal injury, such as erosive esophagitis, peptic stricture, ulceration, Barrett's esophagus, or adenocarcinoma of the esophagus.[8-10] Consequently, endoscopic screening of UCP patients without reported alarm symptoms is a very low-yield procedure.

The impact of UCP on patients' quality of life is likely to match other functional GI disorders, such as IBS. As with other functional bowel disorders, the prognosis of patients with UCP is favorable. Nevertheless, the natural history of UCP in most patients is characterized by the persistence of symptoms, repeated clinic visits or hospital admissions, chronic use of medications, repeated cardiac catheterizations, interruptions to daily activities, and impaired quality of life.

Epidemiology

There are only a few studies that have evaluated the prevalence of UCP in the general population. The mean annual prevalence of UCP in 6 population-based studies was approximately 25%. However, these studies differ in many aspects, such as UCP definition, geography, sample size, sampling order, and ethnic disparities.[4] A population-based survey in the United States assessed the prevalence of GERD in Olmsted County, Minn[11] and reported an overall UCP prevalence of 23%. Unlike other functional GI disorders, gender distribution was similar (24% among males and 22% among females). Drossman et al[12] reported a prevalence of 13.6% in 8250 households in the United States, using the Rome criteria for functional GI disorders. In this study, functional chest pain of presumed esophageal origin was diagnosed rather than UCP. Eslick et al have recently evaluated the prevalence of UCP in Australia by using a mailing of a validated Chest Pain Questionnaire (CPQ) to 1000 randomly selected individuals.[13,14] The study demonstrated a prevalence rate of 33% with almost equal gender distribution (32% in males versus 33% in females). This study also showed that the population prevalence of UCP decreases with increasing age.[13,14] Presently, chest pain is the second most common presentation to hospital emergency departments; however, only 25% of the individuals who experience chest pain actually present to a hospital.[15]

Thus far, it still remains to be elucidated what factors drive UCP patients to seek medical attention and whether the health care-seeking behavior of these patients differs from the health care-seeking behavior of patients with cardiac-related chest pain. Tew et al[16] reported that patients with UCP were younger, consumed greater amounts of alcohol, smoked more, and were more likely to suffer from a psychiatric disorder (anxiety) than their counterparts with ischemic heart disease. These patients continued to seek treatment on a regular basis after diagnosis for both chest pain and other unrelated symptoms. In another study, almost 25% of individuals with UCP had sought health care for chest pain within the previous 12 months. None of the GI (heartburn, dysphagia, acid regurgitation) or psychological (anxiety, depression, neuroticism) risk factors were significantly associated with consultation for UCP.[14]

In general, the prevalence of UCP decreases with increasing age. Females under 25 years of age and those between 45 and 55 years of age were found to have the highest prevalence rates.[14] Kennedy et al[17] reported that females are more likely to present to a hospital emergency department with UCP than males. UCP patients in Asia are more likely than UCP patients in Europe to seek medical care for chest pain. In the United States, African Americans are less likely to report chest pain symptoms than Caucasians.[18]

A recent study by Eslick et al reported that 78% of the patients who presented to a hospital emergency department with acute chest pain had seen a health care provider in the past 12 months.[18] The most common health care provider seen was a general practitioner (85%), followed by a cardiologist (74%), gastroenterologist (30%), pulmonologist (14%), alternative therapist (8%), and psychologist (10%).[18] A multiple logistic regression analysis revealed that patients with chest pain who are also suffering heartburn were 16 times more likely to see a general practitioner (OR 16.40, 95% CI 1.98 to 135.99) and 3 times more likely to consult a gastroenterologist (OR 3.10, 95% CI 1.26 to 7.62). Additionally, work absenteeism rates because of unexplained chest pain were high (29%) as were interruptions to daily activities (63%).[18]

Many patients with UCP report poor quality of life and admit taking cardiac medications despite lack of evidence for a cardiac cause. Only a small fraction of patients feel reassured. Consequently, the economic burden of the disease takes a significant toll on the health care system. In one study, the health care cost for UCP was estimated at over $315 million annually, primarily because of multiple clinic visits, emergency room visits, hospitalizations, and prescription medications.[19] This cost estimate does not include indirect costs such as lost days of work or the impact of symptoms on patients' quality of life, which have been demonstrated to be more significant when evaluating the economic burden of functional bowel disorders. In Australia, the annual costs associated with UCP presentations to the Nepean Hospital amount to approximately $1.4 million.[20] The researchers extrapolated these costs to the Australian health care system and conservatively estimated that UCP accounts for at least $30 million of the health care budget annually.

Pathogenesis

INTRODUCTION

The pathophysiology of UCP remains to be fully elucidated. Identified underlying mechanisms are diverse and often overlap. GERD is by far the most common cause

---

Table 10-1

THE DIFFERENT PROPOSED UNDERLYING MECHANISMS OF UNEXPLAINED CHEST PAIN

- GER
- Esophageal dysmotility
- Abnormal mechano-physical properties
  - * Hyperactive
  - * ↓ compliance
- Sustained longitudinal muscle contractions
- Visceral hypersensitivity due to altered central or peripheral processing of visceral stimuli
- Altered autonomic activity
- Psychological abnormalities
  - * Panic attack
  - * Anxiety
  - * Depression

---

of UCP. Other etiological factors that have been proposed include esophageal motility disorders, abnormal mechanophysical properties of the esophagus, sustained longitudinal muscle contractions, visceral hypersensitivity due to altered central or peripheral processing of intraesophageal stimuli, altered autonomic activity, and psychological comorbidity (Table 10-1). While some of the proposed underlying mechanisms have been well substantiated, others suffer from paucity of data demonstrating clear causality.

GASTROESOPHAGEAL REFLUX DISEASE

GERD has been reported to be the most common underlying mechanism for UCP. Between 25% and 60% of the patients with UCP have demonstrated abnormal 24-hour esophageal pH monitoring and/or positive upper endoscopy findings. Typical GERD symptoms (ie, heartburn and acid regurgitation) were found to be significantly and independently associated with the presence of UCP. Locke et al[11] demonstrated that UCP was reported more often by patients experiencing frequent heartburn symptoms (at least once a week) as compared to those with infrequent heartburn symptoms (less than once a week) and individuals reporting no GERD symptoms. Eslick et al[13] performed a population-based study to determine the prevalence of UCP. The authors found that among subjects with UCP, 53% experienced heartburn and 58% experienced acid regurgitation.

The finding of esophageal erosions on upper endoscopy in patients with GERD-related UCP has been reported to range between 10% and 70%.[21,22] The different patient populations evaluated can explain the wide range of the results.

Abnormal ambulatory 24-hour esophageal pH monitoring is demonstrated in approximately 50% of the patients with UCP. Fass et al[23] reported that 41.1% of 37 patients with UCP had abnormal pH test. Beedassy et al[24] evaluated 104 patients with UCP and reported that 48% had an abnormal pH test. Of the total number of patients in the study, 52 reported chest pain during the pH study, but only 23 (44%) had an abnormal pH test. In this group of UCP patients, only 21% reported chest pain that coincided with an abnormal pH test.

Positive (>50%) symptom index (SI) (percentage of symptoms associated with acid reflux events) in UCP patients with normal pH test has been considered indicative of GERD as the underlying cause for patients' symptoms. Beedassy et al[24] showed that patients with a positive GER were significantly more likely to have an abnormal pH test. Of the 52 patients with chest pain, only 10 had a positive GER. Of those, 80% had an abnormal pH study as compared with 36% of the patients with a negative GER. However, Dekel et al[25] found that a positive GER is a relatively uncommon phenomenon in UCP patients regardless of whether GERD is present or absent. This is primarily due to lack of reported chest pain symptoms during the pH study.

While studies have shown a high association between UCP and GERD, the mere presence of esophageal inflammation (erosive esophagitis) or abnormal acid exposure suggests association only. In contrast, improvement of chest pain symptoms as a result of antireflux treatment supports causality. Studies have demonstrated that up to 80% of UCP patients with either erosive esophagitis or abnormal pH testing responded to potent antireflux treatment.[21,26] Consequently, in the presence of esophageal mucosal injury and/or abnormal esophageal acid exposure, it is highly likely that GERD is the underlying cause of patients' symptoms.

In a subgroup of patients with cardiac-related chest pain, acid exposure may play a role in triggering cardiac angina. Both organs share similar sensory innervation. Additionally, acid exposure may reduce coronary blood flow as shown by Chauhan et al.[27] In this study, the investigators evaluated patients with syndrome X (negative coronary angiogram but positive stress test) and demonstrated that acidification of the distal esophagus significantly reduced the coronary blood flow, resulting in reports of angina.

Acid has also been demonstrated to sensitize esophageal sensory afferents to subsequent mechanical stimuli, such as intraesophageal balloon distension. Further discussion of this topic is presented in the visceral hypersensitivity section.

ESOPHAGEAL DYSMOTILITY

In UCP patients who lack any evidence of GERD, esophageal dysmotility is commonly entertained as the underlying cause. However, the role of esophageal motility abnormalities in non-GERD-related UCP remains to be elucidated. This is primarily due to lack of any relationship between documentation of esophageal dysmotility on manometry and concomitant reports of chest pain. Furthermore, chest pain may be markedly reduced in the absence of any improvement in patients' esophageal motor disorder.

Only 28% of the patients with non-GERD-related UCP who underwent esophageal manometry at a tertiary referral center with a major interest in esophageal motility were found to have an esophageal motility disorder.[28] Similarly, by using the Clinical Outcomes Research Initiative (CORI) database, Dekel et al[29] evaluated

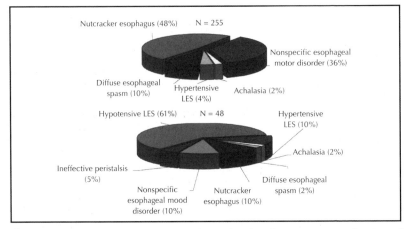

Figure 10-1. Distribution of esophageal dysmotility disorders in patients with UCP and abnormal esophageal manometry.

160 UCP subjects from academic, private, and veterans administration (VA) medical centers and demonstrated that only 30% of the patients with UCP had an abnormal esophageal manometry.

The distribution of esophageal motility disorders in patients presenting with non-GERD-related UCP has been scarcely studied. Figure 10-1 summarizes the 2 currently available studies that assessed distribution of esophageal motility abnormalities among patients with UCP. In the study by Dekel et al,[29] the most common identified motor disorder was hypotensive LES (61%) followed by hypertensive LES, nonspecific esophageal motility disorder (NEMD), and nutcracker esophagus (10% each). It is likely that more patients with GERD ended up in Dekel et al's study due to the higher prevalence rate of hypotensive LES. In contrast, Katz et al[28] reported that the most common motor disorders encountered in patients with non-GERD-related UCP was nutcracker esophagus, followed by NEMDs, diffuse esophageal spasm, hypertensive LES, and achalasia. Regardless, all studies have demonstrated that two thirds of the patients with non-GERD-related UCP have normal esophageal motility.

Overall, the finding of a high prevalence of nutcracker esophagus in UCP patients is common and highly intriguing. Nutcracker esophagus, which is manometrically defined as high-amplitude contractions in the distal esophagus (>180 mmHg) in the presence of a normally functioning LES, remains an area of intense controversy. Investigators have long argued about the clinical relevance of such a manometric phenomenon.[30] However, Achem et al reported that most patients with chest pain associated with nutcracker esophagus responded symptomatically to anti-reflux treatment.[31] Normalization of the nutcracker motility phenomenon was documented only in a minority of the patients, suggesting that GERD was the likely cause of their symptoms rather than the high amplitude contractions in the distal esophagus. Therefore, esophageal motor disorders per se may not be the direct cause of patients' symptoms but may in fact serve as a surrogate marker for esophageal abnormality that is presently poorly understood.[32] Alternatively, esophageal motor disorder in UCP (except achalasia) may have no etiological role in symptom generation and thus should not be pursued diagnostically and therapeutically.

VISCERAL HYPERSENSITIVITY

The mechanisms of pain in patients with non-GERD-related UCP are not fully understood. Numerous studies that focused primarily on this group of patients have consistently documented alteration in pain perception regardless of whether esophageal dysmotility was present. The underlying mechanisms for esophageal hypersensitivity in patients with UCP remain an area of intense research. Peripheral and central sensitization of esophageal sensory afferents and spinal cord neurons has been suggested to result in heightened responses to innocuous and noxious intraesophageal stimuli.[33,34] It has been postulated that inflammation or other injuries to the esophageal mucosa sets off a cascade of events that leads to upregulation of receptors, which in turn induces the development of visceral hypersensitivity through peripheral and central sensitization.[34] The presence of esophageal hypersensitivity can be demonstrated long after the original stimulus has disappeared and the mucosa has healed. It is still unclear what factors determine the long-term persistence of esophageal hypersensitivity.

Acute tissue irritation on visceral afferent pathways has been well characterized in the form of peripheral and central sensitization.[24] Such sensitization manifests as increased background activity of sensory neurons, the lowering of nociceptive thresholds, changes in stimulus response curves, and enlargements of receptive fields. During a noxious event, a series of counter-regulatory mechanisms are activated that are aimed at containing the development of both the acute and any long-lasting sensitization.[24]

Peripheral sensitization involves the reduction of esophageal pain threshold and an increase in the transduction processes of primary afferent neurons.[35] Esophageal tissue injury, inflammation, spasm, or just repetitive mechanical stimulation can sensitize peripheral afferent nerves.

Several seminal studies performed during the mid-1980s were the first to demonstrate that patients with non-GERD-related UCP demonstrate lower perception thresholds for pain. In the first study, a balloon was positioned 10 cm above the LES and distended in a stepwise fashion using a handheld syringe. When air was injected (within 2 seconds) in 1-mL increments to a maximum of 10 mL into the balloon attached to a manometry catheter, patients with UCP were more likely to experience pain (18 of 30) than were normal control subjects (6 of 30).[36] In this study, the intraesophageal volume at the onset of pain also distinguished patients from control subjects, with chest pain patients experiencing pain at balloon volumes of less than 8 mL and the few control subjects experiencing pain at volumes of 9 mL or more. A second report evaluating 50 patients with UCP and 30 healthy volunteers found that 28 (56%) had their "typical" chest pain during balloon inflation as compared to 6 (20%) of the normal controls. Again, most of these patients (24 of 28) had their pain at volumes less than 8 mL.[37] Presence of abnormal motility did not predict a positive test result. When intraballoon pressures were used as a measure of esophageal wall tone, no difference between control subjects and UCP patients were noted.

Rao et al used impedance planimetry, which consists of a probe with 4 ring electrodes, 3 pressure sensors, and a balloon, to evaluate 24 consecutive patients and

12 healthy controls.[38] Stepwise balloon distensions demonstrated lower perception thresholds for first sensation, moderate discomfort, and pain in UCP patients as compared to normal controls. Typical chest pain was reproduced in 83% of the UCP patients. In UCP patients, the reactivity of the esophagus to balloon distension was greater, the pressure elastic modulus was higher, and the tension-strain association showed that the esophageal wall was less distensible.

Rao et al[39] also performed graded balloon distensions of the esophagus using impedance planimetry in 16 consecutive patients with UCP (normal esophageal evaluation) and 13 healthy control subjects. Patients who experienced chest pain during the balloon distension were subsequently restudied after receiving IV atropine. Balloon distensions reproduced chest pain at lower sensory thresholds than controls in most UCP subjects. Similar findings were documented after atropine administration despite a relaxed and more deformable esophageal wall. Thus, the investigators concluded that hyperalgesia, rather than motor dysfunction, is the predominant mechanism for functional chest pain.

Sarkar et al[40] recruited 19 healthy volunteers and seven patients with UCP. Hydrochloric acid was infused into the distal esophagus during a period of 30 minutes. Sensory responses to electrical stimulation were monitored within the acid-exposed distal esophagus and the nonexposed proximal esophagus both before and after infusion. In the healthy subjects, acid infusion into the distal esophagus lowered the pain threshold in the upper esophagus. Patients with UCP already had a lower resting esophageal pain threshold than healthy subjects. After acid perfusion, their pain threshold in the proximal esophagus fell further and for a longer duration than was the case for the healthy subjects. Additionally, there was a decrease in pain threshold after the acid infusion in the anterior chest wall. This study demonstrated the development of secondary allodynia (ie, visceral hypersensitivity to innocuous stimulus in normal tissue that is in proximity to the site of tissue injury) in the proximal esophagus by repeated acid exposure of the distal esophagus. Most likely, the concurrent visceral and somatic pain hypersensitivity is caused by central sensitization (increase in excitability of spinal cord neurons induced by activation of nociceptive C-fibers in the area of tissue injury). The patients with UCP demonstrated both visceral hypersensitivity and amplified secondary allodynia in the esophagus. However, it is unclear from the study what mechanism is responsible for the exaggerated secondary allodynia and what initiates central sensitization in patients with UCP. It is interesting to note that other studies on UCP,[24] using a similar human model of acute tissue irritation by acid infusion, showed no significant effect on pain thresholds.

In one study,[41] healthy subjects underwent perfusion of the distal esophagus with either normal saline or 0.1 N hydrochloric acid. Subsequently, perceptual responses to intraluminal esophageal balloon distension using electronic barostat were evaluated. As compared with saline, acid perfusion reduced the perception threshold (innocuous sensation) and tended to reduce the pain threshold (aversive sensation). This study demonstrated short-term sensitization of mechanosensitive afferent pathways by transient exposure to acid. The authors suggested that in patients with UCP, acid reflux induces sensitization of the esophagus that may subsequently alter the way in which the esophagus perceives otherwise normal esophageal distensions.

Abnormal cerebral processing of esophageal stimuli in patients with UCP has been shown in a study of 12 healthy subjects and 8 patients with UCP.[33] The aim of the study was to compare cortical-evoked potentials and power spectrum analysis of heart rate variability during electrical esophageal stimulation in patients with UCP and healthy subjects. Cortical-evoked potentials were recorded using 22 standard electro-encephalogram scalp electrodes. Patients with UCP perceived lower intensities during electrical esophageal stimulation than did healthy subjects, which was associated with a greater cardiovagal reflex response and decreased sympathetic outflow. Because the cortical-evoked potentials in response to electrical esophageal stimulation were smaller in patients with UCP than in healthy subjects, the authors suggested that the increased perception of esophageal stimuli may result from enhanced cerebral processing of visceral sensory input in patients with UCP, rather than from hyperalgesic responses in visceral afferent pathways.

Several studies have documented altered autonomic function in patients with UCP. In a recent study, Tougas et al[42] assessed autonomic activity using power spectral analysis of heart rate variability before and during esophageal acidification of patients with UCP and matched healthy control subjects. Of the patients with UCP, 68% were considered acid sensitive (ie, they developed angina-like symptoms during esophageal acidification). The acid-sensitive patients had a higher baseline heart rate and lower baseline vagal activity than acid-insensitive patients. During acid infusion, vagal cardiac outflow increased in acid-sensitive but not in acid-insensitive patients. The same investigators have already documented an increase in vagal activity in patients with UCP during other intraesophageal stimuli (mechanical and electrical). The role that altered autonomic function plays in the pathogenesis of UCP remains speculative. As has been stated by Tougas,[43] in most cases in which both central and autonomic factors are involved, it is the effect of the former that most likely leads to the occurrence of the latter.

In addition to cortical-evoked potentials, other techniques have been increasingly used to evaluate the brain-gut relationship in patients with esophageal disorders, including those with UCP. These techniques include positron emission tomography (PET) and functional magnetic resonance imaging (fMRI). The GI tract is intricately connected to the CNS by pathways that are continuously sampling and modulating gut function.[44]

PET scanning is an established method to study the functional neuroanatomy of the human brain.[45,46] Radio-labeled compounds allow the study of biochemical and physiologic processes involved in cerebral metabolism.[44] Tomographic images represent spatial distribution of radioisotopes in the brain. Regional cerebral blood flow is studied with labeled water ($H_2$15O) and glucose metabolism with 18Fl-labeled fluorodeoxyglucose. Unlike PET, fMRI does not require radioisotopes and hence is considered a safer imaging technique. fMRI detects increases in oxygen concentration in areas of heightened neuronal activity.[46-48] This imaging technique is best suited for locating the site but not the sequence or duration of neuronal activity. Overall, fMRI provides both anatomic and functional information.

Thus far, only a few studies have attempted to assess the cortical process of esophageal sensation in humans. Aziz and colleagues examined the human brain loci involved in the process of esophageal sensation using PET and distal esophageal balloon distension in 8 healthy volunteers.[49] Nonpainful stimuli elicited bilateral activation along the central sulcus, insular cortex, and the frontal and parietal operculum. Painful stimuli resulted in intense activation of the same areas and additional activation of the right anterior insular cortex and anterior cingulated gyrus. The former is important in affective processing while the latter is important in pain processing and generating an affective and cognitive response to pain.[50-52]

Further studies are needed to assess cerebral activation in patients with different esophageal disorders. In addition, it would be of great interest to determine whether there are differences in central processing of an intraesophageal stimulus in patients with UCP. It is also important to begin to examine the role of psychophysiologic states such as stress, anxiety, and depression and their effects on central nuclei involved with perception of esophageal stimuli.

PSYCHOLOGICAL COMORBIDITY

The prevalence of psychiatric disorders in UCP appears to be high but has not been fully elucidated. As with other functional bowel disorders, psychological comorbidity is common in patients with UCP. It has been estimated that 17% to 43% of patients with UCP suffer from some type of psychological abnormality, primarily anxiety, depression, panic disorder, and hypochondriasis.[53] Song et al[54] evaluated the psychological profiles of 113 patients with chest pain and a variety of esophageal motility abnormalities, 23 symptomatic control subjects (similar symptoms but without esophageal motility abnormalities), and 27 asymptomatic control subjects. All participants were assessed by the Beck Depression Inventory, Spielberger State-Trait Anxiety Inventory, and the Psychosomatic Symptom Checklist. Symptomatic patients with esophageal dysmotility (hypertensive lower esophageal sphincter, nutcracker esophagus, or hypotensive contractions) exhibited increased prevalence of somatization, anxiety, and depression.

Among all esophageal symptoms, chest pain was shown to closely correlate with psychometric abnormalities. In some patients, chest pain is part of a host of symptoms that characterize panic attack.[15] Panic attack is a common cause for emergency room visits due to chest pain. In a large study that encompassed 441 consecutive ambulatory patients presenting with chest pain to the emergency department of a heart center, 25% were diagnosed as suffering from a panic attack.[55] While the reason for the observed association between UCP and panic disorder is not currently fully understood, hyperventilation was demonstrated to precipitate chest pain in 15% of the patients with UCP.[56] Additionally, it was demonstrated that hyperventilation could provoke reversible esophageal manometric abnormalities such as esophageal spasm (4%) and nonspecific esophageal motor disorder (22%).[56] Furthermore, studies have demonstrated that hyperventilation may precipitate a panic attack.[57]

Anxiety and depression influence reports of pain and thus contribute to the pathophysiology of UCP. Lantinga et al[58] found that patients with UCP had higher levels of neuroticism and psychiatric comorbidity before and after cardiac catheterization than did patients with coronary artery disease. This finding appears to have prognostic significance because these patients display less improvement in pain, more frequent pain episodes, greater social maladjustment, and more anxiety at 1-year follow-up than individuals with relatively low initial levels of psychosocial disturbances. In a large epidemiological study from England, a significant relationship between UCP and psychiatric disorders was demonstrated in young adults.[59] Two independent variables were associated with chest pain: parental illness and fatigue during childhood.[60]

Table 10-2

DIAGNOSTIC TESTS FOR UNEXPLAINED CHEST PAIN

- Gastroesophageal reflux
  * Acid perfusion test (Bernstein test)
  * Ambulatory 24-hour esophageal pH monitoring
  * Barium Swallow
  * PPI test
  * Upper endoscopy
- Esophageal dysmotility
  * Esophageal manometry
  * Edrophonium (Tensilon) test
  * Ergonovine test
- Visceral hypersensitivity
  * Acid perfusion test (Bernstein test)
  * Balloon distension test

Diagnosis

OVERVIEW

Symptoms of UCP patients are clinically indistinguishable from those of cardiac angina patients. Consequently, the burden of making the diagnosis of UCP is currently placed on the cardiologist. Once cardiac cause has been excluded, patients are often referred to a gastroenterologist for further evaluation because the esophagus is one of the most common causes of symptoms in patients with UCP. Other non-esophageal-related abnormalities should be entertained, such as chest wall and other musculoskeletal disorders, pulmonary/pleuritic abnormalities, panic disorder, gastric and biliary diseases, as well as others.

Different tests are currently available to assess patients with UCP (Table 10-2). Essentially, the tests are designed primarily to evaluate for GER, esophageal dysmotility, and visceral hypersensitivity as the potential underlying mechanisms for symptoms.

While GERD is by far the most common underlying esophageal cause for UCP, currently there is no gold standard for diagnosing this disorder. The diagnostic tests available for GERD in patients with UCP include barium esophagogram, upper endoscopy, the acid perfusion test, ambulatory 24-hour esophageal pH monitoring, and the PPI test. The recent introduction of the PPI test has gained general popularity because of its simplicity, reduced cost, and availability at the primary care level. Additionally, the PPI test is highly sensitive and specific and, unlike the other tests for UCP, noninvasive. In patients who failed the PPI test or empirical therapy, pH testing on therapy has been suggested. However, a recent study has questioned the usage of the pH test in these patients because of the low likelihood of having a positive test on high-dose PPI.[61] The role of esophageal manometry has been limited in recent years to solely diagnose achalasia. This is primarily due to lack of association between patients documented with spastic motility disorders and chest pain symptoms. Furthermore, studies have consistently demonstrated that in patients with esophageal motility disorders (except achalasia) pain modulators are more effective in controlling symptoms than therapies directed toward the motility abnormality.

DIAGNOSTIC TOOLS FOR GASTROESOPHAGEAL REFLUX DISEASE-RELATED UNEXPLAINED CHEST PAIN

Barium Esophagogram

Barium esophagogram has a very low sensitivity (20%) for diagnosing GERD-related UCP due to lack of anatomical and mucosal abnormalities in most of these patients.[62] Furthermore, the significance of barium reflux during the procedure as diagnostic of GERD is questionable. Johnston et al[63] found that the proportion of patients with spontaneous barium reflux and abnormal pH test is similar to controls with normal 24-hour esophageal pH monitoring. Furthermore, spontaneous barium reflux has also been demonstrated in up to 20% of healthy subjects.[64] The role of barium esophagogram in patients with GERD-related UCP is likely limited to those with additional dysphagia. In these patients, barium esophagogram may be ordered as the first diagnostic test in order to serve as a "road map" for future upper endoscopy.

Upper Endoscopy

Upper endoscopy is the most accurate diagnostic tool for esophageal mucosal involvement in GERD-related UCP. It is the gold standard for diagnosing erosive esophagitis, stricture, ulcer, and Barrett's esophagus. In patients with UCP and alarm symptoms (weight loss, dysphagia, vomiting, anemia), upper endoscopy should be considered the initial evaluative test to exclude malignancy as well as other mucosal disorders of the upper gut. However, because of the low prevalence of esophageal mucosal injury in UCP, this modality has been considered noncontributory as the initial diagnostic test in UCP.[63] Some authors have even proposed that endoscopy has no role in the diagnostic algorithm of patients with UCP.[64] Interestingly, despite the limited clinical value, community-based gastroenterologists still commonly use endoscopy as the initial diagnostic test in UCP regardless of whether alarm symptoms are reported.[22]

Ambulatory 24-Hour Esophageal pH Monitoring

Ambulatory 24-hour esophageal pH monitoring with symptom correlation is commonly used to diagnose GERD-related UCP.[65] In GERD patients, the sensitivity of this test ranges from 60% to 96%, and the specificity from 85% to 100%.[64] It has been estimated that up to 60% of UCP patients have a pathological acid reflux and a positive GER or a positive GER alone. SI is the percentage of symptoms that correlate with acid reflux events. Hewson et al[65] examined 100 consecutive patients with UCP and detected abnormal esophageal acid exposure in 48 patients (48%). Of the 83 patients with spontaneous chest pain during the pH test, 37 patients (46%) had abnormal reflux parameters and 50 patients (60%) had a positive GER. The authors concluded that 24-hour esophageal pH testing with positive SI is the single best test for evaluating patients with GERD-related UCP.[65] In contrast, Dekel et al[26] found that only a minority of UCP patients experience chest pain during the pH study, and consequently, positive GER is a relatively uncommon phenomenon (19% in GERD-related UCP and 10.6% in non-GERD-related UCP).

The pH test is invasive, costly, inconvenient to most patients, and unavailable for many physicians. Additionally, there are no studies that assessed the sensitivity of the test in UCP patients. A wireless system for pH monitoring was recently introduced into the market. It involves the perioral or transnasal insertion of a radiotelemetry pH capsule and the attachment onto the esophageal mucosa. The pH capsule simultaneously measures pH and transmits recorded data to a pager-size receiver clipped onto the patient's belt, thereby circumventing the need for a nasally-placed catheter, which is uncomfortable for many patients. In comparison with the conventional pH test, the wireless pH monitoring is well tolerated.[66] The wireless pH system may prove to be helpful in further clarifying the extent of GERD in UCP and in better determining the relationship between chest pain symptoms and acid reflux events. Recently, Prakash et al[62] demonstrated that by extending the pH recording period to 48 hours with the wireless pH system in patients with UCP, there was an increase in the number of chest pains reported, resulting in better assessment of the relationship between symptoms and acid reflux events.

Since the introduction of the PPI test, the role of pH testing in UCP has significantly diminished. Unlike the pH test, the PPI test is noninvasive, simple, convenient, readily available, and less costly. Additionally, studies have suggested that the sensitivity of the PPI test is similar to the sensitivity of the pH test.[8]

Acid Perfusion Test (Bernstein Test)

The acid perfusion test was introduced as an objective method to identify esophageal chemosensitivity to acid.[67] The test was originally devised to distinguish between chest pain of cardiac and esophageal origin. However, since the initial description, many modifications have been made to the original Bernstein test. Although the basic principle of the test remained similar, many investigators have tried different acid perfusion rates, concentrations, and durations in the hope of increasing the sensitivity of the test. Furthermore, some have even suggested the addition of bile salts to the acid solution. Additionally, attempts were made to change the test from a qualitative to a quantitative tool. Fass and colleagues[24] placed a manometry catheter 10 cm above the upper border of the LES to ensure sufficient exposure of the esophageal mucosa to acid. Saline was infused initially for 2 minutes, and then without the patient's knowledge, 0.1 N HCl acid was infused for 10 minutes at a rate of 10 mL per minute. Patients were instructed to report whenever their typical symptoms were reproduced. Esophageal chemosensitivity to acid was assessed by both the duration until typical symptom perception was induced (expressed in seconds) and the total sensory intensity rating reported by the subject at the end of acid perfusion by using a verbal descriptor scale.

The acid perfusion test is highly specific but the sensitivity ranges from 6% to 60%. A negative test has no clinical relevance and does not exclude esophageal origin for patients' chest pain.

Presently, the acid perfusion test is rarely performed in clinical practice because of its limited diagnostic value in UCP and other esophageal disorders. Because of the low sensitivity and the emergence of noninvasive and highly sensitive modalities, such as the PPI test and empirical therapy with PPI, many authors have considered the acid perfusion test to be obsolete.

The Proton Pump Inhibitor Test

The limitations of the currently available diagnostic modalities for GERD make a therapeutic trial with a PPI an attractive option. The test uses a short course of high-dose PPI as an aid in diagnosing GERD. Overall, the PPI test is a simple, readily available, and clinically practical diagnostic tool.[68] However, a standardized PPI test is not documented in the literature.

The main requirement of a therapeutic trial is to achieve a significant improvement in the symptoms of as many patients as possible within a relatively short period of drug administration. Thus far, only PPIs have been used in studies assessing therapeutic trials because of their profound and consistent effect on acid inhibition.[22,69-74] Originally, omeprazole was the first PPI used as a test in UCP patients, leading to the term "the omeprazole test."

The sensitivity of the PPI test for GERD-related UCP ranged from 69% to 95% and the specificity from 67% to 86% (Table 10-3).[9,72,73,75-78] The dosages of PPIs used ranged from 60 mg to 80 mg daily for omeprazole, 30 mg to 90 mg daily for lansoprazole, and 40 mg daily for rabeprazole. The trial duration ranged from 1 to 28 days.

In 2 early studies, a single dose of 80 mg omeprazole was tested, resulting in variable sensitivity (69% to 90%).[72,73] However, in these studies, patients were crossed over to the opposite arm after a washout period of 2 to 5 days, which may be too short and result in a carry-over effect. Subsequently, in a double-blind, placebo-controlled trial, 37 patients with UCP were randomized to either placebo or high-dose omeprazole (40 mg in the morning and 20 mg in the evening) for 7 days.[22] After a washout period and repeated baseline symptom assessment, patients crossed over to the opposite arm. The PPI test was considered positive if the chest pain improved by at least 50% after treatment. The combination of upper endoscopy and 24-hour esophageal pH monitoring was used as the gold standard. Sixty-two percent (23 of 37) of the patients had evidence of GERD: 7 had abnormal esophageal acid exposure by pH testing only, 8 had erosive esophagitis only, and 8 had both. Of the GERD-positive group, 78.3% had a positive PPI test, and 22.7% had a positive placebo response. In contrast, of the GERD-negative group, 14.2% had a positive PPI test, and 7.1% had a positive placebo response. Thus, the calculated sensitivity was 78.3%, specificity 85.7%, and positive predictive value 90%.[22] When different reductions in chest pain were evaluated, the greater accuracy of predicting GERD-related UCP was obtained with 65% symptom reduction, resulting in a sensitivity of 85.5% and specificity of 90.9%.[22] Using similar design, other investigators confirmed the usefulness of the PPI test for diagnosing GERD-related UCP.[9,76] Furthermore, in subsequent studies, Fass et al demonstrated that therapeutic trials with PPIs other than omeprazole achieve similar efficacy for the diagnosis of GERD-related UCP.[77] A recent study in the Chinese population showed that the PPI test using lansoprazole 30 mg daily for a period of 4 weeks was useful in diagnosing endoscopy-negative GERD-related UCP (see Table 10-3).[9]

Table 10-3

PROTON PUMP INHIBITOR TESTS IN UNEXPLAINED CHEST PAIN

Author	Dosing Schedule	Number of Patients	Symptom Improvement Threshold (%)	Sensitivity (%)	Specificity (%)
Young	Omeprazole 80 mg/day for 1 day	30	75	90	80
Squillace	Omeprazole 80 mg/day for 1 day	17	50	69	75
Xia	Lansoprazole 30 mg/day for 4 weeks	68	50	92	67
Pandak	Omeprazole 40 mg twice daily for 2 weeks	37	50	90	67
Fass	Omeprazole: 40 mg in the AM and 20 mg in the PM for 7 days	37	50	78	86
Fass	Lansoprazole: 60 mg in the AM and 30 mg in the PM for 7 days	40	50	78	82
Fass	Rabeprazole: 20 mg in the AM and 20 mg in the PM for 7 days	20	50	83	75

When using the PPI test, there was a significant correlation between the extent of esophageal acid exposure in the distal esophagus as determined by ambulatory 24-hour esophageal pH monitoring and the change in symptom intensity score after treatment, suggesting that the higher the esophageal acid exposure, the greater the response to the PPI test in patients with GERD-related UCP.[27]

Economic analysis showed that the PPI test for GERD-related UCP is a cost-saving approach primarily due to a significant reduction in the usage of various costly and invasive diagnostic tests.[22]

DIAGNOSTIC TOOLS FOR ESOPHAGEAL DYSMOTILITY

Esophageal Manometry

Various esophageal motility abnormalities may present with chest pain only or, more commonly, with other esophageal-related symptoms. They include diffuse esophageal spasm, nutcracker esophagus, achalasia, long-duration contractions, multipeaked waves, and hypertensive LES.[79] However, esophageal manometry appears to have a relatively poor sensitivity in evaluating patients with UCP. When evaluated by esophageal manometry, most patients with UCP demonstrate normal esophageal motor function. Furthermore, patients rarely experience chest pain during esophageal manometry regardless of whether esophageal dysmotility was documented.[80] Obviously, this raises the question about the relationship between the documented esophageal dysmotility and patients' chest pain. Unlike GERD, we are still devoid of highly effective drugs that can easily correct patients' motility abnormalities and consequently can be used to demonstrate causal relationship. Some authorities suggest using the motility abnormalities as a marker for an underlying esophageal motor disorder that may be responsible for patients' symptoms.[80] The usage of ambulatory 24-hour esophageal manometry has been suggested to improve the sensitivity of the test in UCP; however, the results varied considerably.[81,82] In fact, in these studies, a significant number of patients reported no symptoms at all during the 24-hour recordings (between 27% to 43%). Moreover, in only 13% and 24% of the patients, the investigators were able to relate the pain episodes to a recorded esophageal dysmotility. These results question the routine usage in clinical practice of ambulatory 24-hour esophageal manometry for the evaluation of patients with UCP.

Presently, patients who did not respond to anti-reflux treatment (non-GERD-related UCP) are likely to undergo manometry. This diagnostic tool has become an integral part of the evaluation of UCP patients. However, with the exception of achalasia, UCP patients with other esophageal motility abnormalities (primarily spastic motor disorders) respond to pain modulators better than any of the smooth muscle relaxants. As a result, the usefulness of esophageal manometry in UCP is limited to excluding achalasia as the underlying cause of patients' chest pain.

Edrophonium (Tensilon) Test

Edrophonium is an anticholinesterase that increases cholinergic activity at muscarinic receptors.[83] A short-acting drug, edrophonium's pharmacologic action is manifested within 30 to 60 seconds after injection and lasts an average of 10 minutes. The aim of the edrophonium test is to induce greater esophageal body amplitude contractions in the hope of provoking the patient's typical chest pain.[84] The test is performed by injecting either 80 mg/kg or 10 mg edrophonium intravenously, immediately followed by 5 to 10 swallows of 5 to 10 mL of water over a period of 5 to 10 minutes. Commonly, subjects experience pain within 5 minutes after administration of the edrophonium test. The pain usually resolves quickly because of rapid metabolism of the drug.

Side effects are chiefly due to excessive cholinergic stimulation and may include increased salivation, nausea, vomiting, and abdominal cramps. Overall, side effects are minimal, and the antidote atropine is rarely needed. The drug seems to have no effect on the diameter of the coronary arteries.[85]

The sensitivity of the edrophonium test in UCP has varied from 9% to 55%.[86,87] The exact sensitivity is unknown because of the lack of a gold standard. The mechanism by which edrophonium induces chest pain in UCP patients is unclear but may be related to hypersensitivity to augmented esophageal motor activity.

Overall, it seems that if the edrophonium test is positive, then the esophagus is the likely origin of chest pain. However, due to lack of differences in esophageal contractile activity after the edrophonium test between UCP patients and normal healthy subjects, several authorities have suggested performing the test with concomitant esophageal manometric studies.

Other Provocative Tests

The bethanechol test is presently rarely performed in clinical practice because of its questionable diagnostic value and frequent side effects.

The IV ergonovine stimulation test has been demonstrated to induce augmentation of esophageal contractions and chest pain in many UCP patients.[20] Ergonovine is a sympathomimetic agent that is used by the cardiologist to diagnose Prinzmetal's angina. The drug has been shown to induce chest pain in patients with non-cardiac chest pain and demonstrated similar sensitivity as edrophonium. Presently, ergonovine is rarely used for esophageal testing due to potential serious side effects, including severe cardiac effects and even death.

DIAGNOSTIC TOOLS FOR VISCERAL HYPERSENSITIVITY

Balloon Distension

Balloon distension has been used primarily for research purposes to determine perception thresholds for pain. This modality has been used extensively in studies of various functional bowel disorders, most notably IBS, functional dyspepsia as well as UCP.[36,88,89]

More than 40 years ago, intraesophageal balloon distension in humans was reported to produce pain referred to the chest.[88] Early data indicated that in patients with documented ischemic heart disease, balloon distension of the esophagus produced pain indistinguishable from anginal pain but without ECG changes.[90] This may be explained by convergence of sensory pathways at the level of the spinal cord or in the midbrain. Despite this similarity in pain, it seems that esophageal balloon distension itself has no effect on coronary function or blood flow.[91]

Balloon distension was reintroduced during the mid-1980s in a seminal study that evaluated perception thresholds for pain in patients with UCP.[36] The latex balloon was attached to a manometric catheter and filled with air. The balloon was positioned 10 cm above the LES and distended in a stepwise fashion using a hand-held syringe.

The introduction of the electronic barostat, a computer-driven volume-displacement device, has helped to ensure proper location of the balloon regardless of the inflation paradigm that was used.[92] The basic principal of the barostat is to maintain a constant pressure within the balloon/bag in the lumen despite muscular contractions and relaxation.[92,93]

Balloon studies are primarily designed to assess the presence of visceral hyperalgesia in various esophageal disorders. Early studies demonstrated that pain develops with balloon distension more frequently in UCP patients than in normal control subjects and that their pain occurs at smaller volumes.[36,37] The usage of balloon distension protocols in clinical practice has been hampered by limited expertise, cost, concerns about adverse events (such as perforation), and unclear clinical value.

Balloon distension has been commonly used to assess the effect of various drugs on esophageal sensory perception. Imipramine, octreotide, and nifedipine have all been shown to increase perception thresholds for pain in normal controls or patients with UCP.[94-98]

PSYCHOLOGICAL EVALUATION

Some of the patients with UCP require psychological evaluation by an expert psychologist or psychiatrist because of the high prevalence rate of psychological abnormalities in this group of patients. Deciding who should be referred is individually determined, but the likely candidates are those who appeared to be refractory to therapeutic interventions or those who display clear features of a psychological disorder. Physicians can use a structured psychiatric interview to determine if psychological comorbidity is present.[99] There are various diagnostic psychological tools, such as the Symptom Checklist-90R (SCL-90R) and the Beck Depression Inventory questionnaires, that can be used at the clinical level but are unlikely to find a place in a busy GI practice. Regardless, when evaluating a patient with UCP, the presence of coexisting psychological comorbidity should always be entertained.

Treatment

OVERVIEW

Treatment of UCP should be directed to the likely underlying mechanism of patients' symptoms. Anti-reflux treatment has been repeatedly shown to be effective in relieving symptoms of patients with GERD-related UCP. For patients with non-GERD-related UCP, pain modulators are the mainstay of therapy. The role of muscle relaxants in patients with esophageal dysmotility has diminished due to limited efficacy. Figure 10-2 provides a suggested treatment algorithm.

TREATMENT OF GASTROESOPHAGEAL REFLUX DISEASE-RELATED UNEXPLAINED CHEST PAIN

Treatment of GERD-related UCP should involve lifestyle modifications and pharmacologic intervention. Elevating the head of the bed at night, reducing fat intake, smoking cessation, and avoiding foods that exacerbate GER have been shown to decrease reflux-related symptoms.[100] Thus far, we are still devoid of studies assessing the specific value of lifestyle modifications in patients with GERD-related UCP.

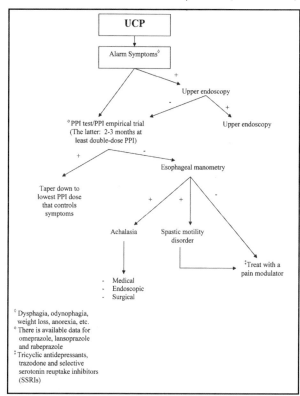

Figure   10-2.
Diagnosis and treatment flow chart for unexplained chest pain—the authors' approach.

In the literature, there have been small, uncontrolled studies comparing histamine-2 receptor antagonists (H2RA) to placebo or omeprazole. The efficacy of H2RAs has ranged from 54% to 83%.[101] As compared with PPIs, they have demonstrated a limited response in patients with UCP. In a small, uncontrolled study by Stahl et al,[102] 13 patients with UCP and GERD were treated with high-dose ranitidine (150 mg orally QID). Seven patients failed lower doses of ranitidine previously. All patients improved with high doses of ranitidine, although 2 patients had to have their dose increased to 300 mg orally QID. DeMeester et al[103] followed 23 UCP patients with abnormal esophageal acid exposure for 2 to 3 years. Twelve patients were treated medically with antacids and cimetidine, and 11 patients were treated with anti-reflux surgical procedure. Of the medically treated patients, 5 (42%) were chest pain free at follow-up. These results are not surprising because H2RA have a limited acid suppressive effect due to a relatively short duration of action. Additionally, tolerance to these drugs generally develops within 2 weeks of repeated administration, resulting in a decline in the acid suppression effect.[104] PPI therapy, on the other hand, produces a more profound and longer duration of acid suppression, and tolerance has not been observed.

When omeprazole 20 mg twice daily was administered over a period of 8 weeks to UCP patients in a double-blind, placebo-controlled trial, the patients who received omeprazole had a significant reduction in the number of days with chest pain and chest pain severity score when compared with patients who received placebo. Although data regarding the efficacy of PPIs in UCP are available only with omeprazole, it is highly likely that all other PPIs will demonstrate similar efficacy.[105] Patients with GERD-related UCP should be treated with at least a double dose of PPI until symptoms remit, followed by dose tapering to determine the lowest dose that can control patients' symptoms. As with other extra-esophageal manifestations of GERD, UCP patients may require more than 2 months of therapy for optimal symptom control. Long-term treatment with a PPI has been shown to be highly efficacious.[106] Borzecki et al[107] developed a decision tree to compare empirical treatment for UCP patients with H2RA or standard dose PPI for 8 weeks with initial investigation (upper endoscopy or upper GI series). Empiric treatment was more cost effective, with a cost of $849 per patient versus $2187 per patient with the initial investigation strategy.

Laparoscopic fundoplication relieves heartburn and acid regurgitation in most patients with GERD, but its effect on chest pain is less clear. DeMeester et al[103] found a temporal correlation in 12 of 23 patients who had acid reflux as a cause of their UCP. Pain resolved in the 12 patients when treated surgically (8 patients) or by acid reducing agents. Patti et al[108] reviewed patients who underwent laparoscopic fundoplication for GERD and complained of chest pain in addition to heartburn and acid regurgitation. Overall, chest pain improved in 85% of the patients after laparoscopic fundoplication. This increased to 96% in patients whose chest pain correlated with GER most of the time. Farrell et al[109] evaluated the effectiveness of anti-reflux surgery for patients with atypical manifestations of GERD. Chest pain improved in 90% of patients after laparoscopic fundoplication with symptom resolution in 50% of the patients. Although surgical studies demonstrated a high success rate of anti-reflux surgery in GERD-related UCP patients, the patients included were carefully selected.

Several endoscopic techniques designed to bolster the anti-reflux barrier at the GEJ are under investigation.[110] There are three basic types of endoscopic treatment: suturing, radiofrequency, and injection.[111] The published data report only short-term outcomes of a limited number of patients with usually mild disease. No studies thus far have specifically evaluated patients with GERD-related UCP. Consequently, these endoscopic methods are considered experimental and should not be routinely performed even in patients with confirmed GERD-related UCP. Their effect in GERD-related UCP patients should be studied primarily because several recent anecdotal reports suggested a good response to endoscopic therapy.

TREATMENT OF ESOPHAGEAL DYSMOTILITY-RELATED UNEXPLAINED CHEST PAIN

Directing treatment to esophageal dysmotility in patients with UCP remains a controversial area. In recent years, it has been recognized that the role of esophageal manometry in patients with non-GERD-related UCP is limited to diagnosing achalasia. It appears that UCP patients with other spastic motility disorders respond better to pain modulators than to medications that alter esophageal motility. Furthermore, response to pain modulators in UCP patients is essentially unrelated to the presence or absence of esophageal dysmotility.

Generally, treating esophageal motility abnormalities in patients with UCP is a less rewarding practice. It is primarily due to the paucity of clinically effective motility related-drugs that are currently available. In patients with nutcracker esophagus, antireflux treatment should be tried first before smooth muscle relaxants are considered.[112] Symptom resolution in these patients is unrelated to improvement in esophageal motility.

Smooth muscle relaxants have a very limited role, if any, in patients with UCP and documented esophageal motor disorder. Data supporting the usage of nitrates are scarce and not uncommonly based on anecdotal experience. Sublingual nitroglycerin and long-acting nitrate preparations appear to have no effect on esophageal amplitude contractions of healthy subjects.[113] However, 0.4 mg sublingual nitroglycerin was reported to have a transient effect on esophageal dysmotility with relief of chest pain in a case report.[114] Reports about the value of long-acting nitrates in patients with UCP and esophageal dysmotility are conflicting. In an old study, the authors reported complete symptom resolution of chest pain during a period of up to 4 years.[115] Others could not document a long-term effect.[116] Calcium-channel blockers, although commonly used in clinical practice, appear to also have a very limited effect on esophageal dysmotility in patients with UCP. Their usage might be affected by side effects, such as hypotension, constipation, pedal edema, and others. Diltiazem in doses of 60 to 90 mg four times daily has been shown to improve chest pain scores significantly better than placebo in small trials of patients with UCP and documented nutcracker esophagus on esophageal manometry.[117,118] Nifedipine in doses of 10 to 30 mg twice daily demonstrated a limited symptomatic response in these patients.[119] Symptom improvement lasted only 2 weeks and was noted after a lag time of 3 weeks. By the end of the sixth week, the drug appeared to completely lose its efficacy. Limited effect of calcium channel blockers was also documented in the other spastic motility disorders that were described in association with UCP.

Data about usage of other therapeutic modalities in UCP patients with esophageal dysmotility are even scarcer. The antispasmodic cimetropium bromide has been shown to be efficacious in 8 UCP patients with nutcracker esophagus.[120] Hydralazine, a hypertensive drug that directly dilates peripheral vessels, has been shown in 5 patients to improve chest pain and dysphagia as well as to decrease the amplitude and duration of esophageal contractions.[116]

Botulinum toxin injection into the LES was used in several uncontrolled trials in patients with UCP and spastic motility disorders.[121] It appears that botulinum toxin injection leads to a significant symptomatic improvement in patients with spastic esophageal motility disorders whose major complaint is chest pain. However, the mean duration of symptom response in one study was only 7 months. The authors used 100 units of botulinum toxin injected in 5 circumferential injections of 20 units each at the GEJ.[121]

Pneumatic dilation and long esophageal myotomy with or without fundoplication are reserved for severely symptomatic patients with well-documented spastic motility disorder, severe dysphagia, and weight loss.

TREATMENT OF VISCERAL HYPERSENSITIVITY

In the past decade, pain modulators (visceral analgesics) have become the mainstay of therapy in non-GERD-related UCP. Tricyclics (TCAs), trazodone, SSRIs, and theophylline have all been shown to improve symptoms in UCP patients.

Several TCAs have been assessed in UCP. The mechanism by which TCAs reduce visceral pain is poorly understood. Some studies suggested a central mediating effect,[122] while others claimed a potential peripheral effect. The TCAs demonstrate a varied receptor affinity (acetylcholine, histamine 1, and an adrenergic).[31] Nortriptyline and desipramine are secondary amines (metabolites of tertiary amines) that have less affinity for receptors that result in bothersome side effects.[123] The tertiary amines include amitriptyline, imipramine, doxepin, and others. Imipramine has been shown to increase esophageal perception thresholds for pain in normal subjects without affecting esophageal tone, suggesting a visceral analgesic effect.[95] Similar effect has been noted in UCP patients, which was independent of cardiac, esophageal, or psychiatric testing at baseline.[94] TCAs provide long-term effect in UCP patients, although the drop-out rate due to side effects may reach 30%.[124]

Treatment with TCAs should be administered at bedtime, starting with a low dose (10 to 25 mg) and then increased by 10 to 25 mg increments per week to a maximal non–mood-altering dose of 50 to 75 mg per day.[123] Because of the varied effect of TCAs on the different respective receptors, failure of one TCA to improve symptoms is not indicative of future failure of other TCAs.

The usage of SSRIs in UCP has been scarcely studied. As with TCAs, a neuromodulatory effect has been proposed to mediate their effect on visceral pain. Varia et al[125] performed a randomized trial that assessed the efficacy, tolerability, and safety of the SSRI sertraline in patients with UCP. This was a double-blind, placebo-controlled trial that included 30 subjects. Patients were randomly selected to receive sertraline or placebo in doses starting at 50 mg and adjusted to a maximum of 200 mg. By using intention-to-treat analysis, investigators have demonstrated that patients receiving sertraline reported a significant reduction in their pain scores compared with those who received placebo, regardless of concomitant improvement in psychological scores.[126] This study further confirms the potential role of SSRIs in treating patients with UCP. As with tricyclic antidepressants, the SSRIs' effect on visceral pain perception appears to be independent of their effect on mood.

Low-dose trazodone (100 to 150 mg/day), an antidepressant and anxiolytic, has been shown to improve symptoms in UCP patients with esophageal contraction abnormalities without affecting esophageal amplitude contractions.[127] Information about other compounds with visceral analgesic effect has been limited to isolated reports in the literature. Infusion of theophylline in an open-labeled trial alleviated chest pain in patients with functional chest pain of presumed esophageal origin.[128] It is assumed that theophylline improves esophageal pain by blocking adenosine receptors. Octreotide, a somatostatin analog, given subcutaneously (100 mg) has been shown to increase esophageal perception thresholds to balloon distension in normal subjects.[129] The effect was unrelated to change in esophageal compliance.

TREATMENT OF PSYCHOLOGICAL COMORBIDITY

Reassurance has been emphasized as an important mode of therapeutic intervention in patients with UCP. However, patients' symptoms are seldom relieved by reassurance only, resulting in the need for an additional therapeutic modality.[130] Several anxiolytics have been evaluated in UCP patients, mostly members of the benzodiazepine family. Alprazolam and clonazepam have been demonstrated to reduce panic attack frequency as well as chest pain episodes and anxiety score, respectively.[131,132] However, benzodiazepines should be cautiously used in UCP patients, primarily due to their addictive effect. Buspirone is an anxiolytic without dependency potential, but reported experience in UCP patients is still unavailable.[123]

Young patients and males with UCP appear to be open to pharmacological treatment.[133] However, management of psychological comorbidity in these patients should be reserved for experts in the field. That includes prescribing medications for panic attack, depression, and anxiety.

Several studies have suggested that behavioral therapy can be effective in patients with noncardiac chest pain. Hegel and colleagues published a report in which 3 patients with chest pain and anxiety disorder were treated with relaxation training and controlled diaphragmatic breathing exercises; these techniques were practiced during increasingly complex activities.[134] Two of the patients had substantial reduction in the frequency and intensity of their chest pain that was maintained for 12 months after treatment. Klimes and associates performed the only controlled study of behavioral treatment in patients with chest pain.[135] This treatment of 31 patients consisted of education, controlled breathing, training in relaxation, diversion of attention from pain, and practice of newly learned skills in their home environment. When compared with the waiting list controls, the treatment program produced significant improvement in chest pain episodes, functional disability, and psychological distress that was maintained for 46 months after treatment.

FUTURE TREATMENT OF UNEXPLAINED CHEST PAIN

Research into the underlying mechanisms that result in the development of UCP ultimately may lead to novel therapeutic modalities in the future. Future research will continue to focus on mechanisms for pain in UCP patients, primarily the role of central and peripheral sensitization in enhancing perception of intraesophageal stimuli. Alosetron, a 5-hydroxytryptamine (5HT) type 3 antagonist, which was previously available for the treatment of female patients with diarrhea-predominant IBS, raised the hope for a therapeutic potential in patients with UCP.[136] This class of drugs appears to have a pain-modulatory effect, probably by altering the initiation, transmission, or processing of extrinsic sensory information from the GI tract. The role of the new partial 5HT type 4 agonist, tegaserod, in modulating pain that originates from the GI tract is less clear.

Phosphorylation of N-methyl-D-asparate (NMDA) receptors expressed by dorsalhorn neurons leads to central sensitization via an increase in their excitability and receptive field size.[40] Potentially, this central sensitization may be prevented or even reversed by antagonism of NMDA receptors within the spinal cord. However, it is important to remember that CNS mechanisms that mediate visceral hyperalgesia are sensitive to both NMDA receptor blockers and non-NMDA receptor antagonists.[137]

Other neuromodulators such as fedotozine and asimadoline; kappa opioid receptor agonists (produce a peripheral anti-nociceptive effect in patients with IBS); neurokinin receptor antagonists NK1 and NK2 (reduce gut motility and pain); and cholecystokinin-A receptor antagonist loxiglumide (visceral analgesic effect in patients with IBS) may all have a future role in non-GERD-related UCP.

Lastly, acid pump inhibitors are likely to be introduced into the market by the end of 2010. This class of drugs, which exhibits a rapid onset of action independent of meal stimulation, predictable dose response effect, and profound acid secretion blockage, may play an important role in GERD-related UCP as a diagnostic tool (the "APA test") or as an improved short- and long-term treatment for GERD-related UCP.

Summary

UCP is the most common atypical/extraesophageal manifestation of GERD. Diagnosis in the past decade has shifted to noninvasive modalities (ie, the PPI test or the PPI empirical trial). The role of pH testing has been questioned, and the role of esophageal manometry has been limited to diagnosing achalasia.

The availability of highly potent anti-reflux medications has improved our capability to treat patients with GERD-related UCP. In those patients with non-GERD-related UCP, regardless of whether esophageal dysmotility is present or absent, pain modulators remain the cornerstone of therapy.

References

1. The Rome II Multinational Working Team. Functional chest pain of presumed esophageal origin. In: Drossman DA, Corazziari E, Talley NJ, Thompson WG, Whitehead WE, eds. *Rome II: The Functional Gastrointestinal Disorders.* 2nd ed. Lawrence, Kan: Allen Press, Inc; 2000:264-274.

2. Nevens F, Janssens J, Piessens J, Ghillebert G, De Geest H, Vantrappen G. Prospective study on prevalence of esophageal chest pain in patients referred on an elective basis to a cardiac unit for suspected myocardial ischemia. *Dig Dis Sci.* 1991;36(2):229-235.

3. Richter JE. Chest pain and GER disease. *J Clin Gastroenterol.* 2000;30(3 Suppl): S39-S41.

4. Katerndahl DA, Trammell C. Prevalence and recognition of panic states in STARNET patients presenting with chest pain. *J Fam Pract.* 1997;45(1):54-63.

5. Faybush EM, Fass R. GER disease in noncardiac chest pain. *Gastroenterol Clin North Am.* 2004;33(1):41-54.

6. Richter JE. Extraesophageal presentations of GER disease: an overview. *Am J Gastroenterol.* 2000;95(8 Suppl):S1-S3.

7. Shrestha S, Pasricha PJ. Update on noncardiac chest pain. *Dig Dis.* 2000;18(3):138-146.

8. Fass R, Ofman JJ, Sampliner RE, Camargo L, Wendel C, Fennerty MB. The omeprazole test is as sensitive as 24-hr oesophageal pH monitoring in diagnosing gastro-oesophageal reflux disease in symptomatic patients with erosive esophagitis. *Aliment Pharmacol Ther.* 2000;14(4):389-396.

9. Xia HH, Lai KC, Lam SK, et al. Symptomatic response to lansoprazole predicts abnormal acid reflux in endoscopy-negative patients with non-cardiac chest pain. *Aliment Pharmacol Ther.* 2003;17(3):369-377.

10. Garcia-Compean D, Gonzalez MV, Galindo G, et al. Prevalence of GER disease in patients with extraesophageal symptoms referred from otolaryngology, allergy, and cardiology practices: a prospective study. *Dig Dis.* 2000;18(3):178-182.

11. Locke G, 3rd, Talley NJ, Fett SL, Zinsmeister AR, Melton LJ, 3rd. Prevalence and clinical spectrum of GER: a population-based study in Olmstead County, Minnesota. *Gastroenterology.* 1997;112(5):1448-1456.

12. Drossman DA, Li Z, Andruzzi E, et al. U.S. householder survey of functional gastrointestinal disorders. Prevalence, sociodemography, and health impact. *Dig Dis Sci.* 1993;38(9):1569-1580.

13. Eslick GD. Noncardiac chest pain: epidemiology, natural history, health care seeking, and quality of life. *Gastroenterol Clin North Am.* 2004;33(1):1-23.

14. Eslick GD, Jones MP, Talley NJ. Non-cardiac chest pain: prevalence, risk factors, impact and consulting—a population-based study. *Aliment Pharmacol Ther.* 2003;17(9):1115-1124.

15. Potokar JP, Nutt DJ. Chest pain: panic attack or heart attack? *Int J Clin Pract.* 2000;54(2):110-114.

16. Tew R, Guthrie EA, Creed FH, Cotter L, Kisely S, Tomenson B. A long-term follow-up study of patients with ischemic heart disease versus patients with nonspecific chest pain. *J Psychosom Res.* 1995;39(8):977-985.

17. Kennedy JW, Killip T, Fisher LD, Alderman EL, Gillespie MJ, Mock M. The clinical spectrum of coronary artery disease and its surgical and medical management, 1974-1979. The Coronary Artery Surgery Study. *Circulation.* 1985;66(5, Pt 2):III16-23.

18. Eslick GD, Talley NJ. Non-cardiac chest pain: predictors of health care seeking, the types of health care professional consultation, work absenteeism and interruption of daily activities. *Aliment Pharmacol Ther.* 2004;20(8):909-915.

19. Richter JE, Bradley LA, Castell DO. Esophageal chest pain: current controversies in pathogenesis, diagnosis, and therapy. *Ann Intern Med.* 1989;110(1):66-78.

20. Eslick GD, Talley NJ. Non-cardiac chest pain: squeezing the life out of the Australian health care system? *Med J Aust.* 2000;173(5):233-234.

21. Fass R, Fennerty MB, Ofman JJ, et al. The clinical and economic value of a short course of omeprazole patients with noncardiac chest pain. *Gastroenterology.* 1998;115(1):42-49.

22. Fass R, Winters GF. Evaluation of the patient with noncardiac chest pain: is GER disease or an esophageal motility disorder the cause? *Medscape Gastroenterol eJournal.* 2001;3(6):1-7.

23. Fass R, Naliboff B, Higa L, et al. Differential effect of long-term esophageal acid exposure on mechanosensitivity and chemosensitivity in humans. *Gastroenterology.* 1998;115(6):1363-1373.

24. Beedassy A, Katz PO, Gruber A, Peghini PL, Castell DO. Prior sensitization of esophageal mucosa by acid reflux predisposes to reflux-induced chest pain. *J Clin Gastroenterol.* 2000;31(2):121-124.

25. Dekel R, Martinez-Hawthorne SD, Guillen RJ, Fass R. Evaluation of symptom index in identifying GER disease-related noncardiac chest pain. *J Clin Gastroenterol.* 2004;38(1):24-29.

26. Fass R, Fennerty MB, Johnson C, Camargo L, Sampliner RE. Correlation of ambulatory 24-hour esophageal pH monitoring results with symptom improvement in patients with noncardiac chest pain due to GER disease. *J Clin Gastroenterol.* 1999;28(1):36-39.

27. Chauhan A, Petch MC, Schofield PM. Cardio-oesophageal reflex in humans as a mechanism for "linked angina." *Eur Heart J.* 1996;17(3):407-413.

28. Katz PO, Dalton CB, Richter JE, Wu WC, Castell DO. Esophageal testing of patients with noncardiac chest pain or dysphagia. Results of three years' experience in 1161 patients. *Ann Intern Med.* 1987;106(4):593-597.

29. Dekel R, Pearson T, Wendel C, De Garmo P, Fennerty MB, Fass R. Assessment of oesophageal motor function in patients with dysphagia or chest pain—the Clinical Outcomes Research Initiative experience. *Aliment Pharmacol Ther.* 2003;18(11-12):1083-1089.

30. Kahrilas PJ. Nutcracker esophagus: an idea whose time has gone? *Am J Gastroenterol.* 1993;88(2):167-169.

31. Achem SR, Kolts BE, Wears R, Burton L, Richter JE. Chest pain associated with nutcracker esophagus: a preliminary study of the role of GER. *Am J Gastroenterol.* 1993;88(2):187-192.

32. Richter JE. Oesophageal motility disorders. *Lancet.* 2001;358(9284):823-828.

33. Hollerbach S, Bulat R, May A, Kamath MV, Upton AR, Fallen EL, Tougas G. Abnormal cerebral processing oesophageal stimuli in patients with noncardiac chest pain (NCCP). *Neurogastroenterol Motil.* 2000;12(6):555-565.

34. Aziz Q. Acid sensors in the gut: a taste of things to come. *Eur J Gastroenterol Hepatol.* 2001;13(8):885-888.

35. Handwerker HO, Reeh PW. Nociceptors: chemosensitivity and sensitization by chemical agents. In: Willis WD, Jr, ed. *Hyperalgesia and Allodynia.* New York: Raven Press; 1992:107.

36. Richter JE, Barish CF, Castell DO. Abnormal sensory perception in patients with esophageal chest pain. *Gastroenterology.* 1986;91(4):845-852.

37. Barish CF, Castell DO, Richter JE. Graded esophageal balloon distention. A new provocative test for noncardiac chest pain. *Dig Dis Sci.* 1986;31(12):1292-1298.

38. Rao SS, Gregersen H, Hayek B, Summers RW, Christensen J. Unexplained chest pain: the hypersensitive, hyperreactive, and poorly compliant esophagus. *Ann Intern Med.* 1996;124(11):950-958.

39. Rao SS, Hayek B, Summers RW. Functional chest pain of esophageal origin: hyperalgesia or motor dysfunction. *Am J Gastroenterol.* 2001;96(9):2584-2589.

40. Sarkar S, Aziz Q, Woolf CJ, Hobson AR, Thompson DG. Contribution of central sensitisation to the development of non-cardiac chest pain. *Lancet.* 2000;356(9236):1154-1159.

41. Hu WH, Martin CJ, Talley NJ. Intraesophageal acid perfusion sensitizes the esophagus to mechanical distension: a Barostat study. *Am J Gastroenterol.* 2000;95(9):2189-2194.

42. Tougas G, Spaziani R, Hollerbach S, et al. Cardiac autonomic function and oesophageal acid sensitivity in patients with non-cardiac chest pain. *Gut.* 2001;49(5):706-712.

43. Tougas G. The autonomic nervous system in functional bowel disorders. *Gut.* 2000;47(Suppl 4):78-80.

44. Aziz Q, Thompson DG. Brain-gut axis in health and disease. *Gastroenterology.* 1998;114(3):559-578.

45. Harshorne MF. Positron emission tomography. In: Orrison WW, Lewine JD, Sanders JA, Hartshorne MF, eds. *Functional Brain Imaging.* St. Louis, Mo: Mosby-Year Book; 1995:187-212.

46. Aine CJ. A conceptual overview and critique of functional neuroimaging techniques in humans: I. MRI/FMRI and PET. *Crit Rev Neurobiol.* 1995;9(2-3):229-309.

47. Smout AJ, DeVore MS, Dalton CB, Castell DO. Cerebral potentials evoked by oesophageal distension in patients with non-cardiac chest pain. *Gut.* 1992;33(3):298-302.

48. Sanders JA, Orrison WW. Functional magnetic resonance imaging. In: Orrison WW, Lewine JD, Sanders JA, Hartshorne MF, eds. *Functional Brain Imaging.* St. Louis, Mo: Mosby-Year Book; 1995:239-326.

49. Aziz Q, Andersson JL, Valind S, et al. Identification of human brain loci processing esophageal sensation using positron emission tomography. *Gastroenterology.* 1997;113(1):50-59.

50. Minshohima S, Morrow TJ, Koeppe RA. Involvement of insular cortex in central autonomic regulation during painful thermal stimulation. *J Cereb Blood Flow Metab.* 1995;15(Suppl 1):1355-1358.

51. Talbot JD, Marrett S, Evans AC, Meyer E, Bushnell MC, Duncan GH. Multiple representations of pain in human cerebral cortex. *Science.* 1991;251(4999):1355-1358.

52. Vogt BA, Sikes RW, Vogt LJ. Anterior cingulate cortex and the medial pain system. In: Vogt BA, Gabriel M, eds. *Neurobiology of Cingulate Cortex and Limbic Thalamus.* Boston, Mass: Birkhauser; 1994:313-344.

53. van Peski-Oosterbaan AS, Spinhoven P, van Rood Y, van der Does JW, Bruschke AV, Rooijmans HG. Cognitive-behavioral therapy for noncardiac chest pain: a randomized trial. *Am J Med.* 2000;106(4):424-429.

54. Song CW, Lee SJ, Jeem YT, et al. Inconsistent association of esophageal symptoms, psychometric abnormalities and dysmotility. *Am J Gastroenterol.* 2001;96(8):2312-2316.

55. Fleet RP, Dupuis G, Marchand A, Burelle D, Arsenault A, Beitman BD. Panic disorder in emergency department chest pain patients: prevalence, comorbidity, suicidal ideation, and physician recognition. *Am J Med.* 1996;101(4):371-380.

56. Stollman NH, Bierman PS, Ribeiro A, Rogers AI, Ribiero A. CO_2 provocation of panic: symptomatic and manometric evaluation in patients with noncardiac chest pain. *Am J Gastroenterol.* 1997;92(5):839-842.

57. Cooke RA, Anggiansah A, Wang J, Chambers JB, Owen W. Hyperventilation and esophageal dysmotility in patients with noncardiac chest pain. *Am J Gastroenterol.* 1996;91(3):480-484.

58. Lantinga LJ, Sprafkin RP, McCroskery JH, Baker MT, Warner RA, Hill NE. One-year psychosocial follow-up of patients with chest pain and angiographically normal coronary arteries. *Am J Cardiol.* 1988;62(4):209-213.

59. Hotopf M, Mayou R, Wadsworth M, Wessely S. Psychosocial and development antecedents of chest pain in young adults. *Psychosom Med.* 1999;61(6):861-867.

60. Orlando RC. Esophageal perception and noncardiac chest pain. *Gastroenterol Clin North Am.* 2004;33(1):25-33.

61. Vaezi MF, Charbel S. Abstract: on-therapy pH monitoring: usually recommended but should we do it? *Gastroenterology.* 2004;126(4, Suppl 2):A-82, #640.

62. Prakash C, Clouse RE. Abstract: extended pH monitoring with the Bravo capsule increases diagnostic yield in chest pain patients. *Gastroenterology.* 2004;126(4, Suppl 2):A-321, #M1376.

63. Johnston BT, Troshinsky MB, Castell JA, Castell DO. Comparison of barium radiology with esophageal pH monitoring in the diagnosis of GER disease. *Am J Gastroenterol.* 1996;91(6):1181-1185.

64. Eslick GD, Fass R. Noncardiac chest pain: evaluation and treatment. *Gastroenterol Clin North Am.* 2003;32(2):531-552.

65. Hewson EG, Sinclair JW, Dalton CB, Richter JE. Twenty-four-hour esophageal pH monitoring: the most useful test for evaluating noncardiac chest pain. *Am J Med.* 1991;90(5):576-583.

66. Wong MM, Bautista J, Dekel R, et al. Feasibility and tolerability of transnasal/peroral placement of the wireless pH capsule vs. traditional 24-h oesophageal pH monitoring—a randomized trial. *Aliment Pharmacol Ther.* 2005;21(2):155-163.

67. Bernstein LM, Baker LA. A clinical test for esophagitis. *Gastroenterology.* 1958;34(5):760-781.

68. Fass R. Empirical trials in treatment of GER disease. *Dig Dis.* 2000;18(1):20-26.
69. Schenk BE, Kuipers EJ, Klinkenberg-Knol EC, et al. Omeprazole as a diagnostic tool in GER disease. *Am J Gastroenterol.* 1997;92(11):1997-2000.
70. Schindlbeck NC, Klauser AG, Voderholzer WA, Muller-Lisner SA. Empiric therapy for GER disease. *Arch Intern Med.* 1995;155:1808-1812.
71. Johnsson F, Weywadt L, Solhaug JH, Hernqvist H, Bengtsson L. One-week omeprazole treatment in the diagnosis of gastro-oesophageal reflux disease. *Scand J Gastroenterol.* 1998;33(1):15-20.
72. Young MF, Sanowski RA, Talbert GA, et al. Abstract: omeprazole administration as a test for GER. *Gastroenterology.* 1992;102:192.
73. Squillace SJ, Young MF, Sanowski RA. Abstract: single dose omeprazole as a test for noncardiac chest pain. *Gastroenterology.* 1992;107:A197.
74. Fass R, Ofman JJ, Gralnek IM, et al. Clinical and economic assessment of omeprazole test in patients with symptoms suggestive of GER disease. *Arch Intern Med.* 1999;159(18):2161-2168.
75. Kahrilas PJ. Editorial: nutcracker esophagus: an idea whose time has gone? *Am J Gastroenterol.* 1993;88(2):167-169.
76. Pandak WM, Arezo S, Everett S, et al. Short course of omeprazole: a better first diagnostic approach to noncardiac chest pain than endoscopy, manometry, or 24-hour esophageal pH monitoring. *J Clin Gastroenterol.* 2002;35(4):307-314.
77. Fass R, Pulliam G, Hayden CW. Abstract: patients with non-cardiac chest pain (NCCP) receiving an empirical trial of high dose lansoprazole, demonstrate early symptom response—a double-blind, placebo-controlled trial. *Gastroenterology.* 2001;122:A580, #W1175.
78. Fass R, Fullerton H, Hayden CW, Garewal HS. Abstract: patients with noncardiac chest pain (NCCP) receiving an empirical trial of high dose rabeprazole demonstrate early symptom response—a double-blind, placebo-controlled trial. *Gastroenterology.* 2002;122:A580, #W1175.
79. Kahrilas PJ, Clouse RE, Hogan WJ. An American Gastroenterological Association medical position statement on the clinical use of esophageal manometry. *Gastroenterology.* 1994;107:1865-1884.
80. DiMarino AJ, Jr., Allen ML, Lynn RB, Zamani S. Clinical value of esophageal motility testing. *Dig Dis.* 1998;16(4):198-204.
81. Breumelhof R, Nadorp JH, Akkermans LM, Smout AJ. Analysis of 24-hour esophageal pressure and pH data in unselected patients with noncardiac chest pain. *Gastroenterology.* 1990;99(5):1257-1264.
82. Lam HG, Dekker W, Kan G, Breedijk M, Smout AJ. Acute noncardiac chest pain in a coronary care unit: evaluation by 24-hour pressure and pH recording of the esophagus. *Gastroenterology.* 1992;102:453-460.
83. London RL, Ouyangm A, Snape WJ, Jr., Goldberg S, Hirshfeld JW, Jr, Cohen S. Provocation of esophageal pain by ergonovine or edrophonium. *Gastroenterology.* 1981;81(1):10-14.
84. Nostrant TT. Provocation testing in noncardiac chest pain. Chest pain of undetermined origin. *Am J Gastroenterol.* 1991;5A:S56-S64.
85. Richter JE, Hackshaw BT, Wu WC, Castell DO. Edrophonium: a useful provocative test for esophageal chest pain. *Ann Intern Med.* 1985;103(1):14-21.
86. De Caestecker JS, Pryde A, Heading RC. Comparison of IV edrophonium and oesophageal acid perfusion during oesophageal manometry in patients with non-cardiac chest pain. *Gut.* 1988;29(8):1029-1034.

87. Ghillebert G, Janssens J, Vantrappen G, Nevens F, Piessens J. Ambulatory 24 hour intraoesophageal pH and pressure recordings v provocation tests in the diagnosis of chest pain of oesophageal origin. *Gut.* 1990;31(7):738-744.

88. Ritchie J. Pain from distension of the pelvic colon by inflating a balloon in the irritable colon syndrome. *Gut.* 1973;14(2):125-132.

89. Mertz H, Walsh JH, Sytnik B, Mayer EA. The effect of octreotide on human gastric compliance and sensory perception. *Neurogastroenterol Motil.* 1995;7(3):175-185.

90. Lipkin M, Sleisenger MH. Studies of visceral pain: measurements of stimulus intensity and duration associated with the onset of pain in esophagus, ileum and colon. *J Clin Invest.* 1958;37:28.

91. Yakshe PN, Tong LJ, Andreini SJ, et al. Abstract: does provocative esophageal testing influence coronary blood flow or coronary flow reserve? Preliminary results of concurrent esophageal can cardiac testing. *Gastroenterology.* 1993;104:A227.

92. Whitehead WE, Delvaux M. Standardization of barostat procedures for testing smooth muscle tone and sensory thresholds in the gastrointestinal tract. The Working Team of Glaxo-Wellcome Research, UK. *Dig Dis Sci.* 1997;42(2):223-241.

93. Azpiroz F, Dapoigny M, Pace F, et al. Nongastrointestinal disorders in the IBS. *Digestion.* 2000;62(1):66-72.

94. Cannon RO, 3rd, Quyyumi A, Mincemoyer R, et al. Imipramine in patients with chest pain despite normal coronary angiograms. *N Engl J Med.* 1994;330(20):1411-1417.

95. Peghnini PL, Katz PO, Castell DO. Imipramine decreases oesophageal pain perception in human male volunteers. *Gut.* 1998;42(6):807-813.

96. Castell DO, Wood JD, Frieling T, Wright FS, Vieth RF. Cerebral electrical potentials evoked by balloon distention of the human esophagus. *Gastroenterology.* 1990;98(3):662-666.

97. DeVault KR. Abstract: nifedipine does not alter barostat determined oesophageal smooth muscle tone. *Gastroenterology.* 1995;108(4):A591.

98. Smout AJ, DeVore MS, Dalton CB, Castell DO. Effects of nifedipine on esophageal tone and perception of esophageal distension. *Dig Dis Sci.* 1992;37(4):598-602.

99. Clouse RE. Psychiatric disorders in patients with esophageal disease. *Med Clin North Am.* 1991;75:1081-1096.

100. Storr M, Meining A, Allescher HD. Pathophysiology and pharmacological treatment of GER disease. *Dig Dis.* 2000;18(2):93-102.

101. Fang J, Bjorkman D. A critical approach to noncardiac chest pain: pathophysiology, diagnosis, and treatment. *Am J Gastroenterol.* 2001;96(4):958-968.

102. Stahl WG, Beton RR, Johnson CS, Brown CL, Waring JP. Diagnosis and treatment of patients with GER and noncardiac chest pain. *South Med J.* 1994;87(7):739-742.

103. DeMeester TR, O'Sullivan GC, Bermudez G, Midell AI, Cimochowski GE, O'Drobinak J. Esophageal function in patients with angina-type chest pain and normal coronary angiograms. *Ann Surg.* 1982;196(4):488-498.

104. Jones R, Bytzer P. Review article: acid suppression in the management of gastro-oesophageal reflux disease—an appraisal of treatment options in primary care. *Aliment Pharmacol Ther.* 2001;15(6):765-772.

105. Fass R. Chest pain of esophageal origin. *Curr Opin Gastroenterol.* 2002;18:464-470.

106. Fass R, Malagon I, Schmulson M. Chest pain of esophageal origin. *Curr Opin Gastroenterol.* 2001;17:376-380.

107. Borzecki AM, Pedrosa MC, Prashker MJ. Should noncardiac chest pain be treated empirically? A cost-effectiveness analysis. *Arch Intern Med.* 2000;160(6):844-852.

108. Patti MG, Molena D, Fisichella PM, Perretta S, Way LW. GER disease (GERD) and chest pain. Results of laparoscopic antireflux surgery. *Surg Endosc.* 2002;16(4):563-566.

109. Farrell TM, Richardson WS, Trus TL, Smith CD, Hunter JG. Response of atypical symptoms of gastro-oesophageal reflux to antireflux surgery. *Br J Surg.* 2001;88(12):1649-1652.

110. Moss SF, Armstrong D, Arnold R, et al. GERD 2003—a consensus on the way ahead. *Digestion.* 2003;67(3):111-117.

111. Waring JP. Surgical and endoscopic treatment of GER disease. *Gastroenterol Clin North Am.* 2002;31(4 Suppl):S89-S109.

112. Fass R. Noncardiac chest pain. In: Fass R, ed. *GERD/Dyspepsia Fast Facts.* Philadelphia: Hanley & Belfus; 2004:703-706.

113. Kikendall JW, Mellow MH. Effect of sublingual nitroglycerin and long-acting nitrate preparations on esophageal motility. *Gastroenterology.* 1980;79(4):703-706.

114. Orlando RC. Clinical and manometric effects of nitroglycerin in diffuse esophageal spasm. *N Engl J Med.* 1973;289(1):23-25.

115. Swamy N. Esophageal spasm: clinical and manometric response to nitroglycerine and long acting nitrites. *Gastroenterology.* 1977;72(1):23-27.

116. Mellow MH. Effect of isosorbide and hydralazine in painful primary esophageal motility disorders. *Gastroenterology.* 1982;83(2):364-370.

117. Sontag SJ, O'Connell S, Khandelwal S, et al. Most asthmatics have GER with or without bronchodilator therapy. *Gastroenterology.* 1990;99(3):613-620.

118. Olson NR. Laryngopharyngeal manifestations of GER disease. *Otolaryngol Clin North Am.* 1991;24(5):1201-1213.

119. Ott DJ, Ledbetter MS, Koufman JA, Chen MY. Globus pharyngeus: radiographic evaluation and 24-hour pH monitoring of the pharynx and esophagus in 22 patients. *Radiology.* 1994;191(1):95-97.

120. Bassotti G, Gaburri M, Imbimbo BP, et al. Manometric evaluation of cimetropium bromide activity in patients with the nutcracker oesophagus. *Scand J Gastroenterol.* 1988;23(9):1079-1084.

121. Jaspersen D, Diehl KL, Geyer P, Martens E. Diagnostic omeprazole test in suspected reflux-associated chronic cough. *Pneumologie.* 1999;53(9):438-441.

122. Mertz H, Fass R, Kodner A, Yan-Go F, Fullerton S, Mayer EA. Effect of amitryptyline on symptoms, sleep and visceral perception in patients with functional dyspepsia. *Am J Gastroenterol.* 1998;93(2):160-165.

123. Clouse RE. Psychotropic medications for the treatment of functional gastrointestinal disorders. *Clin Perspect Gastroenterol.* 1999;2:348-356.

124. Prakash C, Clouse RE. Long-term outcome from tricyclic antidepressant treatment of functional chest pain. *Dig Dis Sci.* 1999;44(12):2373-2379.

125. Varia I, Logue E, O'Connor C, et al. Randomized trial of sertraline in patients with unexplained chest pain of noncardiac origin. *Am Heart J.* 2000;140(3):367-372.

126. Krishnan KR. Selected summary: chest pain and serotonin: a possible link? *Gastroenterology.* 2001;121(2):495-496.

127. Clouse RE, Lustman PJ, Eckert TC, Ferney DM, Griffith LS. Low-dose trazodone for symptomatic patients with esophageal contraction abnormalities. A double-blind, placebo-controlled trial. *Gastroenterology.* 1987;92(4):1027-1036.

128. Rao SS, Mudipalli RS, Mujica V, Utech CL, Zhao X, Conklin JL. An open-label trial of theophylline for functional chest pain. *Dig Dis Sci.* 2002;47(12):2763-2768.

129. Johnston BT, Shils J, Leite LP, Castell DO. Effects of octreotide on oesophageal visceral perception and cerebral evoked potentials induced by balloon distension. *Am J Gastroenterol.* 1999;94(1):65-70.

130. Clouse RE, Carney RM. The psychological profile of non-cardiac chest pain patients. *Eur J Gastroenterol Hepatol.* 1995;7(12):1160-1165.

131. Beitman BD, Basha IM, Trombka LH, et al. Pharmacotherapeutic treatment of panic disorder in patients presenting with chest pain. *J Fam Pract.* 1989;28(2):177-180.

132. Wulsin LR, Maddock R, Beitman BD, Dawaher R, Wells VE. Clonazepam treatment of panic disorder in patients with recurrent chest pain and normal coronary arteries. *Int J Psychiatry Med.* 1999;29(1):97-105.

133. van Peski-Oosterbaan AS, Spinhoven P, van der Does JW, Bruschke AV. Noncardiac chest pain: interest in a medical psychological treatment. *J Psychosom Res.* 1998;458(5):471-476.

134. Hegel MT, Abel GG, Etscheidt M, Cohen-Cole S, Wilmer CI. Behavioral treatment of angina-like chest pain in patients with hyperventilation syndrome. *J Behav Ther Exp Psychiatry.* 1989;20(1):31-39.

135. Klimes I, Mayou RA, Pearce MJ, Coles L, Fagg JR. Psychological treatment for atypical non-cardiac chest pain: a controlled evaluation. *Psychol Med.* 1990;20(3):605-611.

136. Burbige EJ. Abstract: use of a 5-HT3 antagonist in a patient with noncardiac chest pain. *Gastroenterology.* 2001;96(9):S183, #579.

137. Cervero F. Commentary: Visceral hyperalgesia revisited. *Lancet.* 2000;356(9236):1127-1128.

Gastroparesis: Presentation, Evaluation, and Management

Kashyap V. Panganamamula, MD; Frank K. Friedenberg, MD; Robert S. Fisher, MD; and Henry P. Parkman, MD

Introduction

Gastroparesis is a chronic motility disorder of the stomach characterized by delayed gastric emptying in the absence of a mechanical cause of obstruction. Gastroparesis can occur in many clinical settings with varied symptoms and severity of symptoms. Diabetic, postsurgical, and idiopathic etiologies comprise the majority of cases. Diagnostic evaluation in patients with presumed gastroparesis generally consists of upper endoscopy and gastric emptying scintigraphy. Management of this condition can be particularly challenging. Recently, the AGA developed a medical position statement and an accompanying review on gastroparesis.[1,2] This chapter discusses the evaluation and treatment of patients with gastroparesis.

Normal Gastric Emptying and Abnormalities in Gastroparesis

Gastric myoelectrical activity originates from a gastric pacemaker located at the junction of the proximal third and distal two thirds of the gastric corpus along the greater curvature. The ICCs are located in the myenteric plexus and are coupled to gastric smooth muscle cells. These ICCs are now considered to be responsible for generation of gastric slow wave activity. The electrical impulses are transmitted distally in an aboral fashion at a rate of 3 cycles/minute, producing antral contractions. The antral contractions help in triturating the food into small particles, allowing passage across the pylorus. Undigested and larger particles are swept across the pylorus by a series of contractions known as the phase III migrating motor complex that occur in the fasting state in cycles of every 90 minutes.

Normal gastric emptying reflects a coordinated activity of different regions of the stomach and the duodenum. It is regulated by the influence of the CNS predominantly through the vagal efferent pathways and enteric nervous system on gastric smooth muscle. Important events related to normal gastric emptying include postprandial receptive relaxation of the gastric fundus allowing accommodation of food without significantly increasing gastric pressure, rhythmic antral contractions for trituration of large food particles and breakdown into appropriate size, pyloric relaxation to allow food to enter the duodenum, coordination of antropyloroduodenal motor events, and finally neural/hormonal inhibitory feedback from nutrients in the small bowel. Abnormalities in any of these activities can result in the process of delayed emptying of the stomach and may lead to symptoms of gastroparesis.

Etiology of Gastroparesis

Gastroparesis was initially described as an infrequent complication of long-standing diabetes especially in association with other complications of diabetes such as neuropathy. In a recent series of 146 patients with gastroparesis, the 3 major categories of gastroparesis were diabetic (29%), postsurgical (13%), and idiopathic (36%) (Table 11-1).[3]

DIABETIC GASTROPARESIS

Gastroparesis is a well-recognized complication of diabetes mellitus. It is classically considered to occur in patients with long-standing type 1 diabetes mellitus in the presence of other associated complications such as retinopathy, nephropathy, and peripheral neuropathy. Estimated prevalence in one study of gastroparesis in diabetic patients was 40%.[4] Many affected patients may have other signs of autonomic dysfunction, including postural hypotension. Gastroparesis has also been described in approximately 30% of patients with type 2 diabetes mellitus.[5] Individuals with diabetes of relatively short duration may have rapid emptying. In those with accelerated emptying, impairment of fundic receptive relaxation to the meal may be the underlying defect; this may be from vagal dysfunction.[6] Gastroparesis traditionally has been considered to confer a poor prognosis for affected diabetic patients; however, recent investigations suggest that this may be incorrect.[7]

Symptoms in affected patients include nausea, vomiting, early satiety, fullness, and abdominal discomfort. Symptoms of fullness and bloating have some predictive value for gastroparesis in diabetic patients. Symptom severity, however, does not necessarily correlate well with the degree of gastric stasis.[4,5] Some patients with severe symptoms may have near-normal to normal gastric emptying. In these individuals, other abnormalities, including impaired fundic relaxation, gastric slow wave dysrhythmias, or visceral hypersensitivity, may be potentially responsible for the symptoms.[4] The term diabetic gastropathy is occasionally used since symptoms may not predict delayed gastric emptying and response to prokinetic treatment.

Changes in gastric emptying in affected patients may influence the postprandial blood glucose concentrations. Delayed gastric emptying contributes to erratic glycemic control because of unpredictable delivery of food into the duodenum.[8] Impaired gastric emptying with continued administration of exogenous insulin may produce hypoglycemia. Conversely, acceleration of emptying has been reported to cause hyperglycemia.[9] Problems with blood glucose control may be the first indication that a diabetic patient is developing gastroparesis.[10] In type 1 diabetic patients with gastroparesis, prokinetic therapy may potentially benefit glycemic control although this has been shown in only a few studies.[10]

Table 11-1

CAUSES OF GASTROPARESIS

- Diabetes mellitus
- Idiopathic
- Postsurgical
  * Partial gastric resection/vagotomy
  * Nissen fundoplication
  * Transplantation: lung, heart-lung

Gastrointestinal Disorders Associated With Delayed Gastric Emptying

- Diffuse gastrointestinal motor disorders (eg, chronic intestinal pseudo-obstruction)
- GERD
- Functional dyspepsia
- Hypertrophic pyloric stenosis

Nongastrointestinal Disorders Associated With Delayed Gastric Emptying

Neurologic Disorders

- CNS tumors
- Parkinson's disease

Collagen Vascular Disorders

- Scleroderma
- Systemic lupus erythematosus

Endocrine and Metabolic Disorders

- Thyroid dysfunction
- Parathyroid dysfunction

Eating Disorders

- Anorexia nervosa

Other

- Amyloidosis
- Chronic renal insufficiency
- Gastric infection
- Chronic mesenteric ischemia
- Tumor associated (paraneoplastic)
- Medication-associated delayed gastric emptying

Diabetic gastroparesis is likely to result from impaired neural control of gastric motility, possibly at the level of the vagus nerve.[11] Other factors, including impairment of the inhibitory nitric oxide–containing nerves,[12] damage of the pacemaker ICCs,[13] and underlying smooth muscle dysfunction, have been described.[14] In one study, selective loss of pyloric nitric oxide synthase was shown to contribute to gastroparesis in an animal model and was reversible by administration of insulin or agents that restore nitric oxide activity.[15]

Hyperglycemia alone also may reversibly affect gastric motility and reduce the effectiveness of prokinetic agents. Hyperglycemia decreases antral contractility, decreases antral phase III of the migrating motor complex (MMC), increases pyloric contractions, causes gastric dysrhythmias (primarily tachygastria), delays gastric emptying, and even modulates fundic relaxation properties.[16,17] Normalization of serum glucose levels in hyperglycemic patients may stabilize gastric myoelectric activity, improve gastric emptying, and restore antral phase III activity. Hyperglycemia appears to cause a reversible impairment of vagal efferent function.

POSTSURGICAL GASTROPARESIS

Gastroparesis may occur as a complication of a number of abdominal surgical procedures. Historically, most cases have resulted from performance of vagotomy in combination with gastric drainage for medically refractory PUD.[18] With the advent of laparoscopic techniques to treat GERD, more individuals are presenting with gastroparesis as a complication of fundoplication possibly from vagal injury from the surgery. The vagus nerves regulate both meal-evoked fundic relaxations and phasic antral contractions. The effects of complete vagal denervation are to accelerate gastric emptying of liquids and to retard emptying of solids. To avert the gastroparetic effects of vagotomy, a gastric drainage procedure such as a pyloroplasty or gastroenterostomy is often also performed. In most patients, the net result is that vagotomy combined with a drainage procedure produces little alteration in gastric emptying.

Approximately 5% of patients undergoing vagotomy with antral resection and gastrojejunostomy develop severe postsurgical gastroparesis.[18] In these individuals, the antrum is not present to triturate solids and the proximal stomach is unable to generate sufficient pressure to empty solid food residue.

Postprandial abdominal pain, bloating, nausea, and vomiting characterize the Roux-en-Y stasis syndrome. The combination of vagotomy, distal gastric resection, and Roux-en-Y gastrojejunostomy predisposes to severe gastric stasis as a result of both slow emptying from the gastric remnant and delayed small bowel transit in the denervated Roux efferent limb.[18]

IDIOPATHIC GASTROPARESIS

Idiopathic gastroparesis refers to symptomatic disease with no detectable primary underlying abnormality for delayed gastric emptying. This may represent the most common form of gastroparesis.[1] Symptoms may fluctuate, with episodes of pronounced symptoms interspersed with a relatively asymptomatic period. Most patients with idiopathic gastroparesis are women, typically young or middle aged.[19] Symptoms of idiopathic gastroparesis overlap with those of functional dyspepsia and in some patients, it may be difficult to provide a definitive distinction between the two. Abdominal pain/discomfort typically is the predominant symptom in functional dyspepsia, whereas nausea, vomiting, early satiety, and bloating predominate in idiopathic gastroparesis. Gastroparesis can also be seen in patients with GERD in which reflux symptoms may predominate.

The histologic basis of idiopathic gastroparesis is poorly understood. In one case, myenteric hypoganglionosis and reductions in numbers of ICCs were observed.[20] A subset of patients with idiopathic gastroparesis report sudden onset of symptoms after a viral prodrome, suggesting a potential viral etiology for their symptoms. In this patient subset, previously healthy subjects developed the sudden onset of nausea, vomiting, diarrhea, fever, and cramps suggestive of a systemic viral infection. However, instead of experiencing resolution of symptoms, these individuals note persistent nausea, vomiting, and early satiety. Viruses that have been implicated in these cases include cytomegalovirus, Epstein-Barr virus, and varicella zoster. These patients appear to have slow resolution of their symptoms over several years.[21] In contrast, individuals with idiopathic gastroparesis without a viral trigger tend to show less improvement over time.

Clinical Presentation of Gastroparesis

Symptoms of gastroparesis are variable and include early satiety, nausea, vomiting, bloating, and upper abdominal discomfort. In one series of 146 patients with gastroparesis, nausea was present in 92%, vomiting in 84%, abdominal bloating in 75%, and early satiety in 60%.[1] Complications of gastroparesis may contribute to patient morbidity and include esophagitis, Mallory-Weiss tear, and vegetable-laden bezoars.[22]

Symptoms of gastroparesis may simulate the symptoms related to other structural disorders of the stomach and proximal GI tract such as PUD, partial gastric or small bowel obstruction, gastric cancer, and pancreaticobiliary disorders.[22] There is also an overlap between the symptoms of gastroparesis and functional dyspepsia. Indeed, idiopathic gastroparesis can be considered one of the causes of functional dyspepsia.

The majority of patients with gastroparesis are women. In one large investigation, 82% of gastroparetic patients were female.[1] Women tend to exhibit slower emptying rates than men, especially during the later portion of the menstrual cycle (the luteal phase).[23,24] It is believed that gastric muscle contractility is reduced by progesterone.

Symptom correlation with delayed gastric emptying is variable for diabetic gastropathy, idiopathic gastroparesis, and functional dyspepsia. In recent studies, early satiety, postprandial fullness, and vomiting have been reported to predict delayed emptying in patients with functional dyspepsia.[25] In patients with diabetes, abdominal fullness and bloating were found to predict delayed gastric emptying.[5] In individuals with symptoms of gastroparesis who have normal rates of gastric emptying, other motor, myoelectric, or sensory abnormalities may be responsible for the symptoms.

Abdominal discomfort or pain is present in 46% to 89% of patients with gastroparesis but is usually not the predominant symptom, in contrast to its prominence in functional dyspepsia.[3,26] Nevertheless, treatment of abdominal pain in gastroparesis can be challenging. Patients with functional dyspepsia exhibit increased sensitivity to gastric distention suggestive of afferent neural dysfunction as a contributing factor for the symptoms.[27] Similarly, in diabetic patients with dyspeptic symptoms, gastric distention elicits exaggerated nausea, bloating, and abdominal discomfort, suggesting that sensory nerve dysfunction may participate in symptom genesis in some patients with gastroparesis.[28]

Table 11-2

EVALUATION OF PATIENTS WITH SYMPTOMS SUGGESTIVE OF GASTROPARESIS

1. Initial evaluation
   A. History and physical examination
   B. Blood tests
      i. Complete blood count
      ii. Complete metabolic profile
      iii. Amylase, if abdominal pain is significant symptom
      iv. Pregnancy test, if appropriate
   C. Abdominal obstruction radiographic series
2. Evaluate for organic disorders
   A. Upper endoscopy to evaluate for mechanical obstruction or mucosal lesions (alternative: barium UGI series, often with small bowel follow-through)
   B. Biliary ultrasonography if abdominal pain is a significant symptom
3. Evaluate for delayed gastric emptying
   A. Solid-phase gastric emptying test
   B. Screen for secondary causes of gastroparesis
      i. Thyroid function tests (thyroid-stimulating hormone)
      ii. Tests for collagen vascular disease (antinuclear antibody, anti-scleroderma antibody)
      iii. Glycosylated hemoglobin (HbA1C)
4. Treatment trial with prokinetic agent and/or antiemetic agent
5. If no clinical response, consider further investigation
   A. Electrogastrography (EGG)
   B. Antroduodenal manometry
   C. Small bowel evaluation with enteroclysis or small bowel follow-through

Evaluation of Patients With Suspected Gastroparesis

A careful history and careful physical examination is an important part of the initial evaluation (Table 11-2). History should include reviewing all of the patient's medications to help identify and eliminate drugs that can aggravate symptoms. Physical examination may reveal signs of dehydration or malnutrition in patients with long-standing, severe symptoms of gastroparesis. The presence of a succussion splash, detected by auscultation over the epigastrium while moving the patient side to side or rapidly palpating the epigastrium, indicates excessive fluid in the stomach from gastroparesis or mechanical gastric outlet obstruction.

Initial laboratory studies should be performed to identify electrolyte abnormalities such as hypokalemia and metabolic alkalosis, renal insufficiency, anemia, pancreatitis, or thyroid dysfunction. An abdominal obstruction series should be performed to evaluate for mechanical gastric outlet or small bowel obstruction. Most patients will need an upper endoscopy or a radiographic UGI series to exclude mechanical obstruction or ulcer disease. The presence of retained food in the stomach after overnight fasting without evidence of mechanical obstruction is suggestive of gastroparesis. Bezoars may be found in severe cases.

Contrast radiography of the small intestine is performed in those patients with refractory symptoms, those with symptoms suggestive of a small bowel etiology (eg, profound distention, steatorrhea, feculent emesis), or those who exhibit dilated small bowel loops on plain radiography. When UGI radiography is ordered, a small bowel follow-through can be included to screen for small bowel lesions. The small bowel follow-through is accurate for detection of high-grade small bowel obstruction, usually provides an adequate assessment of the terminal ileum, and may rarely suggest superior mesenteric artery syndrome. Enteroclysis (small bowel enema), obtained by placing a nasoduodenal or oroduodenal tube and with contrast instilled directly into the small bowel, provides double-contrast images and is more accurate in detecting small intestinal mucosal lesions, mild to intermediate grades of obstruction, and small bowel neoplasia. Computed tomographic scanning with oral and IV contrast may also be useful for detection and localization of intestinal obstruction.

EVALUATION OF GASTRIC EMPTYING, MOTOR FUNCTION, AND MYOELECTRIC ACTIVITY

Several methods have been proposed for quantification of gastric emptying, motor function, and myoelectric activity (Table 11-3).

Gastric Emptying Scintigraphy

Gastric emptying scintigraphy of a solid-phase meal is considered the gold standard for diagnosis of gastroparesis because it quantifies the emptying of a physiologic caloric meal. Measurement of gastric emptying of solids is more sensitive for detection of gastroparesis because liquid emptying may remain normal even in the presence of advanced disease. Dual solid and liquid phase emptying scans may be useful in symptomatic patients after gastric surgery.

For solid-phase testing, most centers use a 99mTc sulfur colloid-labeled egg sandwich as the test meal with standard imaging at 0, 1, 2, and 4 hours.[29,30] The radiolabel should be cooked into the meal to ensure radioisotope binding to the solid phase. This prevents elution of the radiotracer into the liquid phase, which might produce an erroneous measurement of the faster liquid-phase gastric emptying. Scintigraphic assessment of emptying should be extended to at least 2 hours after meal ingestion.[31] Even with extension of the scintigraphic study to this length, there may be significant day-to-day variability (up to 20%) in rates of gastric emptying. For shorter durations, the test is less reliable due to larger variations of normal gastric emptying. Extending scintigraphy to 4 hours has been advocated to improve the accuracy in determining the presence of gastroparesis.[32]

Table 11-3

TESTS TO ASSESS GASTRIC MOTOR AND MYOELECTRICAL FUNCTION

	Advantages	Disadvantages
Tests Assessing Gastric Emptying		
UGI barium radiographic study	Assess for mucosal lesions	Nonphysiologic Radiation exposure (moderate)
Scintigraphy	Gold standard Noninvasive Able to assess solid and liquid emptying	Radiation exposure (minimal)
Breath tests using ^{13}C	Noninvasive	Not commonly performed Need normal small intestinal absorption, liver metabolism, and pulmonary excretion
Ultrasonography for serial changes in antral area	Noninvasive, physiologic	Requires expertise for imaging and interpretation Primarily measures liquid emptying
Magnetic resonance imaging	Noninvasive	Expensive, time consuming Need specialized centers and software

(continued)

Table 11-3

TESTS TO ASSESS GASTRIC MOTOR AND MYOELECTRICAL FUNCTION (CONTINUED)

	Advantages	Disadvantages
Tests Assessing Gastric Contractile Activity		
Antroduodenal manometry	Assesses contractility in fasting and postprandial periods	Invasive Need expertise to perform and interpret
Gastric barostat	Measures proximal stomach relaxation and contraction	Invasive Research technique
Tests Assessing Gastric Myoelectrical Activity		
EGG	Noninvasive	Movement artifact may make recording difficult to interpret
Tests Assessing Gastric Accommodation		
Gastric barostat	Measures proximal stomach accommodation response	Invasive Research technique Balloon may interfere with accommodation
Satiety test	Measures combination of accommodation and sensitivity	Simple Not well standardized or accepted

Patients should discontinue medications that may affect gastric emptying for an adequate period before this test based on drug half-life. This will be 48 to 72 hours for most medications. The most important groups of medications to stop include opioid analgesics and anticholinergic agents. Prokinetic agents that accelerate emptying may give a falsely normal gastric emptying result. Serotonin receptor antagonists such as ondansetron, which have little effect on gastric emptying, may be given for severe symptoms before performance of gastric scintigraphy. Hyperglycemia delays gastric emptying in diabetic patients. It is not unreasonable to defer gastric emptying testing until relative euglycemia is achieved to obtain a reliable determination of emptying parameters in the absence of acute metabolic derangement.

Emptying of solids typically exhibits a lag phase followed by a prolonged linear emptying phase. A variety of parameters can be calculated from the emptying profile of a radiolabeled meal such as half emptying time and duration of the lag phase. The simplest approach for interpreting a gastric emptying study is to report the percent retention at defined times after meal ingestion usually 2 and 4 hours, with normal being <50% remaining in the stomach at 2 hours and <10% remaining at 4 hours.

Breath Testing for Gastric Emptying

Breath tests using the nonradioactive isotope ^{13}C bound to a digestible substance have been validated for measuring gastric emptying. Most commonly, ^{13}C-labeled octanoate, a medium-chain triglyceride, is bound into a solid meal such as a muffin. Other studies have bound ^{13}C to acetate or to proteinaceous algae (Spirulina). After ingestion and stomach emptying, ^{13}C-octanoate is absorbed in the small intestine and metabolized to $^{13}CO_2$, which is then expelled from the lungs during respiration. The rate-limiting step is the rate of solid gastric emptying. Thus, octanoate breath testing provides a measure of solid-phase emptying.[33] The octanoate breath test provides reproducible results that correlate with findings on gastric emptying scintigraphy.[34,35] Most octanoate breath testing at present is performed as part of clinical research and pharmaceutical studies. Validation of this test in patients with emphysema, cirrhosis, celiac sprue, and pancreatic insufficiency is needed because rates of octanoate metabolism may be impaired in these disorders.

Electrogastrography

EGG records gastric myoelectrical activity, known as the slow wave, using cutaneous electrodes affixed to the anterior abdominal wall overlying the stomach.[36] The slow wave is responsible for controlling the maximal frequency and the controlled aboral propagation of gastric contractions. The normal gastric slow wave frequency is approximately 3 cycles/minute. Meal ingestion increases the amplitude of the EGG signal, which is believed to result from increased antral contractility and distention of the stomach from the ingested meals. EGG testing quantifies the dominant frequency and regularity of gastric myoelectrical activity, quantifies the percentage of time in which abnormal slow wave rhythms are present during fasting and postprandial periods, and assesses the increase in amplitude (or power) after a meal.[37]

Gastric dysrhythmias (tachygastria, bradygastria) and decreased EGG amplitude responses to meal ingestion have been characterized in patients with idiopathic and diabetic gastroparesis.[38] Gastric myoelectric abnormalities have also been described in patients with unexplained nausea and vomiting, motion sickness, and nausea and vomiting of pregnancy. EGG abnormalities are present in 75% of patients with delayed gastric emptying versus 25% of symptomatic patients with normal gastric emptying. Some investigators suggest that EGG abnormalities and delayed gastric emptying may define slightly different patient populations with dyspeptic symptoms.[39] In diabetic patients, hyperglycemia itself can cause gastric arrhythmias.

Clinically, EGG has been used to demonstrate gastric myoelectric abnormalities in patients with unexplained nausea and vomiting or functional dyspepsia. EGG is considered an adjunct to gastric emptying scintigraphy as part of a comprehensive evaluation of patients with refractory symptoms suggestive of an UGI motility disorder.[37,39] However, there has been little investigation to date to validate the utility of EGG in the clinical management of patients with suspected gastric dysmotility.

Antroduodenal Manometry

Antroduodenal manometry provides information about gastric and duodenal motor function in both fasting and postprandial periods.[40] Manometry may be performed in stationary settings over a 5- to 8-hour period or in ambulatory fashion over 24 hours using solid-state transducers. Ambulatory studies afford the advantage of correlating symptoms with abnormal motor patterns; however, catheter migration in these studies may limit interpretation of gastric motility. Indications for antroduodenal manometry include 1) characterization of motor dysfunction in patients with unexplained nausea and vomiting, 2) delineation of the cause of gastric or small bowel stasis (eg, visceral neuropathy or myopathy), and 3) support of a suspected diagnosis of chronic intestinal pseudo-obstruction.[40]

Distinct gastrointestinal motor patterns are present in the interdigestive (fasting) and digestive (fed) periods. The interdigestive (fasting) pattern consists of 3 cyclical phases known as the MMC that recur at approximately 2-hour intervals unless interrupted by a meal. Phase I of MMC is a period of motor quiescence that is followed by a period of intermittent phasic contractions (phase II). The MMC culminates in a burst of regular rhythmic contractions that propagate from the antrum through the proximal small intestine (phase III, activity front). The intense propulsive contractions during phase III have been considered to be a physiologic "intestinal housekeeper" and are responsible for clearance of dietary fiber and indigestible solids from the upper gut. Feeding disrupts the MMC and replaces it with a fed motor pattern of more regular antral and duodenal contractions of variable amplitude that may be either segmental or propagative in character.

In gastroparesis, antroduodenal manometry may identify a decreased frequency/force of antral contractions and origination of most phase III complexes in the duodenum with complete loss of antral component. In some individuals, increased tonic and phasic activity of the pylorus ("pylorospasm") or irregular bursts of small intestinal contractions may be observed.[41] Antroduodenal manometry can help confirm or exclude an underlying dysmotility syndrome when results of gastric emptying testing are normal or borderline. With an accurate stationary recording, reductions in the postprandial distal antral motility index correlate with impaired gastric emptying of solids.[42]

Treatment of Gastroparesis

The treatment goals for patients with symptomatic gastroparesis are control symptoms; correct fluid, electrolyte, and nutritional deficiencies; and identify and treat the underlying cause of gastroparesis if possible.

For relatively mild disease, dietary modifications and a low-dose antiemetic or prokinetic agent might provide satisfactory control of symptoms. Patients with severe manifestations of gastroparesis, such as refractory vomiting, pronounced dehydration, or chaotic glucose control, may require hospitalization for IV hydration, insulin administration, and/or IV administration of antiemetic and prokinetic agents.

DIET

Increasing the liquid nutrient component of the ingested meal should be emphasized because liquid emptying often is preserved. Fats and fiber tend to decrease gastric emptying; thus, their intake should be minimized. Indigestible fiber and roughage may predispose to bezoar formation. Foods that cannot be reliably chewed into smaller constituency should be avoided. Multiple frequent meals are often recommended to limit the caloric intake with each meal.

METABOLIC CONTROL

Diabetic patients with gastroparesis frequently exhibit labile blood glucose concentrations with prolonged periods of significant hyperglycemia. Hyperglycemia itself can delay gastric emptying.[10] Hyperglycemia can counteract the accelerating effects of prokinetic agents on gastric emptying.[43] Improvement of glucose control increases antral contractility, corrects gastric dysrhythmias, and accelerates emptying. To date, there have been no long-term studies confirming the beneficial effects of maintenance of near euglycemia on gastroparetic symptoms. Nevertheless, the consistent findings of physiologic studies in healthy volunteers and diabetic patients provide a compelling argument to strive for near-normal blood glucose levels in affected diabetic patients.

ANTIEMETIC AGENTS

Antiemetic drugs may serve as primary therapy for some patients with gastric dysmotility or as adjuncts to medications that promote gastric emptying (Table 11-4).

Phenothiazines are commonly prescribed antiemetic agents. These dopamine receptor antagonists act at the level of the area postrema of the medulla oblongata, a region termed the chemoreceptor trigger zone. Commonly used antiemetic agents include prochlorperazine, trimethobenzamide, and promethazine. Phenothiazines may be administered as tablets, capsules, or liquid suspensions. For patients with severe symptoms, suppositories or injectable forms may be more efficacious. Side effects from phenothiazines are common and include sedation and extrapyramidal effects.

Serotonin (5-HT3) receptor antagonists, including ondansetron, granisetron, and dolasetron, are useful for prophylaxis of chemotherapy-induced nausea and vomiting as well as symptoms occurring postoperatively or during radiation therapy. 5-HT3 antagonists may act both on the area postrema as well as on peripheral afferent nerve fibers within the vagus. Although these agents are frequently used, there are no studies documenting their efficacy in gastroparesis. If drugs in this class are considered, they are best given on an as-needed basis.

Antihistamines acting on H1 receptors exhibit central antiemetic effects. Commonly prescribed antihistamines include diphenhydramine, dimenhydrinate, and meclizine. There is little evidence that antihistamines serve important roles in symptom control

Table 11-4

ANTIEMETIC THERAPY FOR GASTROPARESIS

Prokinetic agents with antiemetic properties (antagonize dopamine receptors)	Metoclopramide (Reglan [Schwartz Pharma, Inc, Meoquon, Wis])
Phenothiazine derivatives (antagonize dopamine receptors in area postrema)	Prochlorperazine (Compazine [GlaxoSmithKline, Research Triangle Park, NC]) Trimethobenzamide (Tigan [King Pharmaceuticals Inc, Bristol, Tenn])
Antihistamines (H1 receptor antagonists)	Diphenhydramine (Benadryl [Pfizer Inc, New York, NY]) Promethazine (Phenergan [Wyeth Pharmaceuticals, Philadelphia, Pa]) Meclizine (Antivert [Pfizer Inc, New York, NY])
Anticholinergics	Scopolamine
Antiserotoninergic (5-HT3 receptor antagonists)	Ondansetron (Zofran [GlaxoSmithKline, Research Triangle Park, NC]) Granisetron (Kytril [Roche Laboratories Inc, Nutley, NJ]) Dolasetron (Anzemet [Aventis Pharmaceuticals Inc, Bridgewater, NJ]) Palonosetron (Aloxi [MGI Pharma Inc, Bloomington, Minn])
Substance P/neurokinin-1 receptor antagonists	Aprepitant (Emend [Merck & Co Inc, West Point, Pa])

in gastroparesis. These agents are most useful for treatment of motion sickness via their actions on H1 receptors in the vestibular apparatus.

Transdermal hyoscine (scopolamine patch) is occasionally used for nausea and vomiting, primarily from motion sickness and recovery from anesthesia and surgery. This anticholinergic agent may delay gastric emptying.

Benzodiazepines such as lorazepam and diazepam are most commonly used for the prevention of anticipatory nausea and vomiting before administration of chemotherapy. Cannabinoid drugs such as tetrahydrocannabinol have been studied for symptoms from chemotherapy and appear to have potency similar to standard antidopaminergics. A clear role in management of the patient with gastroparesis has not been established. Interestingly, recent reports suggest frequent recreational use of marijuana can aggravate symptoms.

PROKINETIC AGENTS

Prokinetic medications enhance gut contractility and promote the aboral movement of luminal contents (Table 11-5). In the stomach, prokinetic agents increase antral contractility, correct gastric dysrhythmias, and improve antroduodenal coordination. Some prokinetics, notably metoclopramide and domperidone, also exhibit antiemetic properties. Most commonly, prokinetic medications are administered 30 minutes before meals to elicit maximal clinical effects. Bedtime doses often are added to facilitate nocturnal gastric emptying of indigestible solids. The response to treatment is usually judged clinically rather than repeat gastric emptying tests.

Metoclopramide

Metoclopramide, a substituted benzamide structurally related to procainamide, exhibits both prokinetic and antiemetic actions. The drug serves as a dopamine receptor antagonist both in the CNS and in the stomach. It also releases acetylcholine from intrinsic myenteric cholinergic neurons. The prokinetic properties of metoclopramide are limited to the proximal gut. Antidopaminergic actions in the area postrema explain the additional antiemetic actions.

Metoclopramide is approved for use in diabetic gastroparesis and for prevention of postoperative and chemotherapy-induced nausea and vomiting. Controlled trials report that metoclopramide provides symptomatic relief while accelerating gastric emptying of solids and liquids in patients with idiopathic, diabetic, and postvagotomy gastroparesis and in patients with GERD.[44-46] Metoclopramide is effective for the short-term treatment of gastroparesis for up to several weeks. Symptomatic improvement does not necessarily accompany improvement in gastric emptying. Indeed, some investigations have reported extended symptom benefits of metoclopramide without prolonged prokinetic action.[47] The long-term utility of metoclopramide has not been proven.

The usual starting dose of metoclopramide in adults is 10 mg 30 minutes before meals and at bedtime. Dosing can be increased to 20 mg if the response to 10 mg is inadequate. Metoclopramide may be administered intravenously or in a liquid form.

The side effects from metoclopramide result from antidopaminergic actions in the CNS and may restrict its use in up to 30% of patients. Acute dystonic reactions such as facial spasm, oculogyric crisis, trismus, and torticollis occur in 0.2% to 6% of patients; when this occurs, it is often observed within 48 hours of initiating therapy.[48,49] Drowsiness, fatigue, and lassitude are reported by 10% of patients. Metoclopramide can aggravate underlying depression. Other side effects may include restlessness, agitation, irritability, and akathisia. Increased prolactin release may result in breast engorgement, lactation, and menstrual irregularity. Prolonged treatment with metoclopramide can produce Parkinsonian-like symptoms.[50,51] Parkinsonian symptoms usually subside within 2 to 3 months following discontinuation of metoclopramide. Because of this

Table 11-5

PROKINETIC AGENTS FOR GASTROPARESIS

Agent	Mechanism of Action	Comments
Metoclopramide (Reglan)	Dopamine receptor antagonist central/peripheral	FDA approved for gastroparesis CNS side effects in 20% to 30% Prokinetic and antiemetic properties
Erythromycin	Motilin receptor agonist	GI side effects (eg, nausea/vomiting/abdominal pain) in many Tachyphylaxis with chronic oral administration Recently, some cardiac effects reported
Cisapride	5-HT4 receptor agonist facilitates acetylcholine release	Taken off market in March 2000 for prolonging QT interval Was only approved for nocturnal heartburn Currently not available as a prescription in the United States
Domperidone	Dopamine receptor antagonist peripheral	Prokinetic and antiemetic properties Currently not available as a prescription in the United States Available in the United States through FDA IND program
Tegaserod (Zelnorm [Novartis Pharmaceuticals Corp, East Hanover, NJ])	5-HT4 partial agonist	FDA approved for constipation-predominant IBS in women and for constipation in men and women
Bethanechol (Urecholine [Merck & Co, West Point, Pa])	Muscarinic receptor agonist Not a true prokinetic agent	Improves gastric emptying, no data on symptoms Increases amplitude of contractions, not peristalsis

effect, patients with Parkinson's disease should be given metoclopramide cautiously, if at all. Tardive dyskinesia, characterized by involuntary movements of the face, tongue, or extremities, may occur with prolonged use and may not reverse after stopping the medication. The prevalence of tardive dyskinesia ranges from 1% to 15% when taking metoclopramide for at least 3 months, but the complication has been reported to occur with short-term use as well.

Erythromycin

The macrolide antibiotic erythromycin exerts prokinetic effects via action on gastroduodenal receptors for motilin, an endogenous peptide responsible for initiation of the MMC in the upper gut.[52] When administered exogenously, motilin stimulates antral contractility and elicits premature antroduodenal phase III activity. Erythromycin produces effects on gastroduodenal motility similar to motilin.

Clinically, erythromycin has been shown to stimulate gastric emptying in diabetic gastroparesis, idiopathic gastroparesis, and postvagotomy gastroparesis. Erythromycin may be most potent when used intravenously.[53] Limited data exist concerning the clinical efficacy of erythromycin in reducing symptoms of gastroparesis. In a systematic review of studies on oral erythromycin with symptom assessment as a clinical end point, improvement was noted in 43% of patients.[54] One study comparing erythromycin and metoclopramide in an open-label, crossover fashion in diabetic gastroparesis found similar efficacy.[48]

Oral administration of erythromycin should be initiated at low doses (eg, 125 to 250 mg 3 or 4 times daily). Liquid suspension erythromycin may be preferred because it is rapidly and more reliably absorbed. IV erythromycin (100 mg every 8 hours) is used for inpatients hospitalized for severe refractory gastroparesis. Side effects of erythromycin at higher doses include nausea, vomiting, and abdominal pain. Because these symptoms may mimic those of gastroparesis, erythromycin may have a narrow therapeutic window in some patients. There is report that administration of erythromycin chronically may be associated with higher mortality from cardiac disease, especially when combined with agents that inhibit cytochrome p-450, such as calcium channel blockers.

Domperidone

Domperidone is a benzimidazole derivative and is a specific dopamine (D2) receptor antagonist. The effects of domperidone on the upper gut are similar to those of metoclopramide, including stimulation of antral contractions and promotion of antroduodenal coordination. Domperidone does not readily cross the blood-brain barrier; therefore, it is much less likely to cause extrapyramidal side effects than metoclopramide. In addition to prokinetic actions in the stomach, domperidone exhibits antiemetic properties via action on the area postrema, a brainstem region with a porous blood-brain barrier.

Domperidone has been studied primarily in patients with diabetic gastroparesis in whom it increases both solid and liquid emptying. Symptomatic improvement with domperidone does not clearly relate to its motor stimulatory actions; rather, its efficacy may stem from its antiemetic effects. In controlled clinical trials, domperidone provided relief of symptoms and improvement in quality of life to greater degrees than placebo in patients with diabetic gastropathy; symptom improvement was similar to that observed for metoclopramide and cisapride but with fewer CNS side effects.[49,55]

Furthermore, symptomatic diabetic patients with normal gastric emptying reported beneficial effects with domperidone therapy. The prokinetic actions of domperidone may be transitory in nature. Other studies report that improvements in gastric emptying and symptoms were still present after 1 year of treatment. Domperidone has been advocated for therapy of nausea and vomiting in patients with Parkinson's disease, in whom symptoms may be secondary to gastroparesis or to dopaminergic drugs used to treat the disease (eg, L-dopa).

Dosing of domperidone typically begins at 10 mg before meals and at bedtime and can be increased as tolerated to achieve symptom control. In many patients, the dose of domperidone can be more easily increased to improve symptom control because of the near lack of neuropsychiatric and extrapyramidal side effects. The most common side effects of domperidone relate to induction of hyperprolactinemia, with induction of menstrual irregularities, breast engorgement, and galactorrhea. Domperidone is not approved by the Food and Drug Administration (FDA) for prescription in the United States.[56] Fortunately, the FDA has made investigational new drug (IND) applications available for physicians to provide domperidone to patients with gastroparesis refractory to other therapies.

Tegaserod

Tegaserod, an aminoguanidine indole compound, is a partial 5-HT4 receptor agonist approved for the treatment of constipation-predominant IBS and constipation. In healthy volunteers, tegaserod stimulates interdigestive small intestinal motility and postprandial antral and intestinal motility. Tegaserod has been shown to accelerate gastric emptying in some but not all studies of healthy volunteers.[57,58] Tegaserod was shown to accelerate solid-phase gastric emptying in patients with gastroparesis in dose-dependent fashion, with 6 mg 3 times daily and 12 mg twice daily showing greater effect than the standard dose for constipation (ie, 6 mg twice daily).[59] Effects of tegaserod on symptoms has not been as impressive in patients with gastroparesis. However, tegaserod has a marginal effect on symptoms in functional dyspepsia with some improvement in early satiety and postprandial fullness.[60] Clinical studies are ongoing on the effects of tegaserod in patients with functional dyspepsia and gastroparesis.

Management of Refractory Gastroparesis

There is no consensus regarding management of patients with gastroparesis who do not respond to simple antiemetic or prokinetic therapy or who develop medication-induced side effects. Management includes ensuring that gastroparesis is responsible for symptoms, optimizing current therapy, and changing prokinetic agents if maximal doses of the current treatment program are inadequate. It is unclear why some patients respond to one prokinetic agent and not another. Refractory patients often require treatment with both prokinetic and antiemetic agents. For patients who are refractory to all attempts at pharmacotherapy of gastroparesis, placement of a feeding jejunostomy can be considered. Use of TPN should be temporary, if possible, due to the risk of complications. Newer therapies being evaluated are pyloric injection of botulinum toxin and gastric electric stimulation. Gastric resection is usually of limited value for most etiologies of gastroparesis.

COMBINATION PROKINETIC THERAPY

Prokinetic agents act via different mechanisms to enhance gastric emptying. Theoretically, addition of a second prokinetic agent may augment the response of the first drug if the 2 agents act on different receptor subtypes. Dual prokinetic therapy with domperidone and cisapride had been reported to accelerate emptying and reduce symptoms in some patients with refractory gastroparesis.[61] Combinations of available prokinetic agents in the United States, such as domperidone and tegaserod or metoclopramide and erythromycin, have not been specifically studied.

PSYCHOTROPIC MEDICATIONS

Tricyclic antidepressants may have significant benefits in suppressing symptoms in some patients with nausea and vomiting as well as patients with abdominal pain.[62] Doses of tricyclic antidepressants used are lower than used to treat depression. A reasonable starting dose for a tricyclic drug such as amitriptyline is 10 to 25 mg at bedtime. If benefit is not observed in several weeks, doses are increased by 10- to 25-mg increments up to 50 to 100 mg. Side effects are common with use of tricyclic antidepressants and can interfere with management and lead to a change in medication in 25% of patients.[62] The secondary amines, nortriptyline and desipramine, may have fewer side effects. There are limited data on the use of SSRIs in gastroparesis or functional dyspepsia.

PYLORIC BOTULINUM TOXIN INJECTION

Gastric emptying is a highly regulated process reflecting the integration of the propulsive forces of proximal fundic tone and distal antral contractions with the functional resistance provided by the pylorus. Manometric studies of patients with diabetic gastroparesis show prolonged periods of increased pyloric tone and phasic contractions, a phenomenon termed pylorospasm.[41] Botulinum toxin is a potent inhibitor of neuromuscular transmission and has been used to treat spastic somatic muscle disorders as well as achalasia.[63] Several studies have tested the effects of pyloric injection of botulinum toxin in patients with diabetic and idiopathic gastroparesis.[64,65] These studies have all been unblinded in small numbers of patients from single centers and have observed mild improvements in gastric emptying and modest reductions in symptoms for several months. Double-blind controlled studies are needed to support the efficacy of this treatment.

GASTRIC ELECTRIC STIMULATION

Gastric electric stimulation is an emerging treatment for refractory gastroparesis. It involves an implantable neurostimulator that delivers a high-frequency (12 cpm), low-energy signal with short pulses. With this device, stimulating wires are sutured into the gastric muscle along the greater curvature during laparoscopy or laparotomy. These leads are attached to the electric stimulator, which is positioned in a subcutaneous abdominal pouch. Based on the initial studies that have shown symptom benefit especially in patients with diabetic gastroparesis, the gastric electric neurostimulator was granted humanitarian approval from the FDA for the treatment of chronic, refractory nausea and vomiting secondary to idiopathic or diabetic gastroparesis. The main complication of the implantable neurostimulator has been infection, which has necessitated device removal in approximately 5% to 10% of cases. Further investigation is needed to confirm the effectiveness of gastric stimulation in long-term blinded fashion, which patients are likely to respond, the optimal electrode position, and the optimal stimulation parameters, none of which have been rigorously evaluated to date. Future improvements may include devices that sequentially stimulate the stomach in a peristaltic sequence to promote gastric emptying.[66,67]

GASTROSTOMY AND JEJUNOSTOMY PLACEMENT

For patients with gastroparesis who are unable to maintain nutrition with oral intake, placement of a feeding jejunostomy may provide adequate nutrition. Switching from oral to small bowel delivery may decrease symptoms and reduce hospitalizations.[68] Jejunostomy tubes are effective for providing nutrition, fluids, and medications if there is normal small intestinal motor function. Except in cases of profound malnutrition or electrolyte disturbance, enteral feedings are preferable to chronic parenteral nutrition because of the significant risks of infection, thrombosis, and liver disease with TPN. In contrast, home IV hyperalimentation may be needed for individuals with generalized dysmotility unresponsive to diet and changes in medication. The therapeutic response to jejunostomy infusion may be predicted by a trial of nasojejunal feedings, which should precede placement of a permanent jejunostomy tube if small bowel dysmotility is suspected. Jejunostomy tubes usually are surgically placed during laparoscopy or laparotomy, although a few centers place these endoscopically.[69] Carefully regulated enteral nutrient infusion may improve glycemic control in diabetic patients with refractory vomiting. Nocturnal feedings may permit daytime working and functioning. Complications include infection, tube dysfunction, and tube dislodgment.

In refractory patients with severe nausea and vomiting, placement of a gastrostomy tube for intermittent decompression by venting or suctioning may provide symptom relief.[70] This approach also has been suggested for patients with refractory vomiting that responds to nasogastric decompression. Venting gastrostomies may be placed endoscopically, surgically, or by interventional radiology.[70] The use of venting gastrostomies has decreased and is generally avoided with the advent of gastric electrical stimulation as a treatment modality.

New Directions in the Treatment of Gastroparesis and Gastric Dysmotility Syndromes

NOVEL PROKINETIC AGENTS

New prokinetic agents being tested for gastroparesis include 5-HT4 receptor agonists (tegaserod and mosapride), dopamine receptor antagonists (itopride), and motilin receptor agonists (mitemcinal [GM-611]). For each of these, favorable preliminary results have been reported.

FUNDIC RELAXING AGENTS

Agents that relax the fundus and improve accommodation may be helpful in some patients with gastroparesis and functional dyspepsia, especially when early satiety is prominent. 5-HT1 receptor agonists (sumatriptan, buspirone),[71] α-adrenergic receptor agonists (clonidine), and NO donors (nitroglycerin) have been evaluated in physiologic studies. Clonidine reduces proximal gastric tone and pain perception with gastric distention in healthy subjects. In dyspeptic patients, clonidine reduces symptoms by improving gastric accommodation.[71] Clonidine has been reported to decrease symptoms and accelerate gastric emptying in diabetic patients with gastroparesis, although others have observed slowing of emptying with the drug.[72] Sumatriptan allows accommodation of larger volumes before perception or discomfort is reached and improves meal-induced satiety in patients with functional dyspepsia.[73] Buspirone, another oral 5-HT1 agonist, has anxiolytic properties in addition to its fundic relaxant capabilities. Sildenafil augments gastric accommodation by enhancing the effects of NO.[74] In an animal study, sildenafil promoted pyloric relaxation and accelerated gastric emptying. However, a subsequent investigation in rats reported that sildenafil delayed liquid gastric emptying and small bowel transit and an unpublished study in humans also observed delay of gastric emptying.[75]

GASTRIC SLOW WAVE ANTIDYSRHYTHMICS

Many prokinetic drugs (metoclopramide, domperidone, cisapride) also stabilize dysrhythmic slow wave activity in patients with gastroparesis.[76] In some studies, resolution of slow wave rhythm disturbances correlates better with symptomatic improvement than does acceleration of gastric emptying. Prostaglandin inhibitors have been shown to resolve tachygastrias during hyperglycemia.[77] In some patients, indomethacin or ketorolac has reduced symptoms and reversed gastric myoelectrical abnormalities.[78] Unfortunately, indomethacin is also ulcerogenic.

Conclusion

Patients with gastroparesis are being increasingly recognized. Management of this condition can be particularly challenging. Symptoms do not necessarily correlate with gastric emptying, the marker of this disorder. Current management strategies are often suboptimal for adequately improving patient's symptoms. Important advances in the evaluation and treatment of this disorder are being made. Several new treatment modalities are being investigated in this disorder, which makes a favorable outlook for this condition.

References

1. Parkman HP, Hasler WL, Fisher RS. American Gastroenterological Association medical position statement: Diagnosis and treatment of gastroparesis. *Gastroenterology.* 2004;127:1589-1591.
2. Parkman HP, Hasler WL, Fisher RS. American Gastroenterological Association technical review on the diagnosis and treatment of gastroparesis. *Gastroenterology.* 2004;127:1592-1622.

3. Soykan I, Sivri B, Sarosiek I, Kierran B, McCallum RW. Demography, clinical characteristics, psychological profiles, treatment and long-term follow-up of patients with gastroparesis. *Dig Dis Sci.* 1998;43:2398-2404.

4. Horowitz M, Harding PE, Maddox AF, et al. Gastric and oesophageal emptying in patients with type 2 (non-insulin-dependent) diabetes mellitus. *Diabetologia.* 1989;32:151-159.

5. Horowitz M, Harding PE, Maddox AF, et al. Gastric and oesophageal emptying in insulin-dependent diabetes mellitus. *J Gastroenterol Hepatol.* 1986;1:97-113.

6. Frank JW, Saslow SB, Camilleri M, Thomforde GM, Dinneen S, Rizza RA. Mechanism of accelerated gastric emptying of liquids and hyperglycemia in patients with type II diabetes mellitus. *Gastroenterology.* 1995;109:755-765.

7. Kong MF, Horowitz M, Jones KL, Wishart JM, Harding PE. Natural history of diabetic gastroparesis. *Diabetes Care.* 1998;22:503-507.

8. Rayner CK, Samsom M, Jones KL, Horowitz M. Relationships of UGI motor and sensory function with glycemic control. *Diabetes Care.* 2001;24:371-381.

9. Schwartz JG, Green GM, Guan D, McMahan CA, Phillips WT. Rapid gastric emptying of a solid pancake meal in type II diabetic patients. *Diabetes Care.* 1996;19:468-471.

10. Lehmann R, Honegger RA, Feinle C, Fried M, Spinas GA, Schwizer W. Glucose control is not improved by accelerating gastric emptying in patients with type 1 diabetes mellitus and gastroparesis. A pilot study with cisapride as a model drug. *Exp Clin Endocrinol Diabetes.* 2003;111:255-261.

11. Duchen LW, Anjorin A, Watkins PJ, Mackay JD. Pathology of autonomic neuropathy in diabetes mellitus. *Ann Intern Med.* 1980;92:301-303.

12. Takahashi T, Nakamura K, Itoh H, Sima AA, Owyang C. Impaired expression of nitric oxide synthase in gastric myenteric plexus of spontaneously diabetic rats. *Gastroenterology.* 1997;113:1535-1544.

13. He CL, Soffer EE, Ferris CD, Walsh RM, Szurszewski JH, Farrugia G. Loss of ICCs and inhibitory innervation in insulin-dependent diabetes. *Gastroenterology.* 2001;121:427-434.

14. Moscoso GJ, Driver M, Guy RJ. A form of necrobiosis and atrophy of smooth muscle in diabetic gastric autonomic neuropathy. *Pathol Res Pract.* 1986;181:188-194.

15. Watkins CC, Sawa A, Jaffrey S, et al. Insulin restores neuronal nitric oxide synthase expression and function that is lost in diabetic gastropathy. *J Clin Invest.* 2000;106:373-384.

16. Jebbink RJA, Samsom M, Bruijs PPM, et al. Hyperglycemia induces abnormalities of gastric myoelectrical activity in patients with type 1 diabetes mellitus. *Gastroenterology.* 1994;107:1390-1397.

17. Fraser RJ, Horowitz M, Maddox AF, Harding PE, Chatterton BE, Dent J. Hyperglycemia slows gastric emptying in type 1 (insulin-dependent) diabetes mellitus. *Diabetologia.* 1990;33:675-680.

18. Eagon JC, Miedema BW, Kelly KA. Postgastrectomy syndromes. *Surg Clin North Am.* 1992;72:445-465.

19. Stanghellini V, Tosetti C, Paternico A, et al. Risk indicators of delayed gastric emptying of solids in patients with functional dyspepsia. *Gastroenterology.* 1996;110:1036-1042.

20. Zarate N, Mearin F, Wang XY, Hewlett B, Huizinga JD, Malagelada JR. Severe idiopathic gastroparesis due to neuronal and ICCs degeneration: pathological findings and management. *Gut.* 2003;52:966-970.

21. Bityutskiy LP, Soykan I, McCallum RW. Viral gastroparesis: a subgroup of idiopathic gastroparesis—clinical characteristics and long-term outcomes. *Am J Gastroenterol.* 1997;92:1501-1506.

22. Parkman HP, Schwartz SS. Esophagitis and other gastrointestinal disorders associated with diabetic gastroparesis. *Arch Intern Med.* 1987;147:1477-1480.

23. Datz FL, Christian PE, Moore J. Gender-related differences in gastric emptying. *J Nucl Med.* 1987;28:1204-1207.

24. Gill RC, Murphy PD, Hooper HR, Bowes KL, Kingma YJ. Effect of the menstrual cycle on gastric emptying. *Digestion.* 1987;36:168-174.

25. Sarnelli G, Caenepeel P, Geypens B, Janssens J, Tack J. Symptoms associated with impaired gastric emptying of solids and liquids in functional dyspepsia. *Am J Gastroenterol.* 2003;98:783-788.

26. Hoogerwerf WA, Pasricha PJ, Kalloo AN, Schuster MM. Pain: the overlooked symptom in gastroparesis. *Am J Gastroenterol.* 1999;94:1029-1033.

27. Lemann M, Dederding JP, Flourie B, Franchisseur C, Rambaud JC, Jian R. Abnormal perception of visceral pain in response to gastric distension in chronic idiopathic dyspepsia. *Dig Dis Sci.* 1991;36:1249-1254.

28. Samsom M, Salet GAM, Roelofs JMM, Akkermans LM, Vanberge-Henegouwen GP, Smout AJ. Compliance of the proximal stomach and dyspeptic symptoms in patients with type 1 diabetes mellitus. *Dig Dis Sci.* 1995;40:2037-2042.

29. Parkman HP, Harris AD, Krevsky B, Urbain JL, Maurer AH, Fisher RS. Gastroduodenal motility and dysmotility: update on techniques available for evaluation. *Am J Gastroenterol.* 1995;90:869-892.

30. Kim DY, Myung S-J, Camilleri M. Novel testing of human gastric motor and sensory functions: rationale, methods, and potential applications in clinical practice. *Am J Gastroenterol.* 2000;95:3365-3373.

31. Thomforde GM, Camilleri M, Phillips SF, Forstrom LA. Evaluation of an inexpensive screening scintigraphic test of gastric emptying. *J Nucl Med.* 1995;36:93-96.

32. Guo JP, Maurer AH, Fisher RS, Parkman HP. Extending gastric emptying scintigraphy from two to four hours detects more patients with gastroparesis. *Dig Dis Sci.* 2001;46:24-29.

33. Ghoos YF, Maes BD, Geypens BJ, et al. Measurement of gastric emptying rate of solids by means of a carbon-labeled octanoic acid breath test. *Gastroenterology.* 1993;104:1640-1647.

34. Choi MG, Camilleri M, Burton DD, Zinsmeister AR, Forstrom LA, Nair KS. Reproducibility and simplification of 13C-octanoic acid breath test for gastric emptying of solids. *Am J Gastroenterol.* 1998;93:92-98.

35. Bromer MQ, Kantor SN, Wagner DA, Knight LC, Maurer AH, Parkman HP. Simultaneous measurement of gastric emptying with a simple muffin meal using 13C-octanoate breath test and scintigraphy in normal subjects and patients with in dyspeptic symptoms. *Dig Dis Sci.* 2002;47:1657-1663.

36. Chen JZ, McCallum RW. Clinical applications of electrogastrography. *Am J Gastroenterol.* 1993;88:1324-1336.

37. Parkman HP, Hasler WL, Barnett JL, Eaker EY. Electrogastrography: a document prepared by the gastric section of the American Motility Society Clinical GI Motility Testing Task Force. *Neurogastroenterol Motil.* 2003;15:488-497.

38. Chen JD, Lin Z, Pan J, McCallum RW. Abnormal gastric myoelectrical activity and delayed gastric emptying in patients with symptoms suggestive of gastroparesis. *Dig Dis Sci.* 1996;41:1538-1545.

39. Parkman HP, Miller MA, Trate DM, et al. Electrogastrography and gastric empty-ing scintigraphy are complementary for assessment of dyspepsia. *J Clin Gastroenterol.* 1997;24:214-219.

40. Soffer E, Thongsawat S. Clinical value of duodenojejunal manometry. Its usefulness in diagnosis and management of patients with gastrointestinal symptoms. *Dig Dis Sci.* 1996;41:859-863.

41. Mearin F, Camilleri M, Malagelada JR. Pyloric dysfunction in diabetics with recur-rent nausea and vomiting. *Gastroenterology.* 1986;90:1919-1925.

42. Camilleri M, Brown ML, Malagelada JR. Relationship between impaired gastric emptying and abnormal gastrointestinal motility. *Gastroenterology.* 1986;91:94-99.

43. Petiakis IE, Vrachassotakis N, Sciacca V, Vassilakis SI, Chalkiadakis G. Hyperglycemia attenuates erythromycin-induced acceleration of solid phase gastric emptying in idio-pathic and diabetic gastroparesis. *Scand J Gastroenterol.* 1999;34:396-403.

44. Brownlee M, Kroopf SS. Metoclopramide for gastroparesis diabeticorum. *N Engl J Med.* 1974;291:1257-1258.

45. Perkel MS, Moore C, Hersh T, Davidson ED. Metoclopramide therapy in patients with delayed gastric emptying. *Dig Dis Sci.* 1979;24:662-666.

46. McCallum RW, Ricci DA, Rakatansky H, et al. A multicenter placebo-controlled clinical trial of oral metoclopramide in diabetic gastroparesis. *Diabetes Care.* 1983;6:463-467.

47. Ganzini L, Casey DE, Hoffman WF, McCall AL. The prevalence of metoclopramide-induced tardive dyskinesia and acute extrapyramidal movement disorders. *Arch Intern Med.* 1993;153:1469-1475.

48. Erbas T, Varoglu E, Erbas B, Tastekin G, Akalin S. Comparison of metoclopramide and erythromycin in the treatment of diabetic gastroparesis. *Diabetes Care.* 1993;16:1511-1514.

49. Patterson D, Abell T, Rothstein R, Koch K, Barnett J. A double-blind multicenter comparison of domperidone and metoclopramide in the treatment of diabetic patients with symptoms of gastroparesis. *Am J Gastroenterol.* 1999;94:1230-1234.

50. Miller LG, Jankovic J. Metoclopramide-induced movement disorders. Clinical find-ings with a review of the literature. *Arch Intern Med.* 1989;149:2486-2492.

51. Lata PF, Pigarelli DL. Chronic metoclopramide therapy for diabetic gastroparesis. *Ann Pharmacother.* 2003;37:122-126.

52. Peeters TL. Erythromycin and other macrolides as prokinetic agents. *Gastroenterology.* 1993;105:1886-1899.

53. DiBaise JK, Quigley EMM. Efficacy of prolonged administration of IV erythromycin in an ambulatory setting as treatment of severe gastroparesis. *J Clin Gastroenterol.* 1999;28:131-134.

54. Maganti K, Onyemere K, Jones MP. Oral erythromycin and symptomatic relief of gastroparesis: a systematic review. *Am J Gastroenterol.* 2003;98:259-263.

55. Watts GF, Armitage M, Sinclair J, Hill JD. Treatment of diabetic gastroparesis with oral domperidone. *Diabetic Med.* 1985;2:491-492.

56. Jones MP. Access options for withdrawn motility-modifying agents. *Am J Gastroenterol.* 2002;97:2184-2188.

57. Di Stefano M, Vos R, Janssens J, Tack JF. Effect of tegaserod, a 5-HT4 receptor partial agonist, on interdigestive and postprandial gastrointestinal motility in healthy volunteers(abstr). *Gastroenterology.* 2003;124:A163.

58. Degen L, Matzinger D, Merz M, et al. Tegaserod, a 5-HT4 receptor partial agonist, accelerates gastric emptying and gastrointestinal transit in healthy male subjects. *Aliment Pharmacol Ther.* 2001;15:1745-1751.

59. Tougas G, Chen Y, Luo D, Salter J, D'Elia T, Earnest DL. Tegaserod improves gastric emptying in patients with gastroparesis and dyspeptic symptoms (abstr). *Gastroenterology.* 2003;124:A54.

60. Tack J, Delia T, Ligozio G, Sue S, Lefkowitz M, Vandeplassche L. A phase II trial with tegaserod in functional dyspepsia patients with normal gastric emptying (abstr). *Gastroenterology.* 2002;120:A20.

61. Tatsuta M, Iishi H, Nakaizumi A, Okuda S. Effect of treatment with cisapride alone or in combination with domperidone on gastric emptying and gastrointestinal symptoms in dyspeptic patients. *Aliment Pharm Ther.* 1992;6:221-228.

62. Clouse RE. Antidepressants for functional gastrointestinal syndromes. *Dig Dis Sci.* 1994;39:2352-2363.

63. Pasricha PJ, Ravich WJ, Hendrix TR, Sostre S, Jones B, Kallo AN. Intrasphincteric botulinum toxin for the treatment of achalasia. *N Engl J Med.* 1995;332:775-778.

64. Lacy BE, Schettler-Duncan VA, Crowell MD. The treatment of diabetic gastroparesis with botulinum toxin (abstr). *Am J Gastroenterol.* 2000;95:2455-2456.

65. Miller LS, Szych GA, Kantor SB, et al. Treatment of idiopathic gastroparesis with injection of botulinum toxin into the pyloric sphincter muscle. *Am J Gastroenterol.* 2002;97:1653-1660.

66. Mintchev MP, Sanmiguel CP, Amaris M, Bowes KL. Microprocessor-controlled movement of solid gastric content using sequential neural electrical stimulation. *Gastroenterology.* 2000;118:258-263.

67. Jones MP, Maganti K. A systematic review of surgical therapy for gastroparesis. *Am J Gastroenterol.* 2003;98:2122-2129.

68. Fontana RJ, Barnett JL. Jejunostomy tube placement in refractory diabetic gastroparesis: a retrospective review. *Am J Gastroenterol.* 1996;91:2174-2178.

69. Hotokezaka M, Adams RB, Miller AD, McCallum RW, Schirmer BD. Laparoscopic percutaneous jejunostomy for long term enteral access. *Surg Endosc.* 1996;10:1008-1011.

70. Kim CH, Nelson DK. Venting percutaneous gastrostomy in the treatment of refractory idiopathic gastroparesis. *Gastrointest Endosc.* 1998;47:67-70.

71. Thumshirn M, Camilleri M, Cho MG, Zinsmeister AR. Modulation of gastric sensory and motor functions by nitrergic and alpha-2 adrenergic agents. *Gastroenterology.* 1999;116:573-585.

72. Rosa E, Silva L, Troncon LES, et al. Treatment of diabetic gastroparesis with oral clonidine. *Aliment Pharmacol Ther.* 1995;9:179-183.

73. Tack J, Coulie B, Andrioli A, Janssens J. Influence of sumatriptan on gastric fundus tone and of the perception of gastric distension in man. *Gut.* 2000;46:468-473.

74. Sarnelli G, Vos R, Sifrim D, Janssens J, Tack J. Influence of sildenafil on fasting and postprandial gastric tone in man(abstr). *Gastroenterology.* 2001;120:A285-A286.

75. de Rosalmeida MC, Saraiva LD, da Graca JR, et al. Sildenafil, a phosphodiesterase-5 inhibitor, delays gastric emptying and gastrointestinal transit of liquid in awake rats *Dig Dis Sci.* 2003;48:2064-2068.

76. Rothstein RD, Alavi A, Reynolds JC. Electrogastrography in patients with gastroparesis and effect of long-term cisapride. *Dig Dis Sci.* 1993;38:1518-1524.

77. Hasler WL, Soudah HC, Dulai G, Owyang C. Mediation of hyperglycemia-evoked gastric slow-wave dysrhythmias by endogenous prostaglandins. *Gastroenterology.* 1995;108:727-736.

78. Pimentel M, Sam C, Lin HC. Indomethacin improves symptoms and electrogastrographic findings in patients with gastric dysrhythmias. *Neurogastroenterol Motil.* 2001;13:422.

Dumping Syndrome: A Clinician's Guide

Gregg W. Van Citters, PhD and Henry C. Lin, MD

Overview

In this chapter we will focus attention on understanding the constellation of symptoms that comprises dumping syndrome, describing the underlying anatomical perturbation that creates this presentation and outlining the framework for developing a therapeutic strategy. This is a practical guide for the clinician. More traditional reviews of this topic may be found in the major textbooks on gastroenterology.

Symptoms of dumping syndrome include severe postprandial nausea, diarrhea, bloating, and abdominal pain as well as profuse sweating, dizziness, headache, heart palpitations, and shaking. When a patient presents with these symptoms and describes his or her occurrence after a meal, the clinician is faced with the dilemma of developing an appropriate therapeutic strategy to both reduce the symptoms and improve nutrition. The classical framework for understanding dumping syndrome is to consider the postulcer surgery anatomical perturbations such as vagotomy with an antrectomy or a pyloroplasty as a drainage procedure that are strongly associated with dumping syndrome. However, the universe of dumping syndrome extends beyond these traditionally ascribed postulcer surgery anatomical modifications to include any anatomical or physiological dysfunction that may result in accelerated transit of a meal through the tract. For example, the patient who has lost functional terminal ileum to disease (Crohn's disease) or surgical resection may also experience symptoms of dumping syndrome. Immediately following such transit-altering surgery, patients may experience dumping symptoms but may compensate over time, reaching a plateau wherein symptoms are nominal and relatively constant. When the well-compensated patient presents acutely with symptoms of dumping syndrome, the clinician must unravel the reason for the decompensation. What follows is the clinical strategy for considering these issues to determine the appropriate therapeutic strategy for helping the patient with dumping syndrome.

Regulated Transit of a Meal

Digestion and absorption of a meal require prolonged contact time with digestive enzymes and absorptive mucosa. Gastric emptying and intestinal transit are slowed in response to the nutrient content of the meal to ensure that there is adequate time to complete digestion and absorption. Regulated transit of a meal is therefore crucial for optimal nutrition. Transit is controlled when inhibitory feedback signals are generated by nutrients acting on nutrient sensors distributed along the length of the GI tract. This feedback control is triggered by end products of nutrient digestion, including fatty acids. The magnitude of the inhibitory feedback is proportional to the length of the small intestine exposed to nutrients. GI transit becomes uncontrolled with loss of any component of this inhibitory feedback. The resulting rapid movement of a meal limits contact time with digestive enzymes and absorptive mucosa, resulting in diarrhea, maldigestion, malabsorption, and, in some cases, the symptoms of dumping syndrome.

Physical fragmentation (trituration) of a solid meal occurs in the stomach as the ring-like terminal antral contraction carrying the contents of the stomach forward is met with pyloric contractions. Because the pylorus receives the center of the laminar flow where the smallest food fragments are suspended in the gastric juice, liquids and finely triturated particles (<0.1 mm diameter) are ejected into the duodenum, while larger particles fall to the side and are retained for further trituration (gastric sieving). If these larger particles are allowed access to the small intestine, symptoms of dumping syndrome may result because these food fragments resist assimilation to access an exaggerated length of the small intestine. Such an abnormal spread of nutrients may result in symptoms because the corresponding feedback response is similarly exaggerated. Consistent with these ideas is the observation that the majority of dumping episodes occur following a solid meal.

Since gastric emptying is controlled by feedback inhibition arising in the small intestine in response to the nutrient content of the gastric output, liquids devoid of nutrients empty rapidly following first-order kinetics. In contrast, the liquid portion of a nutrient-rich mixed meal empties rapidly at first then the rate of emptying slows as the nutrients activate the inhibitory feedback. Nutrient-rich solids empty very slowly at first. During this lag phase, trituration of solids takes place to prepare food for gastric emptying. The lag phase of solid emptying is then followed by the linear phase. The rate of emptying during the linear phase is determined by the load of nutrients contained in the initial squirt of chyme into the small intestine. More nutrients enter the small intestine with a larger meal during this early postprandial period. Greater inhibitory feedback and, therefore, slower gastric emptying then result when more nutrients spread along a longer length of the small intestine. Acidity, osmolarity, and end products of macronutrient digestion (peptides and peptones, sugars and fatty acids) all serve as triggers of inhibitory feedback to control transit.

Normal regulated control of transit depends then on the appropriate generation of inhibitory feedback. This critical control is governed by events that occur very early in the postprandial period. To reduce the patient's postprandial symptoms, the clinician must remember that dietary intervention should be directed at altering the events during the first 10 to 15 minutes of the postprandial period. It is early in the meal, when there is no inhibitory feedback because the lumen of the gut is empty, that the liquid component of the meal surges out of the stomach at a rate proportional to the meal volume. Because this initial surge of nutrients down the length of the small intestine sets the magnitude of the inhibitory feedback, symptom reduction depends on minimizing the nutrient surge during this period. Thus, additional liquids should be avoided to minimize the volume dependent surge.

With transit so tightly linked to presentation of nutrients, any change in motility or digestive or absorptive capacity can drastically affect nutrient-regulated transit. For example, in the patient with a vagotomy and antrectomy who has impaired gastric sieving, it is the entry into the small intestine of poorly triturated chunks of food that is responsible for symptom generation. Accordingly, to minimize symptoms, eating beef in the form of ground beef (prefragmented solids) would be preferred over steak or roast. By modifying the diet to avoid the mechanism of symptom generation, the triggering of exaggerated inhibitory feedback and thus, dumping symptoms, may be reduced.

Increasing amounts of fatty components of the meal are digested and liberated as a meal progresses down the intestine. Fatty acids, the end products of this digestion, are released to activate transit control mechanisms located in both the proximal and distal intestine. These mechanisms are known as the jejunal[1] and ileal brakes,[2,3] respectively, with the ileal brake being more potent.[4] In the setting of extensive ileal resection or disease, the ileal brake is lost and transit control primarily relies on the jejunal brake. Unfortunately, it is difficult to trigger the jejunal brake in this setting because much less fat hydrolysis occurs in the stomach and duodenum when transit is abnormally accelerated, depriving the jejunum of the end products of fat digestion that are needed to trigger the inhibitory feedback.

Patient History Reveals Rapid Transit

Before determining the therapeutic strategy, it is critical to develop a therapeutic goal. It is often useful to ask whether the symptoms are based on a reversible mechanism or an irreversible mechanism. Proper categorization of the patient, therefore, relies on collecting a thorough and accurate patient history. An important goal of this assessment is to determine whether the symptoms are acute (more likely to be reversible) or chronic (more likely to be irreversible). The therapeutic goals may differ: find and reverse the precipitating factor for the acute presentation, and optimize symptom control in the chronic presentation.

The 2 scenarios differ as follows. The first type of patient may have thoroughly adapted to a surgical perturbation such as a vagotomy and an antrectomy and does not normally experience symptoms of dumping syndrome. This patient is typically well nourished, can enjoy a self-selected diet of wide variety, may lead an active lifestyle, and has infrequent loose stools without undue urgency or incontinence. This well-adapted patient now presents with symptoms suggestive of dumping syndrome. This follows an acute precipitating factor, such as recent travel to a foreign country, that resulted in a suspected decompensation event.

In this setting, it is important to focus the history on determining what event may have led to the acute decompensation. Once the cause is identified and reversed, resolution of symptoms is possible. Begin the history taking by understanding the patient's normal baseline and then the change. These specific changes in symptoms may provide a clue to the decompensation. For example, a history of new travel-related diarrhea would suggest bacterial gastroenteritis. A patient with intestinal resection and baseline mild diarrhea may easily develop symptoms even after a mild case of food poisoning. For other patients with surgically altered anatomy, the precipitating factor may be the development of small intestinal bacterial overgrowth (SIBO). In both of these cases, a course of antibiotics may be warranted to reverse the dumping symptoms and restore the patient to baseline.

The second category of patient is exemplified by someone who undergoes a surgical intervention such as a subtotal gastrectomy or a gastric bypass but presents with chronic and repeated symptoms of dumping syndrome. The clinician should begin by understanding the patient's postprandial symptoms and their usual triggers. Ask what kind of meal he or she ingested recently that preceded a dumping episode. Is the dumping related to the physical state of the meal (liquid vs. solid), the nutrient load of the meal (osmolarity; high fat vs. low fat), or the size of the meal (volume effects)? If the answer to any of these questions is "yes," then the patient may respond well to a nutritional intervention. The clinician should also investigate the possibility of maldigestion or malabsorption. What were the original consistency, frequency, and odor of the stools and how have these stool parameters changed? For those patients with chronic symptoms, it is possible that their symptoms can only be reduced but not eliminated, so it is important to educate these patients in the concepts of their underlying anatomical derangements and the dietary challenges that precipitate symptoms. Therapy would be directed at slowing transit and modifying their diet.

Stomach or Intestine?

Armed with the patient's history, the clinician can now begin to develop a therapeutic strategy. The first step is to determine whether symptoms are triggered by rapid gastric emptying or by rapid intestinal transit. To sort this out, a direct measurement of GI transit such as a scintigraphic transit study is often required since symptoms of rapid gastric emptying are similar to those generated by rapid intestinal transit (ie, pain, bloating, nausea, vomiting, and diarrhea). It is crucial to note that these symptoms of accelerated transit are also indistinguishable from those of delayed gastric emptying. This is important because empiric use of prokinetic agent on the presumption of delayed gastric emptying would certainly make the situation worse. In contrast to the overfilling of the stomach in delayed emptying, rapid emptying triggers symptoms because too much volume or nutrients is delivered to the small intestine per unit time. Since solids are held back by the stomach for fragmentation, dumping is more readily triggered by a nutrient-rich liquid meal. For example, a patient with rapid emptying of liquid fat (not held back by the stomach for trituration) may complain of symptoms of dumping syndrome after a creamy soup but have no symptoms eating the same amount of fat as a solid (such as matrix fat contained within a steak).

The symptoms generated by rapid intestinal transit are similar to those of rapid gastric emptying. The patient's history may help to localize the problem. The patient with history of sprue or intestinal resection is likely to have a small intestinal transit control defect. A routine scintigraphic gastric emptying study may be modified to secure this possibility. The nuclear medicine department should extend image acquisition to the appearance of the radiolabel in the colon and evaluate the time-to-the appearance of tracer in the colon.

In either case, the appropriate treatment is to slow transit to allow more time for digestion and absorption of a meal. This can be done with the established antidiarrheal agents such as narcotics or with a novel, nutrient-based strategy that delivers fatty acids to activate nutrient-triggered inhibitory feedback. Specifically, we have shown that the jejunal brake may be jump-started with end products of fat digestion. This provides a nutrient-based method for slowing GI transit. Specifically, physiologic inhibitory feedback may be activated by giving oleic acid in an emulsion before a meal.[5] This approach may be effective even in patients with poor response to narcotics.

It is also important to consider whether rapid transit is primary or secondary. If rapid transit is the primary problem, then slowing transit is the main treatment. However, if transit were to be secondary to a problem such as gluten intolerance, mucosal inflammation, correcting the underlying problem that is causing the acceleration is the main approach as exemplified by gluten avoidance in the case of celiac sprue, induction of remission in the case of IBD, or eradication of the bacterial overgrowth in SIBO.

The patient with a history of ileal resection illustrates the latter case. A typical patient may have lost the distal, most potent transit mechanism (the ileal brake) but typically adapts following surgery to reach an equilibrium state with relatively minor symptoms. This well-adapted patient appears healthy and well nourished with few adverse effects aside from loose stools once or twice daily and the need for monthly vitamin B_{12} injections. A dramatic change may occur acutely, leading this patient to present with dumping syndrome as highlighted by severe postprandial symptoms of dehydration and rapid weight loss. An important factor in precipitating these changes is the development of SIBO as a secondary complication. Treatment must be directed at eradicating SIBO in order for this secondary cause of accelerated transit to be reversed.

Maldigestion or Malabsorption?

A simple laboratory analysis can shed light upon the issue of maldigestion vs. malabsorption. Digestion of dietary fat is time-consuming, so rapid transit results in reduced gastric, pancreatic, and/or intestinal lipase activity to result in steatorrhea on the basis of fat maldigestion, leading to the presence of undigested neutral fats (triglycerides) in the stool. In the setting of SIBO, bacterial deconjugation of bile salts reduces the capacity for formation of mixed micelles that may itself lead to fat maldigestion.

In addition, the unpleasantness and loss of energy assimilation associated with steatorrhea, a constellation of nutritional deficiencies, may manifest. Hallmarks of chronic steatorrhea include osteoporosis and renal calcium oxalate calculi (caused by loss of calcium in forming fatty acid soaps), essential fatty acid deficiency, vision (vitamin A), and balance (vitamin E) troubles. Dermatitis is a frequent comorbidity resulting from micronutrient deficiency (mainly the water-soluble vitamins and essential fatty acids). Nerve degeneration and megaloblastic anemia are common complications in gastric and ileal resection.

A stool sample collected after a fat challenge (eg, 100 g/day) should be submitted for analysis of neutral (triglyceride) vs. split fat (fatty acids, mono- and diglycerides) content. Another diagnostic test is to try to slow intestinal transit with an opioid peptide or with oleate.[5,6] If transit is slowed by this treatment and symptoms resolve, then the principal problem is most likely that of poorly controlled transit.

Summary and Conclusions

The clinician confronted with a patient complaining of postprandial abdominal pain, bloating, nausea, diarrhea, dizziness, syncope, and/or diaphoresis should consider a diagnosis of dumping syndrome. In addition to alleviating the acute symptoms of dumping syndrome, there is a need to consider the nutritional health of the patient in this clinical setting because dumping syndrome is often associated with a number of important deficiency states.

References

1. Lin HC, Zhao XT, Wang L. Jejunal brake: inhibition of intestinal transit by fat in the proximal small intestine. *Dig Dis Sci.* 1996;41:326-329.

2. Read NW, McFarlane A, Kinsman RI, et al. Effect of infusion of nutrient solutions into the ileum on GI transit and plasma levels of neurotensin and enteroglucagon. *Gastroenterology.* 1984;86:274-280.

3. Spiller RC, Trotman IF, Higgins BE, et al. The ileal brake—inhibition of jejunal motility after ileal fat perfusion in man. *Gut.* 1984;25:365-374.

4. Lin HC, Zhao XT, Wang L. Intestinal transit is more potently inhibited by fat in the distal (ileal brake) than in the proximal (jejunal brake) gut. *Dig Dis Sci.* 1997;42:19-25.

5. Lin HC, Bonorris G, Marks JW. Oleate slows upper gut transit and reduces diarrhea in patients with rapid gut transit and diarrhea. *Gastroenterology.* 1995;108(4):A638.

6. Van Citters GW, Lin HC. Oleic acid improves drug absorption in patients with inflammatory bowel disease. *Gastroenterology.* 1998;114(4):A1105.

Functional Dyspepsia

Alex S. Kuryan, MD and Frank K. Friedenberg, MD

Introduction

Dyspepsia is a term used to describe a constellation of symptoms referable to the UGI tract. The main symptom is episodic or persistent pain/discomfort centered in the upper abdomen. A variety of other associated complaints may be present, including early satiety, fullness, postprandial bloating or distension, belching, nausea, and vomiting. The term dyspepsia should not be used to describe patients with a predominant symptom of heartburn. These patients should primarily be considered as having GERD because their management differs substantially.

It has been estimated that dyspepsia may affect up to 25% of adults annually. However, less than half actually seek medical attention.[1] Nonetheless, dyspepsia is still a common presenting complaint in both the primary care and specialty office. It accounts for up to 7% of office visits and 40% to 70% of GI complaints in the primary care setting.[2] The prevalence of dyspepsia appears to remain stable from year to year, although some patients will lose their symptoms for a period of time, whereas a similar number of patients will experience a relapse of their symptoms.[3] Dyspepsia has a significant impact upon quality of life and cost to society. Limited studies suggest that chronic dyspepsia symptoms interfere with daily activities, working, sleeping, socializing, eating, drinking, and contribute to emotional stress.[4] The cost of dyspepsia includes direct medical costs such as physician visits, diagnostic testing, and medications as well as the indirect costs of absenteeism and diminished productivity in the workplace.[5]

The differential diagnosis of dyspepsia is broad and may include a variety of causative factors and may encompass multiple organ systems (Table 13-1). The majority of patients (50% to 70%) with chronic dyspepsia do not have significant pathology identified by physical examination, routine laboratory assessment, upper endoscopy, or abdominal imaging.[6] These patients are labeled as having functional, or nonulcer, dyspepsia. Functional dyspepsia is, therefore, the most common type of dyspepsia and is considered a diagnosis of exclusion. On the basis of symptoms alone, both

Table 13-1

DIFFERENTIAL DIAGNOSIS OF DYSPEPSIA

- PUD
- Gastroesophageal reflux disease
- Gastroparesis (diabetes, postvagotomy, scleroderma, chronic intestinal pseudo-obstruction)
- Esophageal, gastric, or pancreatic neoplasms
- Infiltrative disorders (Ménétrier's disease, Crohn's disease, sarcoidosis, amyloidosis, eosinophilic gastroenteritis)
- Malabsorption (celiac sprue, lactose intolerance)
- Ischemic bowel disease
- Infections (cytomegalovirus, fungal, tuberculosis, syphilis)
- Intestinal parasites (Giardia or Strongyloides)
- Injury caused by ethanol, aspirin/NSAIDs, antibiotics, iron, glucocorticoids, narcotics, or other substances
- Cholelithiasis or choledocholithiasis
- Sphincter of Oddi dysfunction
- Acute or chronic pancreatitis
- Systemic disorders (diabetes, thyroid and parathyroid disorders, connective-tissue disease, adrenal insufficiency, renal insufficiency, cardiac ischemia, congestive heart failure)
- Pregnancy
- Functional dyspepsia
- IBS
- Food intolerance

Adapted from Fisher RS, Parkman HP. Management of non-ulcer dyspepsia. *N Engl J Med.* 1998;339:1376-1381 and Talley N, Silverstein M, Agreus L, et al. AGA technical review: evaluation of dyspepsia. *Gastroenterology.* 1998;114:582-595.

primary care physicians and gastroenterologists are equally unable to differentiate functional dyspepsia from PUD, which is one of the more common organic causes of dyspepsia.[7] Although often chronic, the symptoms in functional dyspepsia are frequently intermittent, even during a severe symptomatic period.[8] Many patients with functional dyspepsia have multiple somatic complaints, as well as symptoms of anxiety and depression.

The most commonly used criteria to define functional dyspepsia is the Rome II criteria. This criterion has been useful in standardizing the diagnosis of functional dyspepsia in clinical studies. The Rome II criteria defines functional dyspepsia as at least 12 weeks, not necessarily consecutive, within the preceding 12 months of persistent or recurrent dyspepsia, no evidence of organic disease (including an upper endoscopy) that is likely to explain the symptoms, and no evidence that the dyspepsia is exclusively relieved by defecation or associated with the onset of a change in stool frequency or form (ie, not the IBS).[9]

Pathophysiology

Normal GI motor function is a complex series of events requiring coordination of the sympathetic and parasympathetic nervous systems, stomach and intestinal neurons, and intestinal smooth muscle cells.[10] Although several possible mechanisms have been implicated in functional dyspepsia, the pathophysiology is unclear. Some of the proposed mechanisms include delayed gastric emptying, impaired gastric accommodation, abnormal antroduodenojejunal motility, visceral hypersensitivity, autonomic neuropathy, *H. pylori* infection, hypersensitivity to acid or nutrients, CNS dysfunction, and psychosocial factors. A postinfectious etiology has also been proposed.

DELAYED GASTRIC EMPTYING

There are a variety of abnormalities, including vagal interruption, that could lead to delayed gastric emptying. Gastroparesis may be characterized by many of the same symptoms seen in functional dyspepsia, such as early satiety, bloating, nausea, vomiting, and weight loss. It thus seems reasonable to speculate that a disorder of gastric emptying may contribute to certain symptoms seen in functional dyspepsia. In a recent meta-analysis, delayed gastric emptying as measured by scintigraphy, breath tests, or ultrasonography was reported in 40% (studies ranged from 25% to 80%) of patients with functional dyspepsia.[11] In this study, those patients with functional dyspepsia had a 1.5-fold increased risk of delayed gastric emptying as compared to controls. However, whether there is a link between symptoms and delayed gastric emptying in functional dyspepsia remains controversial. Numerous small studies and one larger trial of 551 patients with functional dyspepsia failed to show any specific symptoms that predicted gastric emptying.[12-14] However, two large-scale studies have shown that in a subset of dyspeptic patients with delayed gastric emptying, there was an association with postprandial fullness, early satiety, nausea, and vomiting.[15,16] Therefore, many patients with functional dyspepsia may have delayed gastric emptying, but there remains a lack of convincing evidence of a consistent correlation between symptoms and detected abnormalities.

IMPAIRED ACCOMMODATION

In normal physiology, the stomach is able to expand as it is filled by a meal. This is facilitated by vagally mediated receptive relaxation and gastric accommodation of the proximal stomach (fundus). There is then gradual redistribution of stomach contents into the distal stomach (antrum). Gastric accommodation is controlled by vagal pathways that are mediated through the release of nitric oxide and serotonin.[2] In some patients with functional dyspepsia, an abnormal distribution of food within the stomach has been seen, with a relatively higher proportion of the meal seen in the antrum rather than in the proximal stomach. This results in reduced gastric compliance, which may cause resultant sudden, prolonged distention with postprandial dyspepsia. This phenomenon has been documented using ultrasound, MRI, SPECT, scintigraphy, and barostats.[17-19] Approximately 40% of patients with functional dyspepsia have impaired postprandial fundic accommodation and this may be associated with 2 specific symptoms: early satiety and weight loss.[19] Other groups have not been able to demonstrate such a relationship between the symptom complex in functional dyspepsia and impaired fundic accommodation.[20,21] Therefore, gastric accommodation may be impaired in some patients with functional dyspepsia; however, this has only been shown in a subgroup of patients with meal-related symptoms.

MYOELECTRICAL ABNORMALITIES

The electrical activity of the stomach is controlled by the gastric pacemaker that is located in the proximal body. The basal electrical rhythm (approximately 3 cycles/minute) is generated by the pacemaker and transmitted both longitudinally and circumferentially.[2] The normal EGG shows slow wave (velocity and propagation of gastric contractions) and spike activity (antral contractions).[22] EGG has been used to measure the electrical activity in the stomach in an attempt to determine whether myoelectrical abnormalities can be found in patients with functional dyspepsia. Gastric dysrhythmias have been identified in 40% of patients with functional dyspepsia and 20% of normal controls.[22] Both tachygastrias and bradygastrias have been identified; however, these are not associated with a specific symptom profile or gastric emptying abnormality. Even though an association has been reported between an abnormal EGG and delayed gastric emptying, the relationship to symptoms is inconsistent.[23] In addition, 2 smaller studies found no difference in EGG recordings between patients with functional dyspepsia and healthy controls.[24] However, one study suggested symptomatic improvement in functional dyspeptic patients who had a dysrhythmia (measured by EGG) that responded to cisapride.[25]

ALTERED ANTRODUODENOJEJUNAL MOTILITY

Antroduodenal manometry can be used to assess the contractile activity of the stomach. Several studies have demonstrated postprandial antral hypomotility to be common in patients with functional dyspepsia.[12] However, no clear relationship has been found between antral hypomotility and symptoms.[26] Studies of small bowel manometry in functional dyspepsia have shown hypermotility as well as an increased proportion of contractions propagating from the duodenum to the stomach in a retrograde fashion. Once again, the relevance of these findings with relation to symptoms is unclear.[27]

VISCERAL HYPERSENSITIVITY

An increasing body of evidence points to visceral hypersensitivity as a major pathophysiological mechanism in functional GI disorders. Stimulation of afferent gut mechanoreceptors reaches conscious perception through a 3-neuron chain. In normal neurophysiology, the afferent first-order neuron projects from the GI tract to the prevertebral ganglia and to the cell body in the dorsal root ganglion. The second-order neuron then extends from the dorsal horn via the spinothalamic and spinoreticular tracts to the thalamus and brainstem reticular formation where they then synapse with neurons that project to the limbic system and cerebral cortex. Descending fibers from brainstem centers modulate the sensitivity of the dorsal horn neurons and control the perception of visceral sensation.[28] Most stimuli arising from the GI tract are not consciously perceived.

Visceral hypersensitivity, or visceral hyperalgesia, refers to a lowered threshold for induction of pain by gastric distension in the presence of normal gastric compliance. Both peripheral and central mechanisms have been proposed in visceral hypersensitivity. Mechanoreceptor dysfunction due to inflammation, injury, or intrinsic defect (peripheral mechanism) and aberrant processing of afferent input in the spinal cord or brain (central mechanism) may play a role. Interestingly, somatic sensitivity as measured by transcutaneous electrical hand stimulation is normal in patients with functional dyspepsia.[29]

Several investigators have shown that a significant proportion of patients with functional dyspepsia (ranging from 34% to 65%) have lower sensory thresholds during balloon distention in the proximal stomach and the duodenum as compared to normal controls.[30,31] In a recent large-scale study, a multivariate analysis found gastric hypersensitivity to be associated with the symptoms of postprandial epigastric pain, belching, and weight loss.[30] Delayed gastric emptying and impaired gastric accommodation occurred in 23% and 40% of patients, respectively, in the study but no relationship to visceral hypersensitivity was found. It also appears that visceral hypersensitivity is not related to organic dyspepsia.[31]

Hypersensitivity was also demonstrated in a study of dyspeptic patients who did not seek health care and was unrelated to the presence of psychological abnormalities.[32] This implies that functional dyspepsia is not solely an expression of referral bias or personality factors. This same study also suggested a failure of sensory adaptation in functional dyspepsia. Repeated gastric balloon distention increased the visceral sensory threshold in normal subjects, but the thresholds were unchanged in the patients with functional dyspepsia.

Patients with functional dyspepsia are more sensitive to other forms of luminal stimuli. They are more symptomatic to the dyspeptic effect of aspirin and this is unrelated to the number of erosions. As with the gastric balloon, gastric sensory thresholds only failed to increase following aspirin challenge in the subset that developed symptoms. Thus, failure to increase sensory thresholds during treatment with aspirin may be linked to the development of symptoms in some patients with functional dyspepsia.[33] In summary, visceral hypersensitivity seems to be an independent factor in functional dyspepsia without relation to delayed gastric emptying or impaired gastric accommodation. However, a significant proportion of patients have no such hypersensitivity indicating that other factors must also be involved.

INCREASED SENSITIVITY TO NUTRIENTS

Postprandial symptoms are very common in functional dyspepsia, and many patients report worsened symptoms after a fatty or rich meal. A significant proportion of patients with functional dyspepsia had increased gastroduodenal sensitivity after a high energy or lipid-rich meal. This was not clearly associated with delayed gastric emptying.[34] Additionally, patients with functional dyspepsia are more sensitive to gastric distention after an infusion of lipids but not glucose into the duodenum as compared to controls.[35,36] This response could be diminished by the cholecystokinin (CCK) receptor antagonist dexloxiglumide, indicating a role for CCK–dependent mechanisms in functional dyspepsia.[37]

ACID HYPERSENSITIVITY

Acid exposure may play a role in the pathogenesis of functional dyspepsia. Gastric acid secretion is normal in most patients with functional dyspepsia.[38] The gastric mucosa does not seem to be hypersensitive to acid or duodenal contents.[39] Although patients with functional dyspepsia and controls have similar fasting intragastric and intraduodenal pH levels, dyspeptic patients were found to be more sensitive than controls to acid infusion into the duodenal bulb.[40] These patients developed more nausea and had a reduced acid clearing duodenal motor response compared to controls. Acid suppression seems to provide symptomatic relief in a small subset of patients,[41] and the reduced duodenal motor function was shown to have a modest therapeutic response to PPI therapy.[42] A recent study used 24-hour ambulatory duodenal pH monitoring to compare the duodenal acid exposure of patients with functional dyspepsia and controls.[43] The results showed that patients with functional dyspepsia had an exaggerated and prolonged acid exposure after a meal, but there was no direct relationship between symptoms and acid exposure. Another study in normal subjects showed that duodenal acidification induced proximal gastric relaxation, increased sensitivity to gastric distension, and inhibited gastric accommodation to a meal.[44] Increased duodenal acid exposure may, therefore, be involved in the pathogenesis of dyspeptic symptoms through these mechanisms.

H. PYLORI

The role of H. pylori in the pathophysiology of functional dyspepsia is controversial and has received a great deal of attention over the past decade. The prevalence of H. pylori in patients with functional dyspepsia is similar to that in the general population.[45] However, most of the available data suggest that H. pylori does not play a major role in functional dyspepsia and eradication of the organism likely benefits only a small proportion of patients. Acute infection with H. pylori may lead to transient symptoms of nausea, vomiting, and dyspepsia. Chronic infection with H. pylori can lead to PUD with symptoms of dyspepsia. In addition, the organism may alter smooth muscle function through the induction of an inflammatory response or by the initiation of an antibody response.[46] However, most studies have not found an association between H. pylori and abnormal gastric motor function in patients with functional dyspepsia. A meta-analysis of 30 observational studies involving 3392 patients with functional dyspepsia and 11 observational studies involving 6426 people with uninvestigated dyspepsia concluded that there was not a strong association between H. pylori infection and dyspepsia, although a weak association could not be excluded.[47] A recent study found no correlation between H. pylori infection and symptoms in patients with functional dyspepsia.[48] There was an association with unsuppressed postprandial phasic contractility of the proximal stomach but no affect on gastric emptying, accommodation, or visceral sensitivity. Most importantly, as will be discussed later, eradication of the organism appears to be of marginal benefit with no significant long-term improvement in symptoms.

AUTONOMIC NEUROPATHY

Abnormalities of the autonomic nervous system have been postulated to be of some importance in patients with functional dyspepsia. An efferent dysfunction of the vagus nerve has been observed in some studies. It has been suggested that the vagus nerve can modulate pain perception. Perception thresholds for duodenal distention are lower in patients with a truncal vagotomy than controls, consistent with a vagal antinociceptive effect.[49] In another small study, patients with functional dyspepsia with vagal dysfunction (as evidenced by impaired heart rate variability or plasma levels of pancreatic polypeptide in response to insulin-induced hypoglycemia) also had reduced perception thresholds for duodenal distension.[50] However, another study found vagal dysfunction (measured as pancreatic polypeptide release in response to sham feeding) to be as infrequent in functional dyspepsia patients (2/17) as in healthy controls (1/16).[51] Acute psychological stress has also been shown to alter vagal and sympathetic autonomic function. It has been hypothesized that stress leads to decreased vagal tone, which may give rise to dyspeptic symptoms. However, this mechanism has not yet been established as a cause of dyspepsia.

PSYCHOSOCIAL FACTORS

Psychosocial factors should be explored but not overemphasized in patients with dyspepsia. In contrast to patients with organic causes of dyspepsia, psychological symptoms are commonly seen in patients with functional dyspepsia.[52] Several psychosocial factors including life event stress, psychological morbidity, abuse history, personality, and abnormal illness behavior and beliefs have been shown to be important predictors in which patients with functional dyspepsia seek medical attention.[53] There is evidence for an association between psychopathology and functional dyspepsia, but the relevance to symptom pattern is unknown. It is also important to note that no causal role has been established between psychosocial factors and functional dyspepsia. As compared with healthy subjects, patients with functional dyspepsia have a higher incidence of anxiety disorders, neuroticism, hypochondriasis, depression, and somatoform disorders, but it is unclear whether these traits merely reflect the fact that these patients are more likely to seek health care.[54,55]

The role of life stressors, both acute and chronic, in functional dyspepsia is uncertain and controversial. Theoretically, stress could alter GI motility and autonomic regulation (see above) or reduce visceral pain thresholds. A recent study showed that patients with functional dyspepsia were all experiencing at least one major life stressor.[56] These stressors included marital issues, employment, finances, housing, illness, and death. It is also suggested that these patients have impaired coping styles and less social support.[56] There is also a possible link between self-reported childhood abuse and functional GI disorders.[57]

POSTINFECTIOUS ETIOLOGY

It has been proposed that certain cases of IBS, IBD, and gastroparesis may have a postinfectious etiology. A recent questionnaire study of 400 patients with functional dyspepsia found that 17% had an acute onset of symptoms that was suggestive of a postinfectious origin.[58] There was a high prevalence of impaired gastric accommodation in these patients.

Evaluation

As stated earlier, functional dyspepsia is a diagnosis of exclusion. A careful comprehensive history and physical examination are crucial in order to make the correct diagnosis of dyspepsia and to distinguish it from GERD and IBS. There is a significant amount of overlap seen between functional dyspepsia, GERD, and IBS. Atypical GERD may present as upper abdominal discomfort or pain. In one study, about half of the patients with functional dyspepsia also fulfilled the Rome II criteria for IBS.[59] These patients were also more likely to be female and had greater overall symptom severity. In another study, many patients changed from predominately dyspeptic symptoms to bowel-related symptoms, indicating IBS, or the opposite during a 1-year follow-up period.[3] However, patients with predominant GERD symptoms kept their symptoms to a varying degree and rarely changed their symptom profile to that of dyspepsia or IBS.

An appropriate diagnostic work-up for dyspepsia usually begins with routine laboratory assessment. This should include a complete blood count, electrolyte measurement, calcium level, liver chemistries, and thyroid function tests. In addition, other studies such as amylase, lipase, stool microbiology tests, and pregnancy tests should be ordered as needed. Patients who have alarm symptoms or use NSAIDs should have immediate further diagnostic tests such as endoscopy, abdominal ultrasound, or CT scan. Alarm symptoms include bleeding, anemia, dysphagia, jaundice, significant weight loss, recurrent vomiting, a palpable mass, family history of cancer, or a history of gastric surgery. Other investigations may include small bowel radiography, duodenal biopsy, nuclear scintigraphy studies, 24-hour esophageal pH monitoring, and UGI tract manometry studies. These additional tests should only be performed based on the clinical picture and severity or refractoriness of the patient's symptoms.

The undisputed role of *H. pylori* in the pathophysiology of PUD and gastric cancer has led to empirical eradication therapy in most patients who test positive for the organism with noninvasive testing. Noninvasive testing for *H. pylori* can be performed using serologic evaluation, urea breath testing, or fecal antigen testing. The latter 2 tests should not be used in patients who are taking PPIs or bismuth. Approximately one-third of patients with dyspepsia will test positive for *H. pylori* using noninvasive testing but less than half of these patients will have PUD (ie, most will have functional dyspepsia).[60]

Since PUD is a fairly common cause of dyspepsia, eradication of *H. pylori* has been used as an initial treatment strategy for uninvestigated dyspepsia. In 1998, both the AGA and the American College of Gastroenterology (ACG) recommended the so-called "test and treat" approach as an appropriate first step in exploring and managing dyspepsia without alarm symptoms.[6,61] In this paradigm, patients who have dyspepsia without alarm symptoms are noninvasively tested for *H. pylori* infection and, if positive, then offered eradication therapy. Patients less than 45 years old who are *H. pylori* negative without alarm symptoms are usually offered a trial of antisecretory therapy and/or a prokinetic agent for 4 weeks. Upper endoscopy is only recommended in these younger patients if symptoms persist despite therapy or if they rapidly recur following cessation of therapy. Endoscopy may allow visualization of peptic ulcers, esophagitis, gastritis, and malignancy with high accuracy. However, these findings would not likely alter the initial course of therapy because most patients are given a trial of proton-pump inhibition regardless of endoscopic findings. It has been suggested that a normal upper endoscopy may help relieve the anxiety of some patients; however, this reassurance may only benefit a small number of worried patients.[62]

A number of cost-effectiveness decision analyses have been performed in order to determine the optimal strategy to investigate and treat dyspepsia. Based on the data regarding the efficacy of *H. pylori* eradication in infected patients with functional dyspepsia, which will be presented in the treatment section, most people will continue to be symptomatic after *H. pylori* treatment. These patients should then be offered endoscopy. A recent decision analysis found that empiric PPI therapy was more cost effective than initial endoscopy, either as a first step or following a "test and treat" approach in the patient who did not respond to *H. pylori* eradication therapy.[63] Another study proposed the idea that since the rate of *H. pylori* infection varies widely, it is possible that patients from low prevalence groups would benefit less from the "test and treat" approach compared to patients with a higher chance of infection.[64] Yet another study compared PPI and placebo for 6 weeks in 140 patients. The group on a PPI had a higher early response rate, but a large number of these patients had recurrent dyspepsia after 1 year. This suggests that empiric PPI therapy may only serve to delay further investigation.[65]

By performing an EGD, patients with negative endoscopy findings may reduce the amount of health-related worrying and improve their quality of life. This was shown in one of the larger studies to date on the topic. Five hundred patients were randomly assigned to a "test and treat" strategy or prompt endoscopy. After 1-year follow-up, there was no reported difference in symptoms, quality of life, physician and hospital visits, or sick-leave days. In addition, 60% fewer endoscopies were performed in the "test and treat" group. However, significantly more patients were dissatisfied with their management in the "test and treat" approach (12%) as compared to the early endoscopy group (4%).[62] A subsequent meta-analysis also concluded that there was little support for eradication therapy in patients with functional dyspepsia.[66]

A recent Cochrane systematic review of 17 controlled trials concluded that initial endoscopy was associated with a small reduction in the risk of recurrent dyspeptic symptoms when compared to initial empiric treatment. *H. pylori* testing with endoscopy for a positive result increased costs but did not improve symptoms. *H. pylori* testing followed by eradication of the organism appeared to be as effective as initial endoscopy but reduced costs by decreasing the number of patients that ultimately required endoscopy.[67]

In summary, the evidence does not clearly favor one strategy over another. The currently available data suggest that both the "test and treat" and initial endoscopy approaches are equivalent with regards to symptomatic improvement. Fewer endoscopies are performed with the "test and treat" strategy, but patient satisfaction may be higher with initial endoscopy. A proposed dyspepsia management algorithm is presented in Figure 13-1.

Treatment

There are a wide variety of therapies that have been tried in functional dyspepsia, all of which have had marginal success. This is a reflection of the various possible etiologies of the disease process as well as the current limitations of our understanding of the pathophysiology of functional dyspepsia. Most patients with functional dyspepsia have mild, intermittent symptoms that will respond to reassurance, education, and

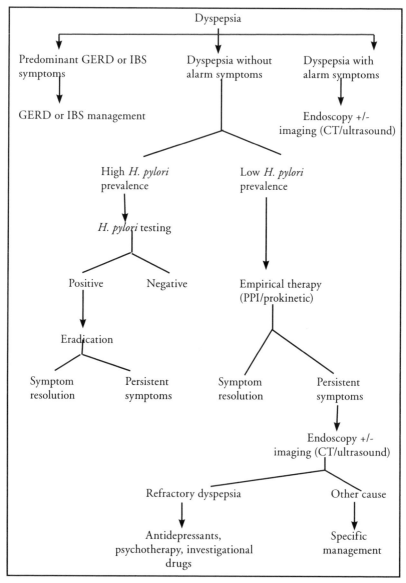

Figure 13-1. Dyspepsia management algorithm. (Adapted from Tack J, Bisschops R, Sarnelli G. Pathophysiology and treatment of functional dyspepsia. *Gastroenterology.* 2004;127:1239-1255.)

lifestyle modifications. The main challenge in all functional diseases is managing the patient who has refractory symptoms. The goal of treatment is to help patients accept, diminish, and cope with symptoms rather than eliminate them.

Once organic disease has been ruled out, the first step is to ensure a therapeutic patient-physician relationship. It is important to address specific concerns or fears that a patient may have. All interactions and data-gathering techniques, including the history and physical, should be nonjudgmental. Recent changes in diet, medications (NSAIDs), stressors, and other symptom triggers should be evaluated as possible causes for symptoms. It seems logical for patients to eat more frequent, smaller meals. Caffeine, excessive alcohol intake, and high fat meals should be avoided. Excessive testing should be avoided because this may erode the patient's confidence in the physician's ability; however, diagnostic testing should address the patient's concerns.

It is important to explain to the patient that functional dyspepsia is a real disease (validation) but to also stress its benign natural history. The patient should be educated on the proposed pathophysiological mechanisms implicated in functional dyspepsia. Realistic treatment goals should be set and lifestyle modifications and coping strategies should be implemented. Patients with psychological or psychiatric problems or a history of physical or sexual abuse with refractory symptoms should be considered for referral to a mental health professional or pain management center. Once all of the preceding elements have been evaluated and optimized, and if the patient continues to have symptoms, pharmacotherapy should be considered.

ACID-SUPPRESSING AGENTS

These agents are the most commonly used drugs in the treatment of dyspepsia. Many studies involving acid-suppressing agents have been conducted even though there is little evidence for the role of abnormal acid secretion or sensitivity in functional dyspepsia. Clinicians often use a trial of histamine-2 receptor antagonists (H2RA) or PPIs as first-line treatment for functional dyspepsia. A meta-analysis found that H2RA's were marginally better than placebo in functional dyspepsia.[68] A recent Cochrane meta-analysis evaluating pharmacological interventions for functional dyspepsia revealed the number needed to treat using H2RA's was 8.[69] However, the quality of most of the analyzed trials was suboptimal and most trials also included patients with reflux disease. PPIs are used more frequently because of their superior acid inhibition, but they have not been shown to be superior to H2RA's in functional dyspepsia. The same Cochrane meta-analysis showed that the number needed to treat functional dyspepsia using PPI therapy was 9.

In most trials, PPIs for functional dyspepsia have marginally superior efficacy when compared to placebo (Table 13-2). The BOND and OPERA studies were 2 large, randomized, double blind, parallel studies that evaluated the use of omeprazole for 4 weeks in functional dyspepsia.[41] The OPERA study alone failed to find a benefit, but when pooled with the BOND study, 1262 patients in total were evaluated. In the combined study, 36% to 38% of patients treated with omeprazole (10 mg and 20 mg, respectively) had complete resolution of symptoms compared to 28% of patients in the placebo group. The response to omeprazole was higher in patients with reflux-like dyspepsia, a subgroup that is no longer considered to belong to functional dyspepsia. There was a lesser response in patients with ulcer-like dyspepsia. The symptoms of patients with dysmotility-like dyspepsia (discomfort, nausea, bloating, etc) did not improve on omeprazole.

Table 13-2

SELECTED RANDOMIZED, PROSPECTIVE, DOUBLE-BLIND, PLACEBO-CONTROLLED TRIALS OF PROTON-PUMP INHIBITOR THERAPY FOR FUNCTIONAL DYSPEPSIA

			Complete Symptom Relief		
Study (Lead author)	N	Treatment Duration	PPI (Low Dose)	PPI (High Dose)	Placebo
Talley[41]	1262	4 weeks	36%* (omeprazole 10 mg/day)	38%* (omeprazole 20 mg/day)	28%
Lauritsen[70]	197	2 weeks	-	31%* (omeprazole 20 mg/day)	16%
Wong[71]	453	4 weeks	23% (lansoprazole 15 mg/day)	23% (lansoprazole 30 mg/day)	30%
Peura[72]	921	8 weeks	47%* (lansoprazole 15 mg/day)	44%* (lansoprazole 30 mg/day)	29%
Blum[73]	598	2 weeks	28%* (omeprazole 10 mg/day)	34%* (omeprazole 20 mg/day)	15%

* p <0.05 compared with placebo.

In a similarly designed trial, 197 patients with functional dyspepsia were randomized to receive omeprazole or placebo. In this study, 31% of those receiving omeprazole had complete symptom relief, compared to 16% of patients receiving placebo.[70] Another large, well-done study from China showed that lansoprazole was not significantly better than, and actually appeared to be inferior to, placebo in terms of symptom relief.[71] There were very few patients considered to have reflux-like dyspepsia in this study (only 18 out of 453 total patients). Interestingly, this was the subgroup that benefited the most in the BOND and OPERA studies. It is possible that patients with NERD or undiagnosed GERD positively influenced the results of the previously discussed PPI trials.

PROKINETIC AGENTS

Besides acid-suppressive agents, prokinetics are the next most widely used drugs in dyspepsia. The possible relationship between delayed gastric emptying and functional dyspepsia has led to trials of prokinetic agents in these patients. A meta-analysis of 17 placebo-controlled trials focused on the use of cisapride and domperidone (neither of which is routinely available in the United States) in functional dyspepsia.[74] Improvement was seen significantly more often with cisapride and domperidone when compared to placebo, with odds ratios of 2.9 and 7.0, respectively. The global assessment of dyspepsia symptoms and the individual symptoms of epigastric pain, early satiety, abdominal distention, and nausea were improved. The Cochrane meta-analysis referenced earlier included 12 trials with a total of 829 patients and showed that prokinetics were associated with a 50% reduction in symptoms when compared to placebo.[69] The number needed to treat using prokinetics was found to be 4 in that analysis. Metoclopramide may also be effective, but it may be associated with potential side effects, especially with long-term use, and has had only limited testing for functional dyspepsia. Mosapride, a newer prokinetic agent, was found to have no benefit over placebo in a recent well-sized, double-blind, placebo-controlled, multicenter trial.[75]

SEROTONERGIC AGENTS

Gastric (fundic) relaxants have been investigated as a possible therapeutic option in functional dyspepsia. Cisapride is a combined 5HT4 receptor agonist and antagonist, which in addition to promoting motility as mentioned above, also enhances the gastric accommodation to a meal.[76] Sumatriptan, used for migraine headaches, is a selective 5-HT1 receptor agonist that has also been shown to relax the proximal stomach in humans.[77] It also restored meal-induced relaxation and decreased meal-induced satiety in patients with impaired accommodation. Buspirone, a partial 5HT1 receptor agonist used to treat anxiety, was superior to placebo in alleviating symptoms of functional dyspepsia, and this was associated with an enhancement of gastric accommodation to a meal.[78] The use of tegaserod (a partial 5-HT4 receptor agonist) in functional dyspepsia is currently being investigated, although phase II studies in functional dyspepsia have yielded promising results.[79] 5HT3 receptor antagonists such as alosetron, tropisetron, and ondansetron have also been studied. Alosetron was recently found to have a potentially beneficial effect in patients with functional dyspepsia. Although the mechanism behind its effects is unclear, it may involve reduction of duodenal lipid sensitivity.[80] Serotonergic agents may eventually be shown to provide benefit, but there is not enough evidence at this time to recommend their use in functional dyspepsia.

Table 13-3

SELECTED RANDOMIZED, PROSPECTIVE, DOUBLE-BLIND, PLACEBO-CONTROLLED TRIALS OF *H. PYLORI* ERADICATION FOR FUNCTIONAL DYSPEPSIA

Study (Lead author)	N	Dyspepsia Resolution at 1 Year		
		H. pylori Treatment	Placebo	p Value
McColl[81]	318	21%	7%	< 0.001
Blum[82]	328	27%	21%	0.17
Talley[83]	279	24%	22%	0.7
Talley[84]	337	28%	23%	0.35

H. PYLORI *THERAPY*

As noted above, the pathogenetic role of *H. pylori* in functional dyspepsia is controversial. Four randomized, prospective, double-blind, placebo-controlled multicenter studies involving *H. pylori*-infected patients with functional dyspepsia have been reported in the past few years (Table 13-3). In one study, 318 patients with dyspepsia and *H. pylori* were randomly assigned to eradication therapy or PPI alone for the same duration. After 1 year of follow-up, dyspepsia resolved significantly more frequently in patients who received eradication therapy (21% vs 7%). Resolution was more common in patients who had symptoms for less than 5 years (27% vs 12%).[81] Three other similarly designed studies involving almost 900 patients reached the opposite conclusion. At the end of 1 year of follow-up, no significant differences in dyspepsia or quality of life were detected between the 2 groups.[82-84] Differences in inclusion criteria and outcome measures were most likely the reason for the conflicting results. Regardless, the observation in all of these studies that eradication of *H. pylori* did not provide symptomatic relief in more than 70% of the patients suggests that *H. pylori* does not have a pathophysiologic role in most cases of functional dyspepsia.

Two meta-analyses have also been conducted in the past few years to evaluate the issue. The most recent Cochrane Systematic Review on this topic concluded that there is a small therapeutic gain from eradication of *H. pylori* with a number needed to treat of 15.[69] A slightly higher benefit favoring treatment was seen in a previous meta-analysis that reported a nonsignificant odds ratio of 1.29 for treatment success after *H. pylori* eradication compared with control groups.[66] However, this study only included 7 trials, whereas the Cochrane review evaluated 12 trials. The following guideline has been proposed for the treatment of *H. pylori* in patients with functional dyspepsia: "There is no conclusive evidence that eradication of *H. pylori* infection will reverse the symptoms of non-ulcer dyspepsia. Patients may be tested for *H. pylori* on a case-by-case basis, and treatment offered to those with a positive result."[61] The risks and uncertain benefit of eradication therapy should be discussed with patients for whom eradication therapy is being considered. Risks include the possibility of *Clostridium difficile* infection, antibiotic-associated side effects, and a possible exacerbation of GERD. In summary, although the role of *H. pylori* in functional dyspepsia is small and probably of minor importance, both the AGA and ACG suggest that eradication of *H. pylori* in infected patients is reasonable after providing an explanation of the risks and limitations of therapy.

ANTIDEPRESSANT THERAPY

Antidepressants are increasingly being used in the treatment of functional disorders. The mechanism of action of these drugs in functional dyspepsia is unclear, but they are believed to affect visceral sensitivity. Although these patients likely have an element of depression, symptom relief from these drugs appears to be independent of the psychiatric effects of the drugs. Experts recommend the use of nortriptyline or desipramine, beginning at 10 to 25 mg/day, increasing slowly to 50 to 75 mg/day.[85] Amitriptyline was associated with improvement of symptoms in functional dyspepsia after 4 weeks in a very small study.[86] The newer SSRIs may prove to be effective treatment alternatives because these drugs increase the availability of serotonin in both the CNS and the enteric nervous system. Fluoxetine reduced symptoms in an open-label study of 40 patients with functional dyspepsia, but only in patients who were depressed at baseline.[87] In another study, paroxetine was shown to increase the meal-induced relaxation of the proximal stomach.[88] Unfortunately, the side effects of SSRIs include nausea and dyspepsia, which may limit the usefulness of these drugs in many patients with functional dyspepsia. Mianserin has also been tested in a broad group of patients with functional digestive disorders with positive results compared to placebo.[89] A meta-analysis of antidepressant therapy for functional GI disorders reported a modest treatment benefit; however, the flawed design of most of its studies limits any firm conclusions.[90]

VISCERAL ANALGESICS

A number of drugs have been postulated to alter visceral sensitivity. These include some of the drugs mentioned earlier such as the various antidepressants and alosetron. Visceral analgesics such as the somatostatin analog octreotide and the kappa receptor opioid agonist fedotozine are also undergoing evaluation in functional digestive disorders. Fedotozine has been evaluated in 2 double-blind, randomized, placebo-controlled trials, which showed that the drug resulted in modest symptom improvement with excellent patient tolerance when compared to placebo.[91,92] Unfortunately, fedotozine is no longer being pursued as a therapeutic agent.

OTHER DRUGS

A variety of other drugs have been tested for use in functional dyspepsia. Simethicone may be of some benefit over placebo.[93] Levosulpiride, a D2 antagonist, reduced dyspeptic symptoms in a small open label study.[94] Oral capsaicin, a substance P modulator, gave better relief in functional dyspepsia than placebo in a very small double-blind study over a 5-week period.[95] The motilin agonist ABT-229 was tested in a large, double-blind, placebo-controlled study in patients with functional dyspepsia but showed no benefit.[96] Other motilin agonists are currently being investigated. As mentioned earlier, CCK receptor antagonists may reduce duodenal lipid sensitivity and might prove useful in the therapy of functional dyspepsia.[37] Sildenafil is another potential therapeutic agent. It relaxes the proximal stomach by blocking phosphodiesterase type 5, which degrades nitric oxide-stimulated 3',5'-cyclic monophosphate, thereby relaxing the smooth muscle in various organs.[97] Nitric oxide donors (nitroglycerin) also relax the proximal stomach, but long-term use may be limited by vascular side effects. Clonidine, an alpha-2 receptor agonist, may also prove to be useful because it has been shown to relax the stomach and reduce gastric sensation.[98]

NONPHARMACOLOGIC THERAPIES

Psychologic treatment alternatives such as psychotherapy, cognitive treatment, and hypnotherapy have undergone evaluation in functional dyspepsia. Psychodynamic intrapersonal psychotherapy was found to have a favorable outcome when compared to supportive therapy in one study of functional dyspepsia.[99] A Cochrane review on psychological interventions in functional dyspepsia reported positive results from only 3 controlled, randomized trials, but a definitive conclusion of the effectiveness of these interventions could not be reached because of varied methodology.[100] A more recent study found that hypnotherapy improved symptoms and quality of life compared to medical therapy with ranitidine or supportive therapy and placebo in both the short and long term.[101] Patients required less medical visits and medication use during the 1-year follow-up period.

Summary

Functional dyspepsia is a very common, yet often frustrating condition to treat. The lack of a clear understanding of the pathogenesis and pathophysiology of the disorder makes it especially challenging. There are likely multiple abnormalities in GI function involved, and it is likely a multifactorial disorder. This makes no one therapeutic option a cure-all for the disorder. Treatment for functional dyspepsia should begin with a discussion of the negative endoscopy results, reassurance, and explanation of the concept of the disorder. Lifestyle modifications should be instituted as discussed earlier. If needed, the next step requires adding medication, keeping in mind the large placebo response. Acid suppression should be given initially to patients, especially those with predominant symptoms of reflux-like or ulcer-like dyspepsia. Prokinetics should be given to patients with symptoms of dysmotility-like dyspepsia. In a patient with refractory symptoms, a trial of a pain-modulating antidepressant should be considered, and, if unsuccessful, nonpharmacologic treatment should be considered. Much more research needs to be conducted to help clarify the many questions that remain unanswered in functional dyspepsia.

References

1. Talley NJ, Zinmeister AR, Schleck CD, et al. Dyspepsia and dyspepsia subgroups: a population based study. *Gastroenterology.* 1992;102:1259-1268.
2. McQuaid KR. Dyspepsia. In: Feldman M, Friedman LS, Sleisenger MH, eds. *Sleisenger and Fordtran's GI and Liver Disease.* Vol 1. 7th ed. Philadelphia: W.B. Saunders; 2002:102-116.

3. Agreus L, Svardsudd K, Talley NJ, et al. Natural history of GERD and functional abdominal disorders: a population based study. *Am J Gastroenterol.* 2001;96:2905-2914.

4. Koloski N, Talley N, Boyce P. The impact of functional GI disorders on quality of life. *Am J Gastroenterol.* 2000;95:67-71.

5. Kurata JH, Nogawa AN, Everhart JE. A prospective study of dyspepsia in primary care. *Dig Dis Sci.* 2002;47:797-803.

6. Talley N, Silverstein M, Agreus L, et al. AGA technical review: evaluation of dyspepsia. *Gastroenterology.* 1998;114:582-595.

7. Byzter P, Talley NJ. Dyspepsia. *Ann Intern Med.* 2001;134:815-822.

8. Agreus L. Natural history of dyspepsia. *Gut.* 2002;50(Suppl 4):2-9.

9. Talley NJ, Stanghellini V, Heading RC, et al. Functional gastroduodenal disorders. *Gut.* 1999;45(Suppl. II):1137-1142.

10. Camilleri M. Autonomic regulation of GI motility. In: Low PA, ed. *Clinical Autonomic Disorders: Evaluation and Management.* Boston, Mass: Little, Brown; 1992:125.

11. Quartero AO, de Wit NJ, Lodder AC, et al. Disturbed solid-phase gastric emptying in functional dyspepsia: a meta-analysis. *Dig Dis Sci.* 1998;43:2028-2033.

12. Stanghellini V, Ghidini G, Maccarini M, et al. Fasting and postprandial GI motility in ulcer and nonulcer dyspepsia. *Gut.* 1992;33:184-190.

13. Talley NJ, Shuter B, McCrudden G, et al. Lack of association between gastric emptying and symptoms in nonulcer dyspepsia. *J Clin Gastroenterol.* 1989;11:625-630.

14. Talley NJ, Verlinden M, Jones M. Can symptoms discriminate among those with delayed or normal gastric emptying in dysmotility-like dyspepsia? *Am J Gastroenterol.* 2001;96:1422-1428.

15. Stanghellini V, Tosetti C, Paternico A, et al. Risk indicators of delayed gastric emptying of solids in patients with functional dyspepsia. *Gastroenterology.* 1996;110:1036-1042.

16. Sarnelli G, Caenepeel P, Geypens B, et al. Symptoms associated with impaired gastric emptying of solids and liquids in functional dyspepsia. *Am J Gastroenterol.* 2003;98(4):783-788.

17. Berstad A, Hauken T, Gilja O, et al. Gastric accommodation in functional dyspepsia. *Scand J Gastroenterol.* 1997;32:193-197.

18. Thurmshirn M, Camilleri M, Saslow S, et al. Gastric accommodation in non-ulcer dyspepsia and the roles of *Helicobacter pylori* infection and vagal function. *Gut.* 1999;44:55-64.

19. Tack J, Piessevaux H, Coulie B, et al. Role of impaired gastric accommodation to a meal in functional dyspepsia. *Gastroenterology.* 1998;115:1346-1352.

20. Kim DY, Delgado-Aros S, Camilleri M, et al. Noninvasive measurement of gastric accommodation in patients with idiopathic nonulcer dyspepsia. *Am J Gastroenterol.* 2001;96:3099-3105.

21. Boeckxstaens GE, Hirsch DP, Kuiken SD, et al. The proximal stomach and postprandial symptoms in functional dyspeptics. *Am J Gastroenterol.* 2002;97:40-48.

22. Leahy A, Besherdas K, Clayman C, et al. Abnormalities of the electrogastrogram in functional GI disorders. *Am J Gastroenterol.* 1999;94:1023-1028.

23. Parkman H, Miller M, Trate D, et al. Electrogastrography and gastric emptying scintigraphy are complementary for assessment of dyspepsia. *J Clin Gastroenterol.* 1997;24:214-219.

24. Holmvall P, Lindberg G. Electrogastrography before and after a high-caloric, liquid test meal in healthy volunteers and patients with severe functional dyspepsia. *Scand J Gastroenterol.* 2002;37:1144-1148.

25. Besherdas K, Leahy A, Mason I, et al. The effect of cisapride on dyspepsia symptoms and the electrogastrogram in patients with non-ulcer dyspepsia. *Aliment Pharmacol Ther.* 1998;12:755-759.

26. Bjornsson E, Abrahamsson H. Contractile patterns in patients with severe dyspepsia. *Am J Gastroenterol.* 1999;94:54-64.

27. Wilmer A, Van Cutsem E, Andrioli A, et al. Ambulatory gastrojejunal manometry in severe motility-like dyspepsia: lack of correlation between dysmotility, symptoms, and gastric emptying. *Gut.* 1998;42:235-242.

28. Camilleri M, Coulie B, Tack J. Visceral hypersensitivity: facts, speculations, and challenges. *Gut.* 2001;48:125-131.

29. Coffin B, Azpiroz F, Guarner F, et al. Selective gastric hypersensitivity and reflex hyporeactivity in functional dyspepsia. *Gastroenterology.* 1994;107:1345-1351.

30. Tack J, Caenepeel P, Fischler B, et al. Symptoms associated with hypersensitivity to gastric distention in functional dyspepsia. *Gastroenterology.* 2001;121:526-535.

31. Mertz H, Fullerton S, Naliboff B, et al. Symptoms and visceral perception in severe functional and organic dyspepsia. *Gut.* 1998;42:814-822.

32. Holtmann G, Gschossmann J, Neufang-Huber J, et al. Differences in gastric mechanosensory function after repeated ramp distensions in non-consulters with dyspepsia and healthy controls. *Gut.* 2000;47:332-336.

33. Holtmann G, Gschossmann J, Buenger L, et al. Do changes in visceral sensory function determine the development of dyspepsia during treatment with aspirin? *Gastroenterology.* 2002;123:1451-1458.

34. Houghton LA, Mangall YF, Dwivedi A, et al. Sensitivity to nutrients in patients with non-ulcer dyspepsia. *Eur J Gastroenterol Hepatol.* 1993;5:109-113.

35. Barbera R, Feinle C, Read NW. Nutrient-specific modulation of gastric mechanosensitivity in patients with functional dyspepsia. *Dig Dis Sci.* 1995;40:1636-1641.

36. Barbera R, Feinle C, Read NW. Abnormal sensitivity to duodenal lipid infusion in patients with functional dyspepsia. *Eur J Gastroenterol Hepatol.* 1995;7:1051-1057.

37. Feinle C, Meier O, Otto B, et al. Role of duodenal lipid and cholecystokinin A receptors in the pathophysiology of functional dyspepsia. *Gut.* 2001;48:347-355.

38. Collen MJ, Loebenberg MJ. Basal gastric acid secretion in nonulcer dyspepsia with or without duodenitis. *Dig Dis Sci.* 1989;34:246-250.

39. George AA, Tsuchiyose M, Dooley CP. Sensitivity of the gastric mucosa to acid and duodenal contents in patients with nonulcer dyspepsia. *Gastroenterology.* 1991;101:3-6.

40. Samsom M, Verhagen M, van Berge Henegouwen G, et al. Abnormal clearance of exogenous acid and increased acid sensitivity of the proximal duodenum in dyspeptic patients. *Gastroenterology.* 1999;116:515-520.

41. Talley NJ, Meineche-Schmidt V, Pare P, et al. Efficacy of omeprazole in functional dyspepsia: double-blind, randomized, placebo-controlled trials (the Bond and Opera studies). *Aliment Pharmacol Ther.* 1998;12:1055-1065.

42. Schwartz MP, Samsom M, Van Berge Henegouwen GP, et al. Effect of inhibition of gastric acid secretion on antropyloroduodenal motor activity and duodenal acid hypersensitivity in functional dyspepsia. *Aliment Pharmacol Ther.* 2001;15:1921-1928.

43. Lee KJ, Demarchi B, Vos R, et al. Comparison of duodenal acid exposure in functional dyspepsia patients and healthy controls using 24-hour ambulatory duodenal pH monitoring. *Gastroenterology.* 2002;122:A-102.

44. Lee KJ, Vos R, Janssens J, et al. Influence of duodenal acidification on the sensorimotor function of the proximal stomach in humans. *Am J Physiol Gastrointest Liver Physiol.* 2004;286(2):G278-G284.

45. Locke R III, Talley N, Nelson D, et al. *Helicobacter pylori* and dyspepsia: a population-based study of the organism and host. *Am J Gastroenterol.* 2000;5:1906-1913.

46. Talley NJ, Hunt RH. What role does *Helicobacter pylori* play in dyspepsia and nonulcer dyspepsia? Arguments for and against *H. pylori* being associated with dyspeptic symptoms. *Gastroenterology.* 1997;113:S67-S77.

47. Danesh J, Lawrence M, Murphy M, et al. Systematic review of the epidemiological evidence on *Helicobacter pylori* infection and nonulcer or uninvestigated dyspepsia. *Arch Intern Med.* 2000;160:1192-1198.

48. Sarnelli G, Cuomo R, Janssens J, et al. Symptom patterns and pathophysiological mechanisms in dyspeptic patients with and without *Helicobacter pylori*. *Dig Dis Sci.* 2003;48(12):2229-2236.

49. Troncon LEA, Thompson DG, Ahluwalia NK, et al. Relations between upper abdominal symptoms and gastric distention abnormalities in dysmotility like functional dyspepsia and after vagotomy. *Gut.* 1995;37:17-22.

50. Holtmann G, Goebell H, Jockenhoevel F, et al. Altered vagal and intestinal mechanosensory function in chronic unexplained dyspepsia. *Gut.* 1998;42:501-506.

51. Thumshirn M, Camilleri M, Saslow S, et al. Gastric accommodation in nonulcer dyspepsia and the roles of *Helicobacter pylori* infection and vagal function. *Gut.* 1999;44:55-64.

52. Wilhelmsen I, Haug TT, Ursin H, et al. Discriminant analysis of factors distinguishing patients with functional dyspepsia from patients with duodenal ulcer: significance of somatization. *Dig Dis Sci.* 1995;40:1105-1111.

53. Koloski NA, Talley NJ, Boyce PM. Predictors of health care seeking for IBS and nonulcer dyspepsia: a critical review of the literature on symptom and psychosocial factors. *Am J Gastroenterol.* 2001;96:1340-1349.

54. Talley NJ, Phillips S, Bruce B, et al. Relation among personality and symptoms in nonulcer dyspepsia and the IBS. *Gastroenterology.* 1990;99:327-333.

55. Drossman D, Creed F, Olden K, et al. Psychosocial aspects of functional GI disorders. *Gut.* 1999;45:II25-II30.

56. Bennett E, Piesse C, Palmer K, et al. Functional GI disorders: psychological, social, and somatic features. *Gut.* 1998;42:414-420.

57. Drossman DA, Talley NJ, Leserman J, et al. Sexual and physical abuse and GI illness. Review and recommendations. *Ann Intern Med.* 1995;123:782-794.

58. Tack J, Demedts I, Dehondt G, et al. Clinical and pathophysiological characteristics of acute-onset functional dyspepsia. *Gastroenterology.* 2002;122:1738-1747.

59. Corsetti M, Caenepeel P, Fischler B, et al. Impact of coexisting IBS on symptoms and pathophysiological mechanisms in functional dyspepsia. *Am J Gastroenterol.* 2004;99(6):1152-1159.

60. Talley N, Axon A, Bytzer P, et al. Management of uninvestigated dyspepsia and functional dyspepsia: a working party report for the World Congresses of Gastroenterology 1998. *Aliment Pharmacol Ther.* 1999;13:1135-1148.

61. Howden CW, Hunt RH. Guidelines for the management of *H. pylori* infection. Ad Hoc Committee on Practice Parameters of the American College of Gastroenterology. *Am J Gastroenterol.* 1998;93:2330-2338.

62. Lassen AT, Pederson FM, Bytzer P, et al. *Helicobacter pylori* test-and-eradicate versus prompt endoscopy for management of dyspeptic patients: a randomized trial. *Lancet.* 2000;356:455-460.

63. Spiegel BM, Vakil NB, Ofman JJ. Dyspepsia management in primary care: a decision analysis of competing strategies. *Gastroenterology.* 2002;122:1270-1285.

64. Silverstein MD, Pettereson T, Talley NJ. Initial endoscopy or empirical therapy with or without testing for *Helicobacter pylori* for dyspepsia: a decision analysis. *Gastroenterology.* 1996;110:72-83.

65. Rabeneck L, Souchek J, Wristers K, et al. A double blind, randomized, placebo-controlled trial of proton pump inhibitor therapy in patients with uninvestigated dyspepsia. *Am J Gastroenterol.* 2002;97:3045-3051.

66. Laine L, Schoenfeld P, Fennerty MB. Therapy for *Helicobacter pylori* in patients with nonulcer dyspepsia. A meta-analysis of randomized, controlled trials. *Ann Intern Med.* 2001;134:361-369.

67. Delaney BC, Innes MA, Deeks J, et al. Initial management strategies for dyspepsia. *Cochrane Database Syst Rev.* 2001;3:CD001961.

68. Finney J, Kinnersley N, Hughes M, et al. Meta-analysis of anti-secretory and gastrokinetic compounds in functional dyspepsia. *J Clin Gastroenterol.* 1998;26:312-320.

69. Moayyedi P, Soo S, Deeks J, et al. Pharmacological interventions for non-ulcer dyspepsia. *Cochrane Database Syst Rev.* 2003;1:CD001960.

70. Lauritsen K, Aalykke C, Havelund T, et al. Effect of omeprazole in functional dyspepsia: a double-blind, randomized, placebo-controlled study. *Gastroenterology.* 1996;110:A702.

71. Wong WM, Wong BC, Hung WK, et al. Double blind, randomized, placebo controlled study of four weeks of lansoprazole for the treatment of functional dyspepsia in Chinese patients. *Gut.* 2002;51:502-506.

72. Peura DA, Kovacs TO, Metz D, et al. Low-dose lansoprazole: effective for non-ulcer dyspepsia. *Gastroenterology.* 2000;118:A439.

73. Blum A, Arnold R, Stolte M, et al. Short course of acid suppressive treatment for patients with functional dyspepsia: results depend on *Helicobacter pylori* status. *Gut.* 2000;47:473-480.

74. Veldhuyzen van Zanten S, Jones M, Verlinden M, et al. Efficacy of cisapride and domperidone in functional (non-ulcer) dyspepsia: a meta-analysis. *Am J Gastroenterol.* 2001;96:689-696.

75. Hallerback B, Bommelaer G, Bredberg E, et al. Dose finding study of mosapride in functional dyspepsia: a placebo-controlled, randomized study. *Aliment Pharmacol Ther.* 2002;16:959-967.

76. Tack J, Broeckaert D, Coulie B, et al. The influence of cisapride on gastric tone and the perception of gastric distension. *Aliment Pharmacol Ther.* 1998;12:761-766.

77. Tack J, Coulie B, Wilmer A, et al. Influence of sumatriptan on gastric fundus tone and on the perception of gastric distension in man. *Gut.* 2000;46:468-473.

78. Tack J, Piessevaux H, Coulie B, et al. A placebo-controlled trial of buspirone, a fundus-relaxing drug in functional dyspepsia: effect on symptoms and gastric sensory and motor function. *Gastroenterology.* 1999;116:G1423.

79. Tack J, Delia T, Ligozio G, et al. A phase II placebo controlled randomized trial with tegaserod (T) in functional dyspepsia (FD) patients with normal gastric emptying (NGE). *Gastroenterology.* 2002;122:154.

80. Talley NJ, Van Zanten SV, Saez LR, et al. A dose-ranging, placebo-controlled, randomized trial of alosetron in patients with functional dyspepsia. *Aliment Pharmacol Ther.* 2001;15:525-537.

81. McColl K, Murray L, El-Omar E, et al. Symptomatic benefit from eradicating *Helicobacter pylori* infection in patients with nonulcer dyspepsia. *N Engl J Med.* 1998;339:1869-1874.

82. Blum AL, Talley NJ, O'Morain C, et al. Lack of effect of treating *Helicobacter pylori* infection in patients with nonulcer dyspepsia. Omeprazole plus Clarithromycin and Amoxicillin Effect One Year after Treatment (OCAY) Study Group. *N Engl J Med.* 1998;339:1875-1881.

83. Talley NJ, Janssens J, Lauritsen K, et al. Eradication of *Helicobacter pylori* in functional dyspepsia: randomized double blind placebo controlled trial with 12 months' follow up. The Optimal Regimen Cures Helicobacter Induced Dyspepsia (ORCHID) Study Group. *BMJ.* 1999;318:833-837.

84. Talley NJ, Vakil N, Ballard ED III, et al. Absence of benefit of eradicating *Helicobacter pylori* in patients with nonulcer dyspepsia. *N Engl J Med.* 1999;341:1106-1111.

85. Clouse R. Psychotropic medications for the treatment of functional GI disorders. *Clin Perspect Gastroenterol.* 1999;50:348-356.

86. Mertz H, Fass R, Kodner A, et al. Effect of amitryptiline on symptoms, sleep, and visceral perception in patients with functional dyspepsia. *Am J Gastroenterol.* 1998;93:160-165.

87. Wu C, Chou L, Chen H, et al. Effect of fluoxetine on symptoms and gastric dysrhythmias in patients with functional dyspepsia. *Hepatogastroenterology.* 2003;50:278-283.

88. Tack J, Schnackers D, Coulie B, et al. 5-hydroxytryptamine is involved in the gastric accommodation reflex in man. *Neurogastroenterol Motil.* 1998;10:475.

89. Tanum L, Malt UF. A new pharmacologic treatment of functional GI disorder: a double-blind placebo-controlled study with mianserin. *Scand J Gastroenterol.* 1996;31:318-325.

90. Jackson J, O'Malley P, Tomkins G, et al. Treatment of functional GI disorders with antidepressant medications: a meta-analysis. *Am J Med.* 2000;108:65-72.

91. Coffin B, Bouhassira D, Chollet R, et al. Effect of the kappa agonist fedotozine on perception of gastric distension in healthy humans. *Aliment Pharmacol Ther.* 1996;10:919-925.

92. Read NW, Abitbol JL, Bardhan KD, et al. Efficacy and safety of the peripheral kappa agonist fedotozine versus placebo in the treatment of functional dyspepsia. *Gut.* 1997;41:664-668.

93. Holtmann G, Gschossmann L, Mayr P, et al. A randomized, placebo-controlled trial of simethicone and cisapride for the treatment of patients with functional dyspepsia. *Aliment Pharmacol Ther.* 2002;16:1641-1648.

94. Distrutti E, Fiorucci S, Hauer S, et al. Effect of acute and chronic levosulpiride administration on gastric tone and perception in functional dyspepsia. *Aliment Pharmacol Ther.* 2002;16:613-622.

95. Bortolotti M, Coccia G, Grossi G, et al. The treatment of functional dyspepsia with red pepper. *Aliment Pharmacol Ther.* 2002;16:1075-1082.

96. Talley NJ, Verlinden M, Snape W, et al. Failure of a motilin receptor agonist (ABT-229) to relieve the symptoms of functional dyspepsia in patients with and without delayed gastric emptying: a randomized double-blind placebo-controlled trial. *Aliment Pharmacol Ther.* 2000;14:1653-1661.

97. Sarnelli G, Vos R, Sifrim D, et al. Influence of sildenafil on fasting and postprandial gastric tone in man. *Gastroenterology.* 2001;120:1478.

98. Thumshirn M, Camilleri M, Choi MG, et al. Modulation of gastric sensory and motor functions by nitrergic and alpha2-adrenergic agents in humans. *Gastroenterology.* 1999;116:573-585.

99. Hamilton J, Guthrie E, Creed F, et al. A randomized controlled trial of psychotherapy in patients with chronic functional dyspepsia. *Gastroenterology.* 2000;119:661-669.

100. Soo S, Moayyedi P, Deeks J, et al. Psychological interventions for nonulcer dyspepsia. *Cochrane Database Syst Rev.* 2001;4:CD002301.

101. Calvert E, Houghton L, Cooper P, et al. Long-term improvement in functional dyspepsia using hypnotherapy. *Gastroenterology.* 2002;123:1778-1785.

Nausea and Vomiting: Etiologies and Treatment

William L. Hasler, MD

Definitions

Nausea is a symptom defined as a subjective feeling of a need to vomit. Vomiting (emesis) is the oral expulsion of GI contents resulting from contractions of gut and thoracoabdominal wall musculature. Symptoms that may be confused with vomiting include regurgitation (ie, the effortless passage of gastric contents into the mouth) and rumination (ie, the repeated regurgitation of stomach contents that may be rechewed and reswallowed). Patients with nausea may report other associated symptoms including epigastric fullness or discomfort, eructation, anorexia, and early satiety.

Pathophysiology

Vomiting is coordinated by the brainstem and is elicited by neuromuscular responses in the gut, pharynx, and thoracoabdominal wall. The mechanisms underlying nausea are poorly understood but likely involve the cerebral cortex because nausea requires conscious perception. Several brainstem nuclei, including the nucleus tractus solitarius; the dorsal vagal and phrenic nuclei; and medullary nuclei, which regulate respiration coordinate the initiation of emesis. Neural pathways involved in this coordination may be mediated by neurokinin NK1, serotonin, and vasopressin receptors. The force required for expulsion of gut contents is generated by somatic muscular events. Inspiratory thoracic and abdominal wall muscles contract, producing high intrathoracic and intra-abdominal pressures that facilitate expulsion of gastric contents. The gastric cardia herniates across the diaphragm and the larynx moves upward to promote oral propulsion of the vomitus. Within the stomach and small intestine, there is disruption or abolition of normal myoelectric slow wave cycling and initiation of orally propagating spike activity, which elicits retrograde contractions that facilitate oral expulsion of gut contents.

Stimulation at a number of anatomic sites can elicit nausea and vomiting. The cerebral cortex mediates symptoms associated with emotional disturbances, depres-

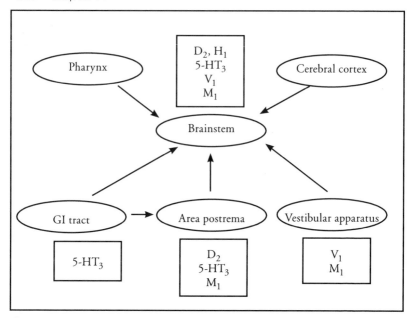

Figure 14-1. Emetic stimuli acting on a variety of sites in the CNS (cerebral cortex, pharynx, vestibular apparatus, and area postrema) activate sites in the brainstem that then evoke the stereotypical somatic motor responses of vomiting. Different neurotransmitter receptors are involved in different regions, including serotonin (5-HT3), dopamine (D2), muscarinic cholinergic (M1), histamine (H1), and vasopressin (V1). The differences in neurotransmitter responses provide a partial explanation for the selective effects of certain antiemetic drugs in varied clinical settings.

sion, eating disorders, and organic diseases, which produce increased intracranial pressure. Cranial nerve pathways mediate vomiting after gag reflex activation. Motion sickness and inner ear disorders act on the labyrinthine apparatus. The area postrema, a medullary nucleus, responds to blood-borne emetic stimuli and has been termed the chemoreceptor trigger zone. Many emetic drugs, including some chemotherapeutic agents, act on the area postrema as do metabolic disorders such as thyroid disease or Addison's disease, endogenous toxins from hepatic failure, and exogenous bacterial toxins. In addition to central neural sites, peripheral regions of the body may also induce nausea and vomiting by activation of visceral afferent nerve pathways. Gastric irritants such as copper sulfate and cytotoxic agents such as cisplatin stimulate gastroduodenal vagal afferent fibers and serve as models of vomiting activated by peripheral pathways.

Neurotransmitters that mediate induction of nausea and vomiting are different for stimuli that act at these distinct sites (Figure 14-1). Labyrinthine processes stimulate vestibular cholinergic muscarinic M1 and histaminergic H1 receptors, whereas vagal afferent stimuli activate serotonin 5-HT3 receptors. The area postrema is richly served by nerve fibers acting on 5-HT3, M1, H1, and dopamine D2 receptor subtypes. Pharmacologic management of vomiting requires understanding of these pathways.

Etiologies

The differential diagnosis of nausea and vomiting includes medications, GI and intraperitoneal diseases, neurologic disorders, metabolic conditions, and infections (Table 14-1).

MEDICATIONS

Drug reactions are among the most common causes of nausea and vomiting, especially within days of initiation of therapy. Chemotherapeutic agents such as cisplatin and cyclophosphamide are potent emetic stimuli that act on central and peripheral afferent neural pathways. Emesis from chemotherapy may be acute, delayed, or anticipatory. Analgesics such as aspirin or NSAIDs induce nausea by direct GI mucosal irritation. Other classes of medications that produce nausea include cardiovascular drugs (eg, digoxin, antiarrhythmics, antihypertensives), diuretics, hormonal agents (eg, oral antidiabetics, contraceptives), antibiotics (eg, erythromycin), and GI medications (eg, sulfasalazine).

ORGANIC DISORDERS OF THE GASTROINTESTINAL TRACT AND PERITONEUM

Organic gut and peritoneal disorders represent prevalent causes of nausea and vomiting. Gastric outlet obstruction often produces intermittent symptoms, whereas small intestinal obstruction is usually acute and associated with abdominal pain. Superior mesenteric artery syndrome, developing after severe weight loss, recent surgery, or prolonged bed rest, occurs when the duodenum is compressed and obstructed by the superior mesenteric artery as it originates from the aorta. Other rare mechanical causes of nausea and vomiting include gastric volvulus and antral webs. Inflammatory conditions (eg, pancreatitis, appendicitis, and cholecystitis) irritate the peritoneal surface, whereas biliary colic produces nausea by activating the afferent neural pathways. Fulminant hepatitis causes nausea, presumably because of accumulation of emetic toxins and increases in intracranial pressure. Nausea is reported by many patients with GER. These effects are sometimes associated with impairments of gastric motor function.

MOTOR AND FUNCTIONAL DISORDERS OF THE GASTROINTESTINAL TRACT

Disorders of gut motor activity such as gastroparesis evoke nausea because of an inability to clear retained food and secretions. Gastroparesis commonly presents with nausea, vomiting, early satiety, fullness, and abdominal discomfort as a consequence of delayed gastric emptying. In more severe cases, patients may develop weight loss, malnutrition, or an inability to maintain adequate intake of food and fluids. The causes of gastroparesis are varied (Table 14-2). Twenty-five percent to 30% of cases result from long-standing diabetes mellitus, usually type I, while >30% are idiopathic. Many cases of idiopathic gastroparesis occur as a consequence of a viral infection, which produces temporary or permanent damage to the gastric myenteric plexus.[1] Less common etiologies of gastroparesis include collagen vascular disease (especially scleroderma), amyloidosis, hereditary visceral smooth muscle or nerve disorders, paraneoplastic visceral neuropathy, and the postvagotomy state. Delays in gastric

Table 14-1

CAUSES OF NAUSEA AND VOMITING

Medications

- NSAIDs
- Cardiovascular drugs (eg, digoxin, antiarrhythmics, antihypertensives)
- Diuretics
- Hormonal agents (eg, oral antidiabetics, contraceptives)
- Antibiotics (eg, erythromycin)
- GI drugs (eg, sulfasalazine)

CNS Disorders

- Tumors
- Cerebrovascular accident
- Intracranial hemorrhage
- Infections
- Congenital abnormalities
- Psychiatric disease (eg, anxiety, depression, anorexia nervosa, bulimia nervosa, psychogenic vomiting)
- Motion sickness
- Labyrinthine causes (eg, tumors, labyrinthitis, Meniere's disease)

Miscellaneous Causes

- Posterior myocardial infarction
- Congestive heart failure
- Excess ethanol ingestion
- Jamaican vomiting sickness
- Prolonged starvation
- Cyclic vomiting syndrome

GI and Peritoneal Disorders

- Gastric outlet obstruction
- Obstruction of the small intestine
- Superior mesenteric artery syndrome
- Gastroparesis
- Chronic intestinal pseudo-obstruction
- Pancreatitis
- Appendicitis
- Cholecystitis
- Acute hepatitis
- Pancreatic carcinoma

(continued)

Table 14-1

CAUSES OF NAUSEA AND VOMITING (CONTINUED)

Endocrinologic and Metabolic Conditions
- Nausea of pregnancy
- Uremia
- Diabetic ketoacidosis
- Thyroid disease
- Addison's disease

Infectious Disease
- Viral gastroenteritis (eg, Hawaii agent, rotavirus, reovirus, adenovirus, Snow Mountain agent, Norwalk agent)
- Bacterial causes (eg, *Staphylococcus spp.*, *Salmonella spp.*, *Bacillus cereus*, *Clostridium perfringens*)
- Opportunistic infection (eg, cytomegalovirus, herpes simplex virus)
- Otitis media

Table 14-2

SOME ETIOLOGIES OF GASTROPARESIS

- Diabetes mellitus
- Idiopathic
- Postsurgical
    * Vagotomy or distal gastric resection
    * Fundoplication
    * Bariatric surgery
- GERD
- Functional dyspepsia
- Chronic intestinal pseudo-obstruction
- Collagen vascular diseases
    * Scleroderma
    * Systemic lupus erythematosus
    * Polymyositis-dermatomyositis
- Amyloidosis
- Anorexia nervosa
- Parkinson's disease

(continued)

Table 14-2

SOME ETIOLOGIES OF GASTROPARESIS (CONTINUED)

- Endocrine and metabolic disorders
  * Hypothyroidism
  * Hyperparathyroidism
  * Gastric infection
- Paraneoplastic
- Gastric ischemia
- Medications

emptying may be a consequence of a variety of motor disturbances. Impairments in fundic tone can contribute to food retention in the proximal stomach. Loss of phasic contractions in the distal stomach and increases in antral diameter reduce the effectiveness of trituration of large food particles. Increases in tone and phasic motor activity in the pylorus, known as pylorospasm, produce a functional outlet obstruction.[2] The correlation of symptoms to rates of gastric emptying is imperfect. The presence of delayed emptying is associated with an increased prevalence of nausea and vomiting in patients with functional dyspepsia, whereas the relation of symptom severity with the degree of gastric retention is poor in diabetics with gastric symptoms.[3,4] Other factors that may influence symptom development in gastroparesis include disruptions of the rhythmic cycling of the gastric electrical pacemaker activity (eg, tachygastria, bradygastria) and development of gastric afferent hypersensitivity in which exaggerated nausea is elicited by minimal gastric distention.[5,6] Finally, metabolic factors may play roles in motor dysfunction in patients with diabetes separate from any organic damage to gastric nerve or muscle tissue. Increasing the blood glucose concentration retards gastric emptying of solids, induces tachygastria, and increases perception of gastric distention.[7]

Chronic intestinal pseudo-obstruction is a motor disorder presenting with impaired transit that may present diffusely throughout the GI tract. Symptoms of intestinal pseudo-obstruction include nausea, vomiting, bloating, bowel disturbances, malnutrition, and malabsorption (as a consequence of small intestinal bacterial overgrowth). Pseudo-obstruction may result from enteric nerve damage (eg, hereditary visceral neuropathy, early scleroderma or amyloidosis, myotonic dystrophy, paraneoplastic response to malignancy such as small cell lung carcinoma) or loss of smooth muscle integrity or function (hereditary visceral myopathy, advanced scleroderma or amyloidosis). Bacterial overgrowth frequently develops due to impaired ability to clear either swallowed organisms or bacteria refluxed from the colon.

Nausea and vomiting are commonly reported symptoms in patients with functional bowel disorders. Approximately 50% of patients with IBS report nausea. Similarly, a sizable fraction of individuals with functional dyspepsia report nausea and vomiting. In both conditions, 25% to 50% of patients exhibit delays in gastric emptying of solid food; however, it is uncertain if these defects represent possible causes of symptoms.[8]

CENTRAL NERVOUS SYSTEM CAUSES

Conditions with increased intracranial pressure, such as tumors, infarction, hemorrhage, infections, or congenital abnormalities, produce emesis with and without nausea. Emotional responses to unpleasant smells or tastes induce vomiting as can anticipation of cancer chemotherapy. Psychiatric causes of nausea include anxiety, depression, anorexia nervosa, and bulimia nervosa. Young women with psychiatric illness or social difficulty may present with psychogenic vomiting. Labyrinthine etiologies of nausea include labyrinthitis, tumors, and Meniere's disease. Motion sickness is induced by repetitive movements that result in vestibular nuclei activation.

ENDOCRINOLOGIC AND METABOLIC CONDITIONS

First trimester pregnancy is the most common endocrinologic cause of nausea. This condition, occurring in 50% to 70% of pregnancies, usually is transitory and is not associated with poor fetal or maternal outcome. However, 1% to 5% of cases progress to hyperemesis gravidarum, which may produce dangerous fluid losses and electrolyte disturbances. Other endocrinologic and metabolic conditions associated with vomiting include uremia, diabetic ketoacidosis, thyroid and parathyroid disease, and Addison's disease.

INFECTIOUS CAUSES

Infectious illness produces nausea and vomiting, usually of acute onset. Viral gastroenteritis may be caused by rotaviruses and the Hawaii, Snow Mountain, and Norwalk agents. Bacterial infection with *Staphylococcus* or *Salmonella* organisms, *Bacillus cereus*, and *Clostridium perfringens* also produces nausea and vomiting, in many cases via toxins that act on the area postrema.[9] Nausea in immunosuppressed patients may result from GI cytomegalovirus or herpes simplex infections. Infections not involving the GI tract, such as hepatitis, otitis media, and meningitis, may also elicit nausea.

MISCELLANEOUS CAUSES OF NAUSEA AND VOMITING

Other conditions may produce nausea and vomiting. Radiation therapy to the upper abdomen elicits vomiting in up to 80% of patients by activation of 5-HT3 on visceral afferent pathways.[10] Nausea and vomiting complicate 17% to 37% of surgical operations, most often in women, more frequently after general anesthesia and after abdominal or orthopedic surgery.[11] Nausea may be a manifestation of posterior wall myocardial infarction as well as of congestive heart failure. Acute graft versus host disease is the dominant cause of nausea and vomiting in bone marrow transplant recipients. Excess ethanol intake evokes nausea by acting on the CNS. Cyclic vomiting syndrome is a condition of unknown etiology characterized by episodes of emesis with intervening asymptomatic periods usually occurring in young childhood and resolving by adolescence. It is now being seen in young adults. An association of cyclic vomiting syndrome and migraine headaches has been reported, suggesting the 2 conditions may share a common pathogenesis.[12] Excess vitamin intake and prolonged starvation also cause nausea. Jamaican vomiting sickness results from ingestion of unripe akee fruit.

Diagnostic Evaluation

HISTORY AND PHYSICAL EXAMINATION

The approach to patients with nausea and vomiting depends strongly on features of the history, including timing, duration, associated symptoms (abdominal pain, fever, weight loss, jaundice, headaches, vertigo), and complications (GI hemorrhage, dehydration, malnutrition). Drugs, toxins, and GI infections commonly cause acute nausea and vomiting, while established illnesses evoke chronic complaints. Pyloric obstruction and gastroparesis produce vomiting within 1 hour of eating, whereas emesis from intestinal obstruction occurs later. In severe cases of gastroparesis, the vomitus may contain food residue ingested hours or days previously. Psychogenic vomiting may occur soon after eating, but most patients control their emesis until gastric contents can be expelled discretely. Early morning nausea characterizes endocrine conditions, such as pregnancy. Meals may relieve nausea associated with peptic ulcer or esophagitis. Vomiting of undigested food is seen with Zenker's diverticulum and achalasia, whereas partial digestion is observed with gastric obstruction and gastroparesis. Bilious vomiting excludes proximal obstruction, whereas vomiting of blood suggests mucosal damage. Feculent emesis occurs with distal intestinal obstructions, bacterial overgrowth, and gastrocolic fistulae. Association of nausea with abdominal pain classically has been considered to reflect organic disease; however, a recent study has reported that 89% of patients with gastroparesis experience some degree of abdominal discomfort or pain.[13] Diarrhea, fever, or myalgias suggest possible infection. Headaches, visual changes, altered mentation, and neck stiffness raise the possibility of CNS etiologies, whereas tinnitus or vertigo indicate labyrinthine causes.

Physical findings in many patients with mild to moderate nausea and vomiting may be minimally abnormal. Demonstration of tachycardia, orthostatic hypotension, and reduced skin turgor indicate intravascular fluid loss from poor oral intake or relentless emesis. The general examination may detect evidence of an unsuspected systemic illness such as scleroderma, liver disease, or malignancy. Careful abdominal examination is critical in patients with unexplained nausea and vomiting. An absence of bowel sounds signifies ileus, whereas high-pitched hyperactive bowel sounds with a distended abdomen are consistent with intestinal obstruction. In some cases of gastroparesis or pyloric obstruction, a succussion splash upon abrupt lateral movement of the patient is found. Abdominal tenderness is noted with inflammation, infection, and luminal distention, whereas gross or occult fecal blood prompts evaluation for ulcer, inflammation, or malignancy.

DIAGNOSTIC TESTING

A thorough history and physical exam will provide sufficient information to diagnose and treat most patients with nausea and vomiting. If there is a clear association of the onset of vomiting with myalgias, cramps, and diarrhea or with initiating a new medication, no further work-up is needed. However, some patients require blood studies, structural evaluation, or assessment of gut function for appropriate management (Figure 14-2).

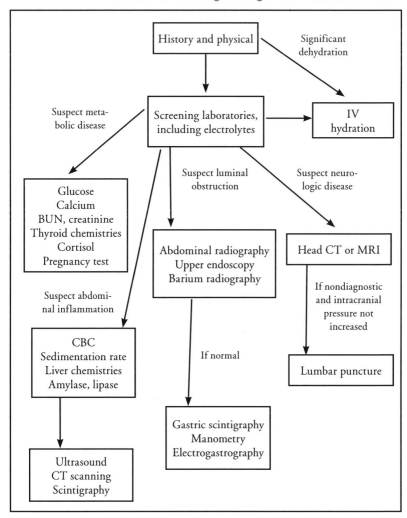

Figure 14-2. A proposed algorithm for the evaluation of the patient with unexplained chronic nausea and vomiting is shown. The decision to proceed with testing is dictated by findings of the history and physical examination and results from initial laboratory testing.

Laboratory Studies

Standard laboratory studies can detect electrolyte abnormalities, anemia, inflammation, metabolic or hormonal disorders, or hepatobiliary and pancreatic disease. With long-standing symptoms or dehydration, serum electrolytes may show hypokalemia or elevated blood urea nitrogen concentrations relative to the creatinine. Metabolic alkalosis may result from loss of hydrogen ions in the acidic vomitus and contraction of the extracellular space from dehydration. Women of childbearing potential should undergo pregnancy testing if nausea of pregnancy is a consideration. If metabolic disease is possible, thyroid chemistries, serum calcium, or fasting morning cortisol levels may be obtained. In unusual cases, rheumatologic serologies or antineuronal antibodies (including antinuclear neuronal antibody-1, anti-Purkinje cell antibody, and antibodies to calcium channels) may suggest collagen vascular disease or a paraneoplastic manifestation of occult malignancy, respectively.[14]

Structural Studies

Structural investigation may be needed to exclude organic illness as a cause of vomiting. Flat and upright abdominal radiographs are obtained as a screening examination. Small intestinal air-fluid levels with absent colonic air suggest obstruction, whereas diffuse distention is consistent with ileus. If a cause of symptoms is not clear from this initial evaluation, contrast radiography or endoscopy may be needed to exclude mechanical obstruction of the gut lumen or other structural disease outside of the GI tract. Suspected partial small intestinal obstruction may be evaluated with a dedicated small bowel follow through or with newer CT enterography techniques, especially if an inflammatory condition such as Crohn's disease is suspected.[15] If testing is negative and suspicion for obstruction remains high, enteroclysis may provide a more detailed assessment of small intestinal luminal processes.[16] For suspected pancreaticobiliary disease, ultrasound, CT, endoscopic ultrasound, hepatobiliary scintigraphy, or magnetic resonance cholangiopancreatography may be useful. CT and MRI scans of the head may be indicated for suspected CNS sources. Angiography or MRI can detect mesenteric ischemia.

Functional Testing

The roles of the different tests of GI motility in the management of dysmotility syndromes including gastroparesis and intestinal pseudo-obstruction have not been validated by controlled studies. Gastroparesis most commonly is diagnosed using gastric scintigraphy, by which emptying of a radiolabeled meal is measured. Recent investigations have attempted to standardize scintigraphic testing by proposing routine use of an egg-substitute meal with imaging performed 1, 2, and 4 hours postprandially.[17] Breath tests using the nonradioactive isotope ^{13}C incorporated within a solid meal have been promoted as office-based alternatives to scintigraphy.[18] The most extensively evaluated test has employed ^{13}C-octanoate in a muffin. With this test, $^{13}CO_2$ exhaled in the breath reflects the intestinal digestion of the triglyceride compound. If no pulmonary disease, maldigestion, or malabsorption is present, the rate of $^{13}CO_2$ liberation is strictly dependent on gastric emptying of the labeled substance into the duodenum. Because of methodological limitations, ultrasound and MRI techniques to quantify rates of gastric emptying have remained largely in the research arena. SPECT, a recently developed technology, has shown special promise in the evaluation of gastric dysmotility because of its ability to quantify postprandial accommodation and intragastric distribution after meal ingestion.[19] Regardless of the method employed, the usefulness of gastric emptying determination in directing patient management is unproved. In a retrospective analysis of 375 patients undergoing gastric scintigraphy, determination of the rate of gastric emptying did not influence therapies offered to patients with possible gastric dysmotility.[20]

Other tests of GI function are performed in selected academic centers. EGG measures gastric slow wave activity using cutaneous electrodes placed over the stomach and has been proposed to evaluate patients with unexplained nausea and vomiting to provide a possible pathophysiologic explanation for symptoms when therapy is ineffective or when gastric scintigraphy is nondiagnostic.[21] EGG has also been promoted as an alternate means of diagnosing gastroparesis, although the correlations between slow wave rhythm or amplitude disturbances and rates of gastric emptying are imperfect. However, acceptance of the technique has been hampered by the lack of available medications that serve as gastric "antiarrhythmics" to normalize slow wave activity.

Antroduodenal manometry provides information on phasic motor activity in the antrum and proximal small intestine during fasting and after a caloric meal. Although manometry can confirm antral hypomotility in patients with gastroparesis, its major indication is to document the presence of a small bowel motor disorder. Intestinal manometry can further characterize the motor abnormality as neuropathic or myopathic based on contractile patterns. Consequently, antroduodenal manometry is considered complementary to gastric scintigraphy as well as small intestinal barium radiography in the evaluation of patients with presumed upper gut dysmotility. Such investigation can obviate the need for surgical full-thickness intestinal biopsy to evaluate for smooth muscle or neuronal degeneration. Analyses of case series suggest that findings of antroduodenal manometry influence patient management decisions in approximately 25% of cases, primarily affecting the choice between enteral and parenteral feedings, including assisting the clinician in the determination to proceed with surgery to place a feeding tube versus chronic venous access.[22]

Treatment Options

GENERAL PRINCIPLES

The treatment of nausea and vomiting from any cause should be directed to the correction of medically or surgically remediable abnormalities if possible. Individuals with severe dehydration or electrolyte disturbances are managed as inpatients, especially if oral fluid replenishment cannot be sustained. The threshold for hospitalization is lower for diabetic patients, those with concurrent diarrhea or other chronic debilitating disease, and very young or old patients. Nasogastric suction may provide benefit in patients with obstruction or ileus. Once oral intake is tolerated, nutrients are restarted as liquids (which are low in fat) because lipids delay gastric emptying. Foods high in indigestible residues are avoided because these also prolong gastric retention. Any medications that delay gastric emptying, including opiates, calcium channel antagonists, and anticholinergics, are discontinued if possible. Diabetics are encouraged to strive for tight glycemic control because of the inhibitory actions of hyperglycemia on gastric emptying.[7] It should be noted, however, that no controlled investigations to date have been performed to support or refute this recommendation.

ANTIEMETIC MEDICATIONS

The most commonly prescribed antiemetic agents act within the CNS to reduce symptoms; however, these actions also are responsible for many of the side effects of these drugs (Table 14-3). Antihistamines such as meclizine and dimenhydrinate and anticholinergic drugs like scopolamine act on labyrinthine-activated pathways and are useful in motion sickness and inner ear disorders such as labyrinthitis and Meniere's disease. Dopamine receptor antagonists in the phenothiazine class treat emesis evoked by area postrema stimuli and are useful for medication, toxic, and metabolic etiologies. CNS side effects of these dopamine antagonists include anxiety, dystonic reactions, hyperprolactinemic effects (galactorrhea and sexual dysfunction), and irreversible tardive dyskinesia.

Other drug classes exhibit antiemetic properties. Serotonin 5-HT3 antagonists such as ondansetron, granisetron, and dolasetron are effective for treatment of vomiting occurring after abdominal irradiation and in the prevention of postoperative nausea and vomiting and cancer chemotherapy-induced emesis. This drug class also plays an important role in treating some cases of cyclic vomiting syndrome. The usefulness of 5-HT3 antagonists for other causes of emesis, including gastroparesis, is not well established.[23] Cannabinoids such as dronabinol, long advocated for cancer-associated emesis, produce significant side effects and exhibit efficacy no better than antidopaminergic agents in many studies.[24] Other drugs that provide antiemetic benefits in patients undergoing cancer chemotherapy include corticosteroids (for delayed emesis) and benzodiazepines (for anticipatory emesis). Low-dose tricyclic antidepressant agents have been reported in uncontrolled retrospective analyses to reduce symptoms in >80% of patients with functional nausea and vomiting.[25] Although traditionally considered to retard gastric emptying, tricyclic drugs also have been observed in preliminary studies to have antiemetic effects in patients with diabetic gastropathy, some with documented gastroparesis. Such agents also exhibit prophylactic effects in some patients with cyclic vomiting syndrome. Selected antimigraine therapies, including sumatriptan, have been reported to reduce symptoms in this disorder, supporting the association between migraine headaches and cyclic vomiting syndrome in some patients.[26]

The newest class of antiemetic drugs, the neurokinin NK1 receptor antagonists, show significant potential for the treatment of a broad range of disorders with nausea and vomiting. The natural ligand for neurokinin receptors, substance P, elicits emesis when injected into specific brainstem structures. In animal models, blockade of NK1 receptor activation prevents vomiting in response to varied stimuli, including chemotherapy, rotatory motion, and gastric irritants. Clinical studies of the NK1 receptor antagonist aprepitant confirm benefits for both acute and delayed nausea and vomiting from highly emetogenic cancer chemotherapy.[27,28] Further investigations will define the spectrum of action of this class of drugs.

PROKINETIC MEDICATIONS

A small number of medications have been shown to enhance GI motor activity and promote aboral movement of luminal contents (Table 14-4). These prokinetic drugs serve as the mainstay for management of gastroparesis. Metoclopramide, a combined 5-HT4 agonist and dopamine antagonist, exhibits efficacy in gastroparesis, but antidopaminergic side effects limit its use in up to 25% of patients. Erythromycin,

Table 14-3

INDICATIONS AND TOXICITY OF ANTIEMETIC MEDICATIONS

Drug Class	Medications	Clinical Uses	Potential Side Effects
Histamine antagonists	Dimenhydrinate Meclizine Promethazine	Motion sickness Labyrinthitis Postoperative vomiting	Sedation Dry mouth
Muscarinic antagonists	Scopolamine Hyoscine	Motion sickness	Sedation Dry mouth Impaired concentration
Dopamine antagonists	Prochlorperazine Thiethylperazine Trimethobenzamide	Extensive indications, including gastroenteritis, toxins, medications, postoperative nausea, postoperative vomiting, radiation-induced vomiting	Sedation Anxiety Mood disturbances Dystonic reactions Tardive dyskinesia Galactorrhea Sexual dysfunction
Serotonin antagonists	Ondansetron Granisetron Dolasetron	Chemotherapy-induced vomiting Radiation-induced vomiting Postoperative vomiting Vomiting in AIDS	Constipation Headache

(continued)

Table 14-3

INDICATIONS AND TOXICITY OF ANTIEMETIC MEDICATIONS (CONTINUED)

Drug Class	Medications	Clinical Uses	Potential Side Effects
Neurokinin antagonists	Aprepitant	Chemotherapy-induced nausea and vomiting	Sedation Fatigue
Tricyclic antidepressants	Amitriptyline Nortriptyline Desipramine	Functional vomiting Diabetic gastropathy	Sedation Constipation Urinary retention
Cannabinoids	Dronabinol	Chemotherapy-induced vomiting	Tachycardia Dizziness Euphoria Paranoia Depression Impaired cognition
Corticosteroids	Dexamethasone Methylprednisolone	Delayed chemotherapy-induced vomiting, postoperative vomiting	Agitation Depression Insomnia Hypertension Hyperglycemia
Benzodiazepines	Lorazepam	Anticipatory nausea and vomiting	Sedation Amnesia

Table 14-4

PROKINETIC MEDICATIONS FOR DYSMOTILITY SYNDROMES

Medication	Mechanism of Action	Potential Side Effects
Metoclopramide	5-HT4 agonist, dopamine antagonist, 5-HT3 antagonist (weak)	Sedation, anxiety, mood disturbance, sleep disruption, dystonic reaction, tardive dyskinesia, galactorrhea, sexual dysfunction
Erythromycin	Motilin receptor agonist	Abdominal pain, nausea and vomiting, diarrhea
Domperidone	Peripheral dopamine antagonist	Galactorrhea, gynecomastia, sexual dysfunction
Tegaserod	5-HT4 agonist	Diarrhea, headache
Bethanechol	Muscarinic agonist	Abdominal pain, salivation, nausea, diaphoresis
Octreotide	Somatostatin analog	Diarrhea, altered glycemic control, gallstones, thyroid disease

a macrolide antibiotic, increases coordinated gastroduodenal motility by action on receptors for motilin, an endogenous stimulant of fasting motor complexes. Both medications are available in IV form for delivery to inpatients with refractory symptoms. Each drug also can be given as an oral liquid to facilitate its delivery and subsequent absorption in the small intestine, and metoclopramide may be injected subcutaneously in patients who cannot tolerate oral therapy.[29] Newer investigational macrolide derivatives without antimicrobial activity are in advanced testing and show promise for treatment of gastroparesis.[30] Domperidone, a dopamine antagonist not approved for prescription in the United States, exhibits prokinetic and antiemetic effects but does not cross into most other brain regions, thus anxiety and dystonic reactions are rare. The main side effects of domperidone relate to induction of hyperprolactinemia via effects on pituitary regions served by a porous blood-brain barrier. Cisapride, a 5-HT4 agonist that stimulates enteric cholinergic nerves, was withdrawn from the US market because it predisposed patients to potentially fatal cardiac arrhythmias. The newer 5-HT4 agonist, tegaserod, at high doses is a potent stimulant of gastric emptying in patients with gastroparesis; however, its clinical utility in reducing symptoms in affected patients is unproved.[31] The muscarinic receptor agonist, bethanechol, is infrequently used. This drug potently stimulates nonpropagating contractions that have little prokinetic effect. Furthermore, significant side effects limit its tolerance. These prokinetic drugs may be tried for patients with intestinal pseudo-obstruction, although their effectiveness in this condition may be limited. Some cases of intestinal pseudo-obstruction may respond to the somatostatin analog octreotide, which selectively induces propagative small intestinal motor complexes.[32]

Botulinum toxin is an inhibitor of neuromuscular transmission that has demonstrated efficacy in a number of spastic somatic muscular conditions as well as GI disorders with increased visceral motor activity, including achalasia and chronic anal fissure. Because some patients with gastroparesis exhibit increased tone and phasic contractions in the pylorus, investigators have considered therapies to reduce pressure at the gastric outlet to facilitate gastric emptying. In an unpublished study, one group reported symptom reductions in diabetics with gastroparesis with performance of surgical pyloromyotomy.[33] More recently, several small case series have reported that pyloric injection of 80 to 200 units of botulinum toxin reduces nausea and vomiting in patients with diabetic or idiopathic gastroparesis.[34,35] Correlative functional studies observe acceleration of gastric emptying and reductions in spastic pyloric motor activity with pyloric botulinum toxin injection.

SURGICAL THERAPY

Surgery is the therapy of choice for a number of organic conditions that produce nausea and vomiting. Lysis of adhesions is commonly performed for small intestinal obstructions not responsive to conservative care, including fasting and nasogastric suction. Some inflammatory conditions (eg, cholecystitis) are best managed by operative intervention.

In carefully selected cases, patients with refractory dysmotility syndromes may respond to surgical treatment. Placement of a feeding jejunostomy reduces hospitalizations and improves overall health in some gastroparesis patients who do not respond to drug therapy, while addition of a gastrostomy may be used to vent the stomach thereby relieving symptoms secondary to overdistention.[36] Patients with postvagotomy gastroparesis may improve with near total resection of the stomach.[37] Although small series have suggested benefits from subtotal gastrectomy for other etiologies of gastroparesis, this approach is not universally accepted due to significant postoperative morbidity. Pancreatic transplantation does not clearly improve symptoms in patients with severe diabetic gastroparesis. In patients with intestinal pseudo-obstruction in whom enteral feedings exacerbate symptoms, placement of a permanent central venous access may be needed for home TPN. Decompressive stomata also may reduce symptoms when prokinetic drugs are ineffective for intestinal pseudo-obstruction.

A goal of researchers for many years has been to devise an electrical device to stimulate defective gastric motor activity in patients with gastroparesis. An initial human study of gastric pacing involved delivery of high energy, electrical stimulation at a rate slightly higher than the normal slow wave frequency through surgically implanted electrodes in open label fashion to nine patients with prokinetic medication-resistant gastroparesis (5 diabetic, 3 idiopathic, 1 postvagotomy).[38] When delivered just before and after meals, the pacing stimuli entrained the slow wave in all individuals, stimulated gastric emptying, and improved gastroparetic symptoms to the point that 8 patients no longer required jejunal tube feedings. Although benefits were suggested by this uncontrolled study, this method has not yet proven to be practical in clinical practice because it relies on external current sources that are unwieldy and are too large for implantation. Early series using an implantable neurostimulator with a compact battery that delivered brief, low energy impulses to the stomach at a frequency 4 times that of the intrinsic slow wave (12 cpm) reported impressive improvements in nausea and vomiting in patients with medication refractory gastroparesis. Because of these apparent benefits, the US FDA approved the gastric neurostimulator as a humanitarian use device and granted it a humanitarian device exemption for treatment of patients with refractory diabetic or idiopathic gastroparesis. Recently, investigations have been published that support the utility of the gastric neurostimulator in such individuals. In several uncontrolled trials, gastric neurostimulation produces marked reductions in nausea and vomiting, increases in weight, and improvements in serum markers of nutrition that persist for up to 10 years.[39-41] To date, only one controlled trial of gastric neurostimulation has been published. In this investigation, 33 patients with refractory gastroparesis (16 idiopathic, 17 diabetic) completed an initial 2-month double-blind, crossover, sham stimulation-controlled trial of neurostimulation followed by a long-term uncontrolled period of observation with the device activated.[42] During the blinded phase, vomiting frequencies were 14% lower when the device was on compared to times when the device was deactivated (P<0.05). In the open trial, nausea and vomiting showed impressive improvements for at least 1 year after surgery. The mechanism of action of gastric electrical neurostimulation at 12 cpm is uncertain, but probably does not relate to stimulation of motor activity because little acceleration of solid phase emptying has been observed in clinical testing. In animal models, gastric neurostimulation increases vagal activity, indicating activation of long-reflex arcs, and elicits significant reductions in proximal gastric tone.[43,44] Furthermore in humans with gastroparesis, electrical neurostimulation enhances the tolerance of noxious fundic balloon inflation, indicating a possible action on visceral afferent transmission.[45]

OTHER TREATMENTS

Nontraditional therapies are often used by patients with nausea or gastroparesis. Ginger and pyridoxine may produce benefits in motion sickness and nausea of pregnancy. Acupressure and acustimulation have also been promoted for nausea of pregnancy, motion sickness, and post-operative nausea and vomiting. Biofeedback techniques are being assessed in patients with gastroparesis, with promising initial results.[46]

Grant support: This work was supported in part by grant 1 K24 DK02726-01 from the National Institutes of Health.

References

1. Bityutskiy LP, Soykan I, McCallum RW. Viral gastroparesis: a subgroup of idiopathic gastroparesis—clinical characteristics and long-term outcomes. *Am J Gastroenterol.* 1997;92:1501-1504.

2. Mearin F, Camilleri M, Malagelada JR. Pyloric dysfunction in diabetics with recurrent nausea and vomiting. *Gastroenterology.* 1986;90:1919-1925.

3. Sarnelli G, Caenepeel P, Geypens B, et al. Symptoms associated with impaired gastric emptying of solids and liquids in functional dyspepsia. *Am J Gastroenterol.* 2003;98:783-788.

4. Horowitz M, Maddox AF, Wishart JM, et al. Relationships between oesophageal transit and solid and liquid gastric emptying in diabetes mellitus. *Eur J Nucl Med.* 1991;18:229-234.

5. Parkman HP, Miller MA, Trate D, et al. Electrogastrography and gastric emptying scintigraphy are complementary for assessment of dyspepsia. *J Clin Gastroenterol.* 1997;24:214-219.

6. Samsom M, Salet GA, Roelofs JM, et al. Compliance of the proximal stomach and dyspeptic symptoms in patients with type I diabetes mellitus. *Dig Dis Sci.* 1995;40:2037-2042.

7. Fraser RJ, Horowitz M, Maddox AF, et al. Hyperglycemia slows gastric emptying in type 1 (insulin-dependent) diabetes mellitus. *Diabetologia.* 1990;33:675-680.

8. Wilmer A, Van Cutsem E, Andrioli A, et al. Ambulatory gastrojejunal manometry in severe motility-like dyspepsia: lack of correlation between dysmotility, symptoms, and gastric emptying. *Gut.* 1998;42:235-242.

9. Su YC, Wong AC. Identification and purification of a new staphylococcal enterotoxin, H. *Appl Environ Microbiol.* 1995;61:1438-1443.

10. Scarantino CW, Ornitz RD, Hoffman LG, Anderson RF. On the mechanism of radiation-induced emesis: the role of serotonin. *J Radiat Oncol Biol Phys.* 1994;30:825-830.

11. Larsson S, Lundberg D. A prospective survey of postoperative nausea and vomiting with special regard to incidence and relations to patient characteristics, anesthetic routines and surgical procedures. *Acta Anaesthesiol Scand.* 1995;39:539-545.

12. Li BU, Murray RD, Heitlinger LA, et al. Is cyclic vomiting syndrome related to migraine? *J Pediatr.* 1999;134:567-572.

13. Hoogerwerf WA, Pasricha PJ, Kalloo AN, et al. Pain: the overlooked symptom in gastroparesis. *Am J Gastroenterol.* 1999;94:1029-1033.

14. Lee HR, Lennon VA, Camilleri M, et al. Paraneoplastic GI motor dysfunction: clinical and laboratory characteristics. *Am J Gastroenterol.* 2001;96:373-379.

15. Raptopoulos V, Schwartz RK, McNicholas MM, et al. Multiplanar helical CT enterography in patients with Crohn's disease. *AJR.* 1997;169:1545-1550.

16. Maglinte DD, Peterson LA, Vahey TN, et al. Enteroclysis in partial small bowel obstruction. *Am J Surg.* 1984;147:325-329.

17. Tougas GH, Eaker EY, Abell TL, et al. Assessment of gastric emptying using a low fat meal: establishment of international control values. *Am J Gastroenterol.* 2000;95:1456-1462.

18. Choi MG, Camilleri M, Burton DD, et al. 13C-octanoic acid breath test for gastric emptying of solids: accuracy, reproducibility, and comparison with scintigraphy. *Gastroenterology.* 1997;112:1155-1162.

19. Kuiken SD, Samsom M, Camilleri M, et al. Development of a test to measure gastric accommodation in humans. *Am J Physiol.* 1999;277:G1217-G1221.

20. Galil MA, Critchley M, Mackie CR. Isotope gastric emptying tests in clinical practice: expectation, outcome, and utility. *Gut.* 1993;34:916-919.

21. Parkman HP, Hasler WL, Barnett JL, et al. Electrogastrography: a document prepared by the gastric section of the American Motility Society Clinical GI Motility Testing Task Force. *Neurogastroenterol Motil.* 2003;15:488-497.

22. Soffer E, Thongsawat S. Clinical value of duodenojejunal manometry. Its usefulness in diagnosis and management of patients with GI symptoms. *Dig Dis Sci.* 1996;41:859-863.

23. Abell TL, Werkman R, Voeller G, et al. Long-term therapy with ondansetron is effective in patients with refractory nausea and vomiting (abstract). *Gastroenterology.* 1995;108:A1.

24. Frytak S, Moertel CG, O'Fallon JR, et al. Delta-9-tetrahydrocannabinol as an antiemetic for patients receiving cancer chemotherapy. A comparison with prochlorperazine and a placebo. *Ann Intern Med.* 1979;91:825-830.

25. Prakash C, Lustman CJ, Freedland KE, et al. Tricyclic antidepressants for functional nausea and vomiting: clinical outcome in 37 patients. *Dig Dis Sci.* 1998;43:1951-1956.

26. Benson JM, Zorn SL, Book LS. Sumatriptan in the treatment of cyclic vomiting. *Ann Pharmacother.* 1995;29:997-999.

27. Navari RM, Reinhardt RR, Gralla RJ, et al. Reduction of cisplatin-induced emesis by a selective neurokinin-1-receptor antagonist. L-754,030 Antiemetic Trials Group. *N Engl J Med.* 1999;340:190-195.

28. Sorbera LA, Castaner J, Bayes M, et al. Aprepitant and L-758298—antiemetic—antidepressant—tachykinin NK1 antagonist. *Drugs Future.* 2002;27:211-222.

29. McCallum RW, Valenzuela G, Polepalle S, et al. Subcutaneous metoclopramide in the treatment of symptomatic gastroparesis: clinical efficacy and pharmacokinetics. *J Pharmacol Exp Ther.* 1991;258:136-142.

30. Fang J, McCallum R, DiBase J, et al. Effect of mitemcinal fumarate (GM-611) on gastric emptying in patients with idiopathic or diabetic gastroparesis (abstract). *Gastroenterology.* 2004;126:T1387.

31. Tougas G, Chen Y, Luo D, et al. Tegaserod improves gastric emptying in patients with gastroparesis and dyspeptic symptoms (abstract). *Gastroenterology.* 2003;124:A54.

32. Soudah HC, Hasler WL, Owyang C. Effect of octreotide on intestinal motility and bacterial overgrowth in scleroderma. *N Engl J Med.* 1991;325:1461-1467.

33. Abouezzi ZE, Melvin WS, Ellison EC, et al. Functional and symptomatic improvement in patients with diabetic gastroparesis following pyloroplasty (abstract). *Gastroenterology.* 1998;114:A1374.

34. Miller LS, Szych GA, Kantor SB, et al. Treatment of idiopathic gastroparesis with injection of botulinum toxin into the pyloric sphincter muscle. *Am J Gastroenterol.* 2002;97:1653-1660.

35. Lacy BE, Zayat EN, Crowell MD, Schuster MM. Botulinum toxin for the treatment of gastroparesis: a preliminary report. *Am J Gastroenterol.* 2002;97:1548-1552.

36. Fontana RJ, Barnett JL. Jejunostomy tube placement in refractory diabetic gastroparesis: a retrospective review. *Am J Gastroenterol.* 1996;91:2174-2178.

37. Eckhauser RE, Conrad M, Knol JA, et al. Safety and long-term durability of completion gastrectomy in 81 patients with postsurgical gastroparesis syndrome. *Am Surg.* 1998;64:711-717.

38. McCallum RW, Chen JD, Lin Z, et al. Gastric pacing improves emptying and symptoms in patients with gastroparesis. *Gastroenterology.* 1998;114:456-461.

39. Abell TL, Van Cutsem E, Abrahamsson H, et al. Gastric electrical stimulation in intractable symptomatic gastroparesis. *Digestion.* 2002;66:204-212.

40. Forster J, Sarosiek I, Lin Z, et al. Further experience with gastric stimulation to treat drug refractory gastroparesis. *Am J Surg.* 2003;186:690-695.

41. Abell T, Lou J, Tabbaa M, et al. Gastric electrical stimulation for gastroparesis improves nutritional parameters at short, intermediate, and long-term follow-up. *JPEN.* 2003;27:277-281.

42. Abell T, McCallum R, Hocking M, et al. Gastric electrical stimulation for medically refractory gastroparesis. *Gastroenterology.* 2003;125:421-428.

43. Liu J, Qiao X, Chen JD. Vagal afferent is involved in short-pulse gastric electrical stimulation in rats. *Dig Dis Sci.* 2004;49:729-737.

44. Xing JH, Brody F, Brodsky J, et al. Gastric electrical stimulation at proximal stomach induces gastric relaxation in dogs. *Neurogastroenterol Motil.* 2003;15:15-23.

45. Tack, J, Coulie, B, Van Cutsem E, et al. The influence of gastric electrical stimulation on proximal gastric motor and sensory function in severe idiopathic gastroparesis (abstract). *Gastroenterology.* 1999;116:G4733.

46. Rashed H, Cutts T, Abell T, et al. Predictors of response to a behavioral treatment in patients with chronic gastric motility disorders. *Dig Dis Sci.* 2002;47:1020-1026.

Small Intestinal Dysmotility

Ann Ouyang, MB, BS and Ian Roy Schreibman, MD

Introduction

One of the small intestine's major functions is to propel chyme in a coordinated fashion into the large intestine. Proper peristalsis is required to insure adequate mixing of chyme with digestive enzymes, absorption of nutrients, and "clearance" of the small intestine of undigested material. Proper motility requires an intricate coordination of multiple factors, including hormonal release, activation of both enteric and extrinsic neurons, and subsequent contraction of intestinal smooth muscle. A defect in any one of these components can result in dysmotility.[1]

Dysmotility can be present in a completely asymptomatic individual or result in a severely ill patient with a physical exam consistent with a complete small bowel obstruction with tympanitic distention, absent bowel sounds, and exquisite pain. However, the typical presentation of a patient with a small bowel motility disorder is one of chronic abdominal pain, distention, and constipation or diarrhea secondary to bacterial overgrowth and malabsorption.[1]

Although the number of disorders that can affect small bowel motility is quite large, there are a limited number of diagnostic tools and therapeutic options available for the clinician. Our understanding of the exact pathophysiology of these diseases is only just beginning. Hopefully, in the future, more knowledge and therapies will be gained. This chapter will review the current diagnostic tools used for evaluating small intestinal motility, and the clinical presentation and available treatment of motility disorders affecting the small bowel.

Diagnostic Tools

The first indication that a patient may have a motility disorder is gained from the history and physical. Typical symptoms include abdominal pain, bloating, excess flatus, diarrhea, weight loss, nausea, and vomiting. A key point is that these patients may present exactly the same way as a small bowel obstruction. This life-threatening condition must be ruled out before a small bowel motility disorder is considered.[1]

Figure 15-1. UGI series of a patient with idiopathic chronic small intestinal pseudo-obstruction. Note the massive dilation of the duodenum.

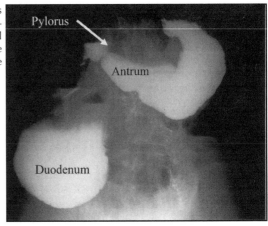

RADIOGRAPHIC STUDIES

Plain radiographic films are often the first indication that a motility disorder is present. They can document any diffuse or localized intestinal dilation with or without air fluid levels. Barium studies (small bowel follow through/enteroclysis) can definitively rule out an obstruction if suspected and also confirm dilation (megaduodenum, megajejunum) or diverticula (Figure 15-1).[2]

The major limitation to radiographic studies is that they are usually nonspecific. Although many of the small bowel motility disorders can have the same appearance, there are several specific findings that can alert the clinician to a specific diagnosis. For example, scleroderma may show a dilated esophagus and dilated jejunal loops that have narrow valvulae conniventes, giving an "accordion" and "hide-bound" appearance,[3,4] and jejunal diverticulosis is easily identifiable and specific. The major benefit of a small bowel contrast study is to definitively rule out a mechanical obstruction, IBD, or some other treatable mucosal abnormality that would change the management of the patient.[2]

LABORATORY STUDIES

As will be discussed below, a number of systemic diseases and metabolic disorders can result in small bowel dysmotility. After a mechanical obstruction has been ruled out and a motility disorder is suspected, the next step in management should be routine laboratory studies to evaluate for malabsorption or malnutrition: CBC, folate, B12, iron profile, albumin, and cholesterol. Electrolytes should also be checked for disturbances because hypocalcemia, hypophosphatemia, and hypokalemia may result in dysmotility. If a systemic disease (such as diabetes, hypothyroidism, or scleroderma) is suspected, the appropriate screening test should be ordered.[1]

MOTILITY STUDIES

If a true obstruction or mucosal abnormality has been excluded and a small bowel motility disorder is suspected, the next diagnostic step is to assess intestinal motor activity. There are 3 parameters that may be measured to assess motor activity:

1. Small bowel transit time.
2. Contractile activity (by manometry).
3. Electromyographic (EMG) activity.

Measuring Small Bowel Transit Time

Three techniques have been described for the assessment of small intestinal transit. The hydrogen breath test is a simple study in which a nonabsorbable, nondigestible carbohydrate, such as lactulose, is ingested by the patient. The principle behind this study is that colonic flora will metabolize the carbohydrate to form hydrogen, which then diffuses into the mucosal blood vessels and is exhaled in the breath, increasing the hydrogen concentration above the values typically observed. Two peaks of hydrogen concentration are seen in this study. The first peak occurs within the first hour of the test and is secondary to fermentation of the ingested carbohydrate by bacteria localized to the oral cavity. The onset of the second peak corresponds to the arrival of the head of the meal in the cecum. Thus, the time from ingestion of the meal to the second peak of breath hydrogen concentration is the orocecal transit time.[5] While noninvasive and readily available, the hydrogen breath test can give several false results.[6] Lactulose itself may decrease small bowel transit time by promoting motility because it is an osmotic laxative. In the setting of small bowel bacterial overgrowth, the increased numbers of bacteria in the proximal small intestine will rapidly metabolize the carbohydrate and increase the hydrogen breath concentration prematurely, resulting in a falsely reduced transit time. As almost all patients with dysmotility have bacterial overgrowth, this is a significant issue.[7,8]

Some investigators feel that the "most cost-effective, reliable and readily available test of gastric emptying and small intestinal transit is scintigraphy."[2] Scintigraphy is a non-invasive test in which a radiolabeled meal is ingested followed by imaging at regular intervals and measuring radioactivity over specific regions of interest. Small bowel transit is calculated indirectly as the difference between the onset of colonic filling and the gastric emptying time.[9,10] While scintigraphic techniques are based on the same principles as those described for the measurement of gastric emptying, accurate definitions of small intestinal transit are more difficult; defining a region of interest (ROI) is less straightforward, and overlap of bowel loops may cause considerable confusion.

Another method available to measure transit time uses sulfasalazine. A 2-g dose of sulfasalazine is administered orally. This drug passes unchanged into the cecum where colonic bacteria cleave the sulfasalazine into sulfapyridine and the 5-aminosalicylate moieties. Serum levels of sulfapyridine can then be checked at regular intervals in the same way that hydrogen concentration is checked in the breath as an indirect measure of orocecal transit time. Again, small bowel bacterial overgrowth can alter these measurements.[11]

All 3 methods are excellent in documenting delayed or accelerated small bowel transit; however, all 3 are also nonspecific. They cannot distinguish a neuropathic process from a myopathic process. To make this distinction, the actual contractile activity of the small intestine must be measured.

Measuring Contractile Activity (Manometry)

When measuring small bowel motility contractions, there are 2 catheters available for use: perfused catheters with external transducers and solid-state probes with transducers mounted on the catheter. Each has advantages and limitations when compared to the other. The perfused catheters are less expensive and more easily designed to allow a greater number of recording sites than the solid-state catheter. However, they require a system to perfuse water through the catheter along with external transducers, which results in cumbersome, stationary equipment, necessitating that the study be non-ambulatory. In practice, these probes are most useful to characterize the motor patterns of short duration such as the fed state pattern that immediately follows a meal.[12-14]

The solid-state probe is more expensive than the perfused catheter and is of wider caliber. The diameter of the probe is related to the number of sensors, which limits their number. Trying to measure a specific area of the intestinal system is more difficult with the solid-state probe because the limited number of sensors increases the likelihood of sensor displacement from the site of interest. However, solid-state probes can provide the benefit of a prolonged ambulatory study and are thus better suited to observe the longer fasting patterns of motility (the migrating motor complex cycles).[12-14]

Both probes share the common limitation of only detecting lumen-occluding contractions. Nonlumen-occluding contractions will not be recorded. Furthermore, it may be difficult to advance either probe into the duodenum in the setting of gastroparesis, which is common in many conditions leading to small intestinal dysmotility. The impaired gastric contractions may prevent advancement of the probe into the duodenum.[12-14]

A brief review of the normal manometric patterns is needed before considering deviations that may be seen in pathologic states. The fasting or interdigestive period is characterized by a classic pattern known as the MMC. The MMC is comprised of 3 phases that cycle every 90 to 120 minutes (Figure 15-2). In phase I (approximately 34 to 40 minutes), there is motor quiescence that progresses through phase II, a period of increasing, irregular contractions lasting 45-55 minutes. The cycle culminates in phase III, the most distinctive pattern, in which there are uninterrupted rhythmic phasic contractions lasting about 5 minutes that migrate slowly along the intestine in an oral to aboral direction. The frequency of contractions during phase III reflects the myoelectric slow wave frequency. The slow wave frequency is distinctive for the specific site in the alimentary canal (3 cycles per minute in the antrum and 11 to 12 cycles per minute in the duodenum).[15-17]

When the small intestinal fasting motor pattern is recorded, there are several features that are examined. Each phase and cycle duration is recorded and the amplitude, velocity, and frequency of contractions in phase III are measured (the most regular and rhythmic phase). Abnormal bursts of activity, retrograde propulsion of phase III, and low amplitude contractions are all possible findings suggesting a motility disorder.[14]

In the postprandial state, the MMC is abolished and the fed motor complex is seen; this represents random, intense motor activity. Contractions of variable amplitude are seen as shown in Figure 15-3. These begin shortly after eating and continue for a variable length of time dependent upon the caloric content of the ingested meal. The apparently random intense nature of these contractions serves a physiologic basis to mix and propel the intestinal contents following a meal. Failure to induce the fed motor complex, rapid return to the fasting MMC, and low amplitude contractions may all be seen in motility disorders.[13]

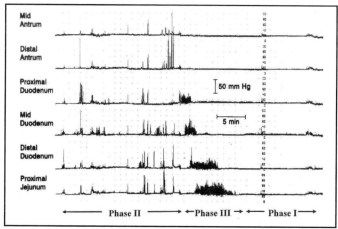

Figure 15-2. A typical MMC in a normal subject. The end of phase II leading into the propagated phase III is seen followed by the quiescent phase I (seen in the most proximal lead). The intense contractile activity propagating down the duodenum and jejunum characterizes phase III.

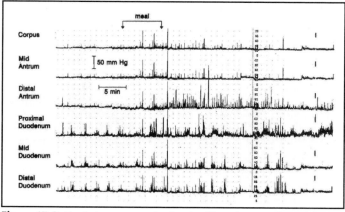

Figure 15-3. The fed motor complex in a healthy volunteer subject following ingestion of a meal. Note that random, intense motor activity is seen.

Despite the "classical" manometric patterns, interpretations of antroduodenal and small intestinal motility recordings remain limited in nature. For one, manometry is not readily available and is usually confined to tertiary care centers. Secondly, there are multiple recording catheters and devices available. Variability from device to device may be seen and standardization has not yet been done. Secondly, a broad consensus has not yet been reached to define true normal and abnormal patterns. Indeed, there are a diverse variety of patterns seen in healthy, control subjects and within an individual patient. The fed pattern in particular has been very difficult to define. The main use of manometry at present is to support the suspected diagnosis by documenting an abnormal pattern in the fasting MMC; it is not a gold standard.[17]

Electromyographic Activity

EMG recordings from the small intestine have been performed from either surgically placed serosal electrodes or from electrodes mounted on an intraluminal catheter. Neither has gained a place in clinical practice, and this approach remains confined to clinical research studies.[1]

Small Bowel Dysmotility Disorders

Small bowel motility disorders encompass a vast array of diseases that may represent a primary disturbance of the intestinal tract or a manifestation of a more diffuse systemic disease. These disorders mimic a true obstruction with symptoms of abdominal pain, nausea, vomiting, constipation, or diarrhea. The motility disorder leads to dilation of the small intestinal lumen with subsequent bacterial overgrowth further contributing to patients' symptoms. Bacterial overgrowth results in steatorrhea, malabsorption, malnutrition, and Vitamin B_{12} deficiencies.[1]

A patient may present with a broad spectrum of symptoms. Some individuals are completely asymptomatic whereas others present with a tense distended abdomen, high-pitched bowel sounds, and exquisite abdominal pain. Motility symptoms may have a chronic, insidious onset or may present acutely within a matter of hours. This distinction is critical because the 2 different presentations suggest different pathologies and have general implications for treatment.[1]

ACUTE PSEUDO-OBSTRUCTION

Acute intestinal pseudo-obstruction or ileus refers to the development of acute intestinal dilation primarily involving the colon but also involving the small intestine as well. When the syndrome only involves the colon, it is termed Ogilvie's syndrome; this distinction is critical in terms of management. The symptoms mimic obstruction with patients complaining of colicky lower abdominal pain and constipation. Signs include a distended, tympanitic abdomen with decreased or absent bowel sounds. X-rays will document massive dilation of the colon and small intestine with air fluid levels often seen.[18]

Acute pseudo-obstruction is most commonly seen following abdominal and other surgical procedures; however, it may also occur in severe medical disorders such as pneumonia, pancreatitis, cholecystitis, myocardial infarction, and neurological conditions such as multiple sclerosis. Other risk factors include ventilated patients, heavy narcotic or sedative use, and metabolic/electrolyte abnormalities. Ileus may also occur without an identifiable cause.[18]

The treatment of acute small bowel pseudo-obstruction requires aggressive supportive care with correction of any metabolic abnormalities and IV resuscitation (Table 15-1). Serum calcium, phosphorous, and potassium levels should all be optimized. The stomach should be decompressed with a NG tube. All anticholinergic agents, narcotics, and sedatives should be discontinued or limited as much as possible. In extreme cases, surgical enterotomy may be required. If an underlying condition is identified, reversal of the condition is associated with a return to normal intestinal functioning.[18]

Table 15-1

MANAGEMENT OF ACUTE PSEUDO-OBSTRUCTION

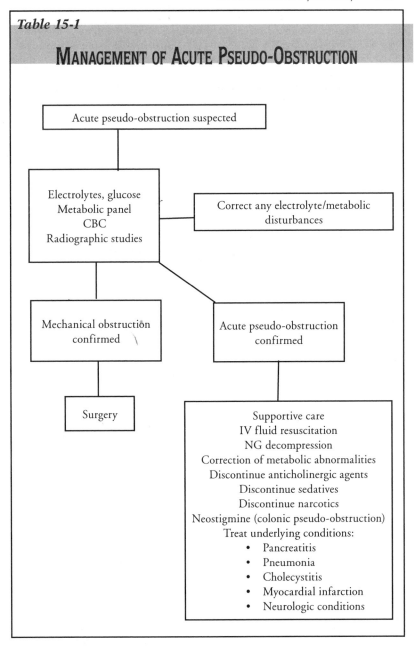

Acute pseudo-obstruction suspected

Electrolytes, glucose
Metabolic panel
CBC
Radiographic studies

Correct any electrolyte/metabolic
disturbances

Mechanical obstruction
confirmed

Acute pseudo-obstruction
confirmed

Surgery

Supportive care
IV fluid resuscitation
NG decompression
Correction of metabolic abnormalities
Discontinue anticholinergic agents
Discontinue sedatives
Discontinue narcotics
Neostigmine (colonic pseudo-obstruction)
Treat underlying conditions:
- Pancreatitis
- Pneumonia
- Cholecystitis
- Myocardial infarction
- Neurologic conditions

Neostigmine is an acetylcholinesterase inhibitor and has been shown to be effective in producing rapid colonic decompression within a short period time (3 to 30 minutes) with a long-standing response. Note that neostigmine is only indicated for those patients with colonic pseudo-obstruction and has no place in the management of small bowel pseudo-obstruction.[19] Another option available for patient's with Ogilvie's syndrome is colonoscopic decompression with placement of a decompression tube within the transverse colon; again, this has no place for small intestinal pseudo-obstruction.

CHRONIC PSEUDO-OBSTRUCTION

Primary or Idiopathic Causes of Chronic Pseudo-Obstruction

Primary or idiopathic intestinal pseudo-obstruction refers to a motility disorder in the absence of a systemic disease. These disorders typically have a chronic presentation. The disease can result from abnormalities of the autonomic innervation or enteric nerves (neuropathies) or of the intestinal muscle layers themselves (myopathies) and may also involve the urinary bladder (Table 15-2). The typical presentation is of recurrent abdominal pain, distention, and vomiting. Intestinal stasis results in bacterial overgrowth.[20-24]

The familial visceral myopathies comprise a number of inherited diseases characterized by degeneration, loss, and fibrosis of smooth muscle cells in the intestines. Familial visceral neuropathies are characterized by myenteric plexus degeneration and subsequent denervation. In contrast to the familial visceral myopathies, the muscle layers are preserved. Occasionally rare cases of myopathy and neuropathy are diagnosed that appear to have no genetic predisposition. Clinically, they are indistinguishable from the inherited disorders.[20-24]

Intestinal myopathies may result in a pronounced duodenal and intestinal hypomotility pattern seen on manometry. Figure 15-4 illustrates minimal, if any, contractile activity in a patient with chronic pseudo-obstruction. Intestinal myopathies may also have a manometry pattern with a normal propagation of phase III of the MMC but with marked suppression of the amplitude of phasic contractions. These disorders will also typically have a normal fed pattern on manometry with decreased pressures. In a visceral neuropathy, there is an abnormal or even absent MMC and loss of the fed pattern.[15,16]

The only definitive way to diagnose a visceral myopathy or neuropathy is to perform a surgical full thickness biopsy. Trichrome staining will reveal that patients with an intestinal myopathy will have complete replacement of the circular muscle layer by fibrosis. Biopsy specimens of the skeletal striated muscle can detect muscular dystrophy. Silver staining of whole mount preparations will assess the myenteric plexus.[18] Biopsies may also be stained for c-kit positive cells using immunohistochemistry. This technique assesses the number of ICCs, the pacemaker cells of the intestine; a decrease in this cell type may lead to neuropathies and has been described in patients with diabetes (see discussion below).[25]

The prognosis of idiopathic intestinal pseudo-obstruction is quite poor in part due to the progressive nature of the disease and the lack of adequate treatment options. Fortunately, all of the idiopathic dysmotilities are quire rare. Death from malnutrition, dehydration, and steatorrhea is common. The only intervention is low residue, low fat, liquid diets and parenteral nutrition if significant malnutrition develops. Promotility agents such as cholinergic agents and metoclopramide have not been useful. Surgery

Table 15-2

THE PRIMARY CAUSES OF INTESTINAL PSEUDO-OBSTRUCTION

Disease	Pattern of Inheritance	Clinical Features
Familial visceral myopathy type I	Autosomal dominant	Esophageal dilation
		Megacolon (surgically treatable)
		Redundant colon
		Megacystitis
		Mostly female
		Present after menarche
Familial visceral myopathy type II	Autosomal recessive	Presents in adolescence to middle age
		Gastroparesis
		Small intestinal dilation
		Neuropathy
		Deafness/ophthalmoplegia
Familial visceral myopathy type III	Autosomal recessive	Diffuse intestinal dilation
		Presents in middle age
		Requires TPN
Familial visceral neuropathy type I	Autosomal dominant	Dilation of distal small intestine/colon
		Requires TPN
Familial visceral neuropathy type II	Autosomal recessive	Hypertrophic pyloric stenosis
		Dilation/malrotation of small intestine
		CNS abnormalities
		Present in infancy

(continued)

Table 15-2

THE PRIMARY CAUSES OF INTESTINAL PSEUDO-OBSTRUCTION

Disease	*Pattern of Inheritance*	*Clinical Features*
Sporadic visceral myopathy	None identified	Esophageal dilation
		Megaduodenum
		Redundant colon
		Megacystitis
		Gastroparesis
		Small intestinal dilation
Sporadic visceral neuropathy	None identified	Diffuse intestinal dilation
		Chronic pseudo-obstruction

Adapted from Anuras S, Chokhavatia S. Dysmotility of the small intestine. In: Yamada T, Alpers DH, Owyang C, Powell DW, Silverstein FE, eds. *Textbook of Gastroenterology.* New York: J.B. Lippincott, Co: 1991.

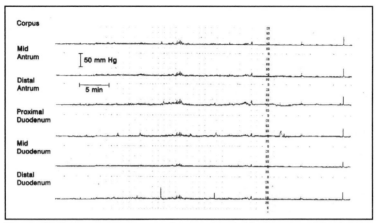

Figure 15-4. A manometry tracing from a patient with chronic pseudo-obstruction. There is minimal contractile activity and an absence of phase III of the MMC.

must be avoided because this condition may actually worsen following operations as a result of adhesion formation. In addition, extensive resections will compromise patients' ability to absorb and digest nutrients (ie, the short gut syndrome).[18]

Secondary Pseudo-Obstruction

As its name implies, secondary pseudo-obstruction results as a consequence of systemic disease. Dysmotility develops from either a myopathy, neuropathy, endocrinologic disorder, pharmacologic side effect, or some other identifiable process. Unlike primary pseudo-obstruction, patients with secondary pseudo-obstruction have a better prognosis. In addition to treating the pseudo-obstruction (which follows the same general principles as acute and primary pseudo-obstruction), it is critical to treat the underlying disease.[1]

Myopathic Causes of Secondary Pseudo-Obstruction

Scleroderma results in smooth muscle degeneration with collagen replacement resulting in fibrosis of the circular muscle layer. While classically described as an esophageal motility problem (>70% of patients), scleroderma results in small bowel symptoms in up to 40% of cases. Intestinal stasis results in bacterial overgrowth and malabsorption.[26] Small intestinal manometric studies typically show diminished contraction amplitude with an absence of phase III contractions.[27] While the myenteric plexus is preserved, some studies in symptomatic patients have also shown an altered, uncoordinated manometric pattern, indicating that a neuropathy is also present.[18]

Other connective tissue disorders (dermatomyositis, polymyositis, and systemic lupus erythematosus) can also result in smooth muscle dysfunction, leading to dilation and ileus of the small intestine. This results primarily from inflammation and subsequent atrophy.[28] Amyloidosis disrupts motility via the infiltration of the smooth muscle layers; however, it also causes malabsorption by infiltrating the mucosal layers of the intestines.[15] Muscular dystrophies cause smooth muscle degeneration, atrophy,

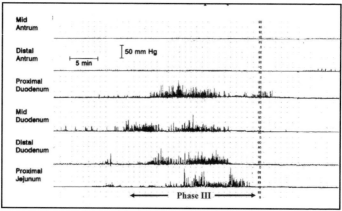

Figure 15-5. An abnormal manometry of a patient with a neuropathic motility disorder secondary to diabetes. Note that there is no clear propagation of phase III of the MMC; antegrade and retrograde propagation is seen. In addition, there is an absence of gastric contractions consistent with diabetic gastroparesis.

and fibrosis. It typically affects the esophagus and stomach; rarely small intestinal dysmotility will be seen. In some patients, the abdominal symptoms will even predate the skeletal symptoms. Manometric studies of all these disorders are similar to those seen in a primary visceral myopathy: low amplitude or absent contractions.[29,30]

Neuropathic Causes of Secondary Pseudo-Obstruction

Diabetes, in addition to causing gastroparesis, may cause small intestinal motility disturbances presumably through autonomic neuropathy as shown in Figure 15-5. There have been several other mechanisms proposed to explain the dysmotility in patients with diabetes. The ICCs are considered the "pacemaker cells" of the stomach and for intestinal motility as well. These cells express the c-kit receptor tyrosine kinase and are readily identifiable using immunohistochemistry. Nakahara et al showed that in healthy control subjects, c-kit positive cells were located at the myenteric plexus region and in the circular muscle layer of the colon.[25] Patients with diabetes only had about 40% of the c-kit positive cells compared to healthy controls. Thus, deficiency of ICC may lead to small bowel dysmotility.[25] Nitric oxide has been shown to be an inhibitory neurotransmitter in the gut and is a major factor in regulating motility. Watkins et al showed in mice models, using streptozotocin to induce diabetes, that the neuronal nitric oxide synthase (nNOS) gene and protein were markedly reduced, presumably leading to delayed gastric emptying.[31] Administration of sildenafil, a phosphodiesterase inhibitor, restored normal gastric emptying; furthermore insulin increased the levels of nNOS.[31] Our lab has also shown a decrease in nNOS expression in the antrum of streptozotocin- induced diabetic rats compared with controls. However, nNOS expression in the duodenum, ileum, and colon of the animal models was not statistically different from controls.[32] A more recent study argues that it is the increase in nNOS levels that leads to impaired gastric emptying in animal models of diabetes.[33] Clearly, this issue needs more investigation. The small intestinal manifestations are not as pronounced as the gastric and colonic manifestations of the disease. While biopsies of the myenteric and submucosal plexuses appear morphologically normal, the manometric pattern observed is consistent with a neuropathy and this remains the best explanation to date.

In addition to causing CNS degeneration, Parkinson's disease can also cause enteric nervous system degeneration, leading to dysmotility and small bowel distention. Other neurologic diseases (multiple sclerosis and stroke) are also associated with hypomotility and distention. Chagas' disease is classically thought to cause megaesophagus and megacolon. However, infection can also result in megaduodenum and megajejunum by destroying the myenteric plexus; megaureter is also seen. Other infections have been implicated in causing GI symptoms. Herpes zoster, cytomegalovirus, Epstein Barr, and the HIV virus have all been documented to cause chronic pseudo-obstruction.[18]

Various cancers (such as small cell lung cancer and epidermoid lip carcinoma) can infiltrate the myenteric and submucosal neurons resulting in chronic pseudo-obstruction. Another proposed mechanism for this paraneoplastic process is that the tumor somehow induces the production of antineuronal nuclear antibodies. The antibodies are thought to be directed against an epitope shared between the underlying malignancy and neuronal elements in the GI tract, leading to nerve damage.[34,35] In many cases, the pseudo-obstruction may predate the diagnosis of the cancer itself.[36]

Neuropathic processes result in failure of the MMC to propagate in the expected fashion. Various patterns can be seen, including slowing the rate of progression of the phase III of MMC and failure to convert to the fed state following a meal.[14]

Miscellaneous Causes of Secondary Pseudo-Obstruction

Hypoparathyroidism leads to impaired contractile activity as a result of hypocalcemia. Hypothyroidism prolongs intestinal transit, leading to intestinal stasis and constipation. It is important to identify these problems because their treatment will result in complete resolution of the intestinal symptoms.[1] Abdominal irradiation following treatments of lymphoma or other intra-abdominal malignancies can lead to impaired motility.

Multiple drugs (ie, narcotics, anticholinergics, antiparkinsonian medications, phenothiazines, clonidine, tricyclic antidepressants, and calcium channel blockers) can also alter intestinal motility. It is presumed that all of the aforementioned pharmacologic agents exert their effects through an anticholinergic mechanism.[37]

Although diverticulosis is most common in the large intestine, it has been known to affect the small intestine. The pathophysiology of small bowel diverticulosis differs from colonic diverticulosis. Colonic diverticula are felt to be herniations of tissue limited to the mucosa and muscularis mucosa only (these are acquired throughout life and form at the site of a penetrating artery). Small bowel diverticula are sac-like herniations that involve the entire bowel wall and are usually congenital. Small bowel follow through and CT scan will readily establish the presence of small intestinal diverticulosis.[38]

While diverticula may be seen throughout the small intestine, they are most common in the duodenum. These duodenal diverticula are rarely symptomatic and almost never associated with a motility disorder; however, they have been associated with small bowel bacterial overgrowth, biliary pigment stones, and cholangitis. Jejunal diverticula are also asymptomatic for the most part (>50% of cases) and diagnosed incidentally in the workup for other conditions. Multiple jejunal diverticula can result in a syndrome of intestinal stasis. As a result of this stasis, bacterial overgrowth can occur, leading to mucosal damage, malabsorption, vitamin B_{12} deficiencies, etc. Meckel's diverticulum is located in the distal small intestine approximately 60 cm from the ileocecal valve. It represents a persistent omphalomesenteric duct and may cause obstruction and hemorrhage if it intussuscepts into the adjacent ileal lumen. Meckel's diverticulum is diagnosed with a technetium scan that is taken up by the gastric tissue that lines the diverticulum. The treatment is surgical excision when symptomatic.[38]

TREATMENT OF CHRONIC PSEUDO-OBSTRUCTION

Just as in the management of acute pseudo-obstruction, several general principles should be followed (Table 15-3 and Table 15-4). Patients should be assessed for any metabolic derangements with appropriate correction and aggressive fluid resuscitation. Potential offending drugs should be discontinued or have dosages reduced. Finally, the underlying disorder should be optimally managed (ie, euthyroid state, excellent glucose control).[1]

Nutritional support is clearly the most important goal of therapy. Some patients may not require any additional support other than simply altering their diet (ie, removing carbonated beverages; smaller, more frequent meals; and low residual meals). If additional support is required, enteral nutrition is ideally preferred. In severe cases, patients may not be able to tolerate any oral intake. These patients require parenteral support and may need NG decompression. A venting G tube may also be required if symptoms are particularly refractory.[18]

There are a number of prokinetic agents available commercially that may be of limited use in patients with chronic pseudo-obstruction. In the past, cisapride was the mainstay therapy; however, the fatal cardiac arrhythmias associated with this drug led to its suspension. Erythromycin is available in both an oral and IV form. It is a partial motilin agonist and stimulates motility by acting upon this receptor. It has been shown to stimulate phase III of the MMC. The IV form of the drug would seem to make it particularly useful for acute exacerbations of pseudo-obstruction. While few studies have shown erythromycin to be of use in chronic therapy, it has only been tried in a small number of patients. As more studies are done, it may yet find a place in practice for small motility disorders. For now, it remains most useful in promoting gastric emptying and treating gastroparesis.[18,39] Metoclopramide is a dopamine agonist that also promotes motility of the stomach and gastric emptying. However, a metoclopramide may be useful in the treatment of pseudo-obstruction. Furthermore, metoclopramide's use is limited by the extrapyramidal side effects of the drug. Up to 10% of patients may develop tardive dyskinesia or a parkinsonian-type syndrome.[18]

Octreotide is typically used as an antisecretory agent and to reduce mesenteric vascular pressures. Several small studies have recently shown that it may also be of benefit in promoting motility.[40-42] The exact mechanism of action is unclear but Haruma et al have shown that subcutaneous octreotide induces a brisk induction of the phase III MMC.[40] It has been of particular use in patients with scleroderma. Soudah et al have shown that in addition to inducing migrating motor complexes, octreotide reduced symptoms of nausea, vomiting, bloating, and pain in patients with scleroderma and chronic intestinal pseudo-obstruction.[41] Verne et al also showed improvement in symptoms in patients with idiopathic intestinal pseudo-obstruction using octreotide in combination with erythromycin.[42]

Table 15-3

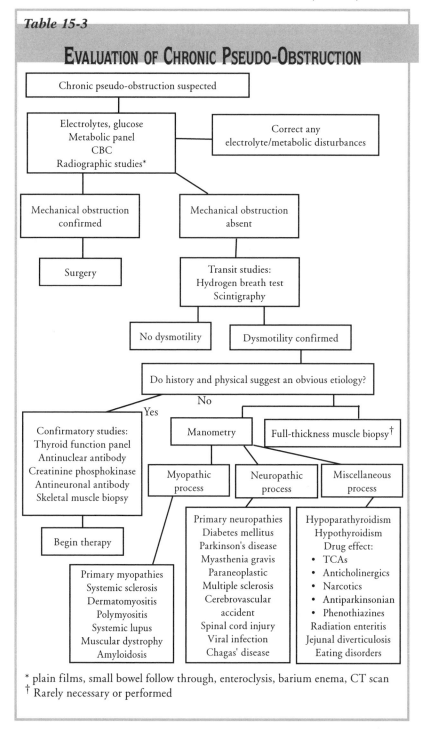

EVALUATION OF CHRONIC PSEUDO-OBSTRUCTION

Chronic pseudo-obstruction suspected

Electrolytes, glucose
Metabolic panel
CBC
Radiographic studies*

Correct any
electrolyte/metabolic disturbances

Mechanical obstruction
confirmed

Mechanical obstruction
absent

Surgery

Transit studies:
Hydrogen breath test
Scintigraphy

No dysmotility

Dysmotility confirmed

Do history and physical suggest an obvious etiology?

Yes   No

Confirmatory studies:
Thyroid function panel
Antinuclear antibody
Creatinine phosphokinase
Antineuronal antibody
Skeletal muscle biopsy

Manometry

Full-thickness muscle biopsy†

Myopathic
process

Neuropathic
process

Miscellaneous
process

Begin therapy

Primary myopathies
Systemic sclerosis
Dermatomyositis
Polymyositis
Systemic lupus
Muscular dystrophy
Amyloidosis

Primary neuropathies
Diabetes mellitus
Parkinson's disease
Myasthenia gravis
Paraneoplastic
Multiple sclerosis
Cerebrovascular
accident
Spinal cord injury
Viral infection
Chagas' disease

Hypoparathyroidism
Hypothyroidism
Drug effect:
• TCAs
• Anticholinergics
• Narcotics
• Antiparkinsonian
• Phenothiazines
Radiation enteritis
Jejunal diverticulosis
Eating disorders

* plain films, small bowel follow through, enteroclysis, barium enema, CT scan
† Rarely necessary or performed

Table 15-4

TREATMENT APPROACH TO CHRONIC PSEUDO-OBSTRUCTION

- Supportive care
- Maintenance of adequate hydration
- Optimize nutritional status
  - * Reduce meal volume; increase meal frequency
  - * Supplementation with elemental liquid diets
  - * In severe cases, elemental liquid diets only or TPN
- NG decompression
  - * If needed for symptoms of nausea/bloating
  - * Consider "venting" percutaneous endoscopic gastrostomy tube
- Maintenance of normal metabolic parameters
- Avoid anticholinergic agents
- Avoid sedatives
- Avoid narcotics
- Optimize management of underlying conditions
- Consider promotility agent†
  - * Erythromycin
  - * Metoclopramide
  - * Tegaserod
  - * Octreotide (especially for scleroderma)[40-42]
- Consider intestinal transplantation for severe cases

† The current literature does not suggest that any of these agents is of particular benefit in the long-term management of chronic small intestinal pseudo-obstruction.

Serotonin (5-hydroxtryptamine, 5-HT) is an important neurotransmitter in regulating intestinal motility. 5-HT is released by the enterochromaffin cells in the intestine in response to a meal. 5-HT then activates specific receptors in afferent neurons that, in turn, activate the myenteric plexus. The specific 5-HT receptor can result in a variety of motility responses. For example, alosetron is a 5-HT3 receptor antagonist that decreases motility and is useful in treating diarrhea predominant IBS.[43,44] Conversely, it has been shown that stimulating the 5-HT4 receptor promotes motility and accelerates transit time.[45,46] Partial agonists of the 5-HT4 receptor (eg, tegaserod) may be useful in treating chronic pseudo-obstruction. However, further studies are needed before this potential use can be validated.

Paradoxically, narcotic use may be required for symptom control but, as with acute pseudo-obstruction, it should be avoided because it inhibits motility and can lead to substance dependence.[1]

Small intestinal transplantation has recently come into medical practice for severe cases of chronic intestinal pseudo-obstruction. It is generally reserved for those patients who have required TPN and developed complications, such as severe pancreatitis or recurrent line infections. This complicated procedure requires great technical expertise and is not widely available. Nevertheless, it is an acceptable option in appropriate patients.[47-49]

SMALL BOWEL BACTERIAL OVERGROWTH

As previously discussed, small bowel bacterial overgrowth is a consequence of small bowel motility disorders. The loss of phase III activity of the MMC leads to increased numbers and species of bacteria in the small intestine. The consequences of bacterial overgrowth are diverse. The increased number of bacteria deconjugates the bile acids present in the intestine, leading to malabsorption of fatty acids. Bacteria can also consume carbohydrates, peptides, vitamin B_{12}, iron, and all the other micro- and macronutrients, leading to malnutrition. As a result, patients have increased caloric requirements and weight loss. The actions of bacteria on carbohydrates produce increased quantities of gas, leading to further dilation of the intestines with subsequent pain. Finally, the bacteria may provoke an inflammatory response, leading to mucosal damage and an inflammatory arthritis.[50]

The treatment of small bowel bacterial overgrowth is to correct the underlying problem if at all possible. In the case of the small intestinal motility disorders, this is unfortunately not usually the case. Motility should be maximally stimulated. Then, a program of rotating antibiotics on a cyclical basis may be beneficial. Multiple drug regimens have been tried and shown to be efficacious. The basic underlying principle of all these regimens is to have a drug-free interval to prevent the development of bacterial resistance.[51]

Conclusion

Motility disorders of the small intestine are a significant problem facing all clinicians. An intricate coordination of hormonal release, neural activation, and the subsequent contraction of intestinal smooth muscle is required to achieve adequate peristalsis.

Dysmotility can result in chronic abdominal pain, distention, and constipation. Diarrhea secondary to bacterial overgrowth and malabsorption may also be seen. It is important to identify and treat underlying causes of dysmotility because this will improve the morbidity and mortality of these disorders. Although the etiologies for dysmotility are vast, there are only a limited number of diagnostic tools and therapeutic options available for the practicing gastroenterologist. Our understanding of the pathophysiology of these diseases has broadened dramatically over the past few years. Hopefully, in the future, there will be even more options to treat these difficult disorders.

References

1. Ouyang A. Small bowel motility disorders. In: Fisher RS, Krevsky B, eds. *Motor Disorders of the Gastrointestinal Tract: What's New and What To Do.* New York: Academy Professional Information Services, Inc; 1993.

2. Kuemmerle JF. Motility disorders of the small intestine: new insights into old problems. *J Clin Gastroenterol.* 2000;31:276-281.

3. Cohen S, Laufer I, Snape WJ Jr. The gastrointestinal manifestation of scleroderma: pathogenesis and management. *Gastroenterology.* 1980;79:155-166.

4. Horowitz AL, Meyers MA. The 'hide-bound' small bowel of scleroderma: characteristic mucosal fold pattern. *Am J Roentgenol.* 1973;119:332-334.

5. Bond JH, Levitt MP. Investigation of small bowel transit time in man utilizing pulmonary hydrogen (H2) measurements. *J Lab Clin Med.* 1975;85:546-555.

6. Read MW, Al-Janabi MN, Bates TE, et al. Interpretation of the breath hydrogen profile obtained after ingesting a solid meal containing nonabsorbable carbohydrate. *Gut.* 1985;26:834-842.

7. Miller MA, Parkman HP, Urbain JL, et al. Comparison of scintigraphy and lactulose breath hydrogen test for assessment of orocecal transit: lactulose accelerates small bowel transit. *Dig Dis Sci.* 1997;42:10-18.

8. Rhoades JM, Middleton P, Jewell DP. The lactulose hydrogen breath test as a diagnostic test for small bowel bacterial overgrowth. *Scand J Gastroenterol.* 1979;14:333-336.

9. Camilleri M, Zinsmeister AR, Greydanus MP, et al. Towards a less costly but accurate test of gastric emptying and small bowel transit. *Dig Dis Sci.* 1991;36:609-615.

10. von der Ohe MR, Camilleri M. Measurement of small bowel and colonic transit: indications and methods. *Mayo Clin Proc.* 1992;67:1169-1179.

11. Stainforth DH, Coates P, Clarke JG. An HPLC assay for sulfapyridine in plasma and its use to assess small bowel transit time after the administration of sulphasalazine. *International Journal of Clinical Pharmacology, Therapy, & Toxicology.* 1987;25(7):406-409.

12. Soffer EE, Thongswat S. Small bowel manometry: short or long recording sessions? *Dig Dis Sci.* 1997;42:873-877.

13. Samsom M, Fraser R, Smout AJ, et al. Characterization of small intestinal pressure waves in ambulant subjects recorded with a novel portable manometric system. *Dig Dis Sci.* 1999;44:2157-2164.

14. Kellow JE. Manometry. In: Schuster MM, Crowell MD, Koch KL, eds. *Schuster Atlas of Gastrointestinal Motility in Health and Disease.* 2nd ed. Hamilton, Ontario: BC Decker, Inc; 2002.

15. Malagelada JR, Camilleri M, Stanghellini V. *Manometric Diagnosis of Gastrointestinal Motility Disorders.* New York: Thieme; 1986.

16. Husebye E. The patterns of small bowel motility: physiology and implications in organic disease and functional disorders. *Neurogastroenterol Motil.* 1999;11:141-161.

17. Ouyang A, Sunshine AG, Reynolds JC. Caloric content of a meal affects duration but not contractile pattern of duodenal motility in man. *Dig Dis Sci.* 1989;34:528-536.

18. Anuras S, Chokhavatia S. Dysmotility of the small intestine. In: Yamada T, Alpers DH, Owyang C, Powell DW, Silverstein FE, eds. *Textbook of Gastroenterology.* New York: JB. Lippincott, Co; 1991.

19. Ponec RJ, Saunders MD, Kimmey MB. Neostigmine for the treatment of acute colonic pseudo-obstruction. *N Engl J Med.* 1999;341:137-141.

20. Schuller MD, Pope CE. Studies of idiopathic intestinal pseudoobstruction. II. hereditary hollow visceral myopathy: family studies. *Gastroenterology.* 1977;73:339-344.

21. Anuras S, Mitros FA, Nowak TV, et al. A family visceral myopathy with external ophthalmoplegia and autosomal recessive transmission. *Gastroenterology.* 1983;84:346-356.

22. Jacobs E, Ardichvili D, Perissimo A, et al. A case of familial visceral myopathy with atrophy and fibrosis of the longitudinal muscle layer of the entire small bowel. *Gastroenterology.* 1979;77:745-750.

23. Mayer MA, Schuffler MD, Rotter JI, et al. Familial visceral neuropathy with autosomal dominant transmission. *Gastroenterology.* 1986;91:1528-1535.

24. Kern IB, Harris MJ. Congenital short bowel. *Aust N Z J Surg.* 1973;42:283-285.

25. Nakahara M, Isozaki K, Hirota S, et al. Deficiency of KIT-positive cells in the colon of patients with diabetes mellitus. *J Gastroenterol Hepatol.* 2002;17:666-670.

26. Reinhardt JF, Barry WF. Scleroderma of the small bowel. *Am J Roentgen.* 1962;88:687-692.

27. Rees WD, Leigh RJ, Christofides ND, et al. Interdigestive motor activity in patients with systemic sclerosis. *Gastroenterology.* 1982;83:575-580.

28. Kleckner F. Dermatomyositis and its manifestations in the gastrointestinal tract. *Am J Gastroenterol.* 1970;53:141-146.

29. Nowak T, Anuras S, Brown B. Small intestinal motility in myotonic dystrophy patients. *Gastroenterology.* 1984;86:808-813.

30. Nowak T, Ionasescu V, Anuras S. Gastrointestinal manifestations of the muscular dystrophies. *Gastroenterology.* 1982;82:800-810.

31. Watkins CC, Sawa A, Jaffrey S, et al. Insulin restores neuronal nitric oxide synthase expression and function that is lost in diabetic gastropathy. *J Clin Invest.* 2000;106(3):373-384.

32. Wrzos HF, Cruz A, Polavarapu R, et al. Nitric oxide synthase (NOS) expression in the myenteric plexus of streptozotocin-diabetic rats. *Dig Dis Sci.* 1997;42(10):2106-2110.

33. Adeghate E, al-Ramadi B, Saleh, AM, et al. Increase in neuronal nitric oxide synthase content of the gastroduodenal tract of diabetic rats. *Cell Mol Life Sci.* 2003;60(6):1172-1179.

34. Simpson DA, Pawlak AM, Tegmeyer L, et al. Paraneoplastic intestinal pseudo-obstruction, mononeuritis multiplex, and sensory neuropathy/neuronopathy. *J Am Osteo Assoc.* 1996;96:125-128.

35. Briellmann RS, Sturzenegger M, Gerber HA, et al. Autoantibody-associated sensory neuronopathy and intestinal pseudo-obstruction without detectable neoplasia. *Euro Neurol.* 1996;36:369-373.

36. Sodhi N, Camilleri M, Camoriano JK, et al. Autonomic function and motility in intestinal pseudoobstruction caused by paraneoplastic syndrome. *Dig Dis Sci.* 1989;34:1937-1942.

37. Neitlich JD, Burrell MI. Drug induced disorders of the small bowel. *Abdom Imaging.* 1999;24:17-22.

38. Isselbacher KJ, Epstein A. Diverticular, vascular, and other disorders of the intestine and peritoneum. In: Braunwald E, Fauci AS, Kasper DL, et al, eds. *Harrison's Principles of Internal Medicine.* 15th ed. New York: McGraw-Hill; 2001.

39. Catnach SM, Fairclough PD. Erythromycin and the gut. *Gut.* 1992;33:397-401.

40. Haruma K, Wiste JA, Camilleri M. Effect of octreotide on gastrointestinal pressure profiles in health and in functional and organic gastrointestinal disorders. *Gut.* 1993;35:1064-1069.

41. Soudah HC, Hasler WL, Owyang C. Effect of octreotide on intestinal motility and bacterial overgrowth in scleroderma. *N Engl J Med.* 1991;325:1461-1467.

42. Verne GN, Eaker EY, Hardy E, Sninsky CA. Effect of octreotide and erythromycin on idiopathic and scleroderma-associated intestinal pseudoobstruction. *Dig Dis Sci.* 1995;40:1892-1901.

43. Grider JR, Foxx-Orenstein AE, Jin J-G. 5-hydroxytryptamine4 receptor agonists initiate the peristaltic reflex in human, rat, and guinea pig intestine. *Gastroenterology.* 1998;115:370-380.

44. Foxx-Orenstein AE, Jin JG, Grider JR. 5-HT4 receptor agonists and α-opioid receptor antagonists act synergistically to stimulate colonic propulsion. *Am J Physiol.* 1998;275:G979-G983.

45. Prather CM, Camilleri M, Zinsmeister AR, et al. Tegaserod accelerates orocecal transit in patients with constipation-predominant irritable bowel syndrome. *Gastroenterology.* 2000;118:463-468.

46. Bouras EP, Camilleri M, Burton DD, et al. Prucalopride accelerates gastrointestinal and colonic transit in patients with constipation without a rectal evacuation disorder. *Gastroenterology.* 2001;120:354-360.

47. DiMartini A, Rovera GM, Graham TO, et al. Quality of life after small intestinal transplantation and among home parenteral nutrition patients. *Journal of Parenteral & Enteral Nutrition.* 1998;22:357-362.

48. Goulet O, Lacaille F, Jan D, Ricour C. Intestinal transplantation: indications, results and strategy. *Curr Opin Clin Nutr Metab Care.* 2000;3:329-338.

49. Coulie B, Camilleri M. Intestinal pseudo-obstruction. *Ann Rev Med.* 1999;50:37-55.

50. Sherman P, Lichtman S. Small bowel bacterial overgrowth syndrome. *Dig Dis.* 1987;5:157- 171.

51. Vanderhoof JA, Young RJ, Murray N, Kaufman SS. Treatment strategies for small bowel bacterial overgrowth in short bowel syndrome. *J Pediatr Gastroenterol Nutr.* 1998;27:155-160.

Small Bowel
Bacterial Overgrowth

Kathleen Lukaszewski, DO; Marianne T. Ritchie, MD;
and Dilip Bearelly, MD

Introduction

Small bowel bacterial overgrowth is a syndrome of nutrient malabsorption, malnutrition, diarrhea, and weight loss that is associated with an excessive number of bacteria within the proximal small intestine. The syndrome may also be known as blind loop syndrome, stagnant loop syndrome, and small bowel stasis. One must first understand the role that the normal GI flora has in the metabolism of nutrients and vitamins in order to fully appreciate the impact of small bowel bacterial overgrowth. This chapter will briefly review the normal microbial flora of the GI tract and then focus on the etiology and pathogenesis of small bowel bacterial overgrowth. Lastly, the methods of diagnosis of bacterial overgrowth will be discussed and the various treatment modalities will be reviewed.

Normal Microbial Flora
of the Gastrointestinal Tract

The human GI tract is sterile at birth. Shortly thereafter, it becomes colonized by microorganisms from the environment and from the mother's fecal flora. Initially, the intestine is populated by coliforms and streptococci.[1-4] As these bacteria multiply, they consume oxygen and create an environment suitable for the growth of anaerobic bacteria.[3] Bacteroids and clostridia become the predominant organisms in the colon within the first few weeks of life. Later in infancy, lactobacilli, peptostreptococci, and peptococci are acquired and populate the GI tract.

The actual microbiology of the GI tract is influenced by luminal pH, motility, and the structural integrity of the alimentary tract. The stomach and duodenum contain few microorganisms due to gastric acidity and peristalsis. The literature reports colony counts of 10^3 to 10^4 colony-forming units may be present for these organisms.[4] The jejunum contains approximately 10^4 colony-forming units consisting primarily of aerobes and facultative anaerobes. The terminal ileum has been described as a transition zone between the aerobic colonization of the UGI tract and the anaerobic population of the colon. Colony counts in the ileum have been reported to be as high as 10^9 colony-forming units.[4] An intact ileocecal valve serves as a barrier to the backflow of colonic flora. If the valve is dysfunctional or has been changed surgically, the microbiology of the ileum is consistent with that of the colon. The normal enteric flora influence a variety of functions of the intestine, including nutrient and vitamin production, as well as bile acid, lipid, carbohydrate, and protein metabolism. Enteric bacteria are known to produce nutrients and vitamins such as folate and vitamin K. Colonic bacterial enzymes are required for normal bile acid metabolism. The bacteria deconjugate unabsorbed bile acids and convert the primary bile acids to the secondary bile acids that are eventually excreted.[4-6] Short chain fatty acids are produced by bacterial degradation of lipids, as well as by fermentation of unabsorbed carbohydrates.[6,7] Protein metabolism is also influenced by enteric bacteria such that these bacteria are involved in the degradation of protein and urea into ammonia.[4] Lastly, enteric bacteria are involved in the metabolism of several pharmacologic agents and are also involved in the production of carcinogens.[4]

There are several defense mechanisms that control against bacterial overgrowth within the normal functioning alimentary tract. As mentioned above, luminal pH, peristalsis, and an intact ileocecal valve are a few of these mechanisms.[1] Additional protective mechanisms include the destruction of bacteria by proteolytic enzymes in the small intestine, trapping of bacteria by the intestinal mucous layer, and the secretion of IgA immunoglobulins in the GI tract.[8]

Etiology

It is reasonable that any perturbation in the normal defense mechanisms protecting against bacterial overgrowth can lead to its occurrence. Intestinal stasis, gastric acid disorders, structural changes within the intestinal tract, and immunodeficiency states are among the most common conditions favoring bacterial overgrowth (Table 16-1).

Intestinal stasis can result from both anatomic changes in the intestinal tract and from motility disorders. Surgeries such as the Billroth II gastrojejunostomy, end-to-side enteroenterostomies, ileoanal anastomoses, and jejunoileal bypasses have all been associated with bacterial overgrowth in the stagnant loop and pouches.[9,10] Diverticula of the small intestine can also serve as stagnant pouches and facilitate bacterial overgrowth. Obstruction of the small bowel from strictures, radiation changes, and adhesions can also foster overgrowth of bacteria.[4] Motility disorders secondary to scleroderma, pseudo-obstruction, and neuropathies can also predispose to overgrowth.[11,12]

Conditions of achlorhydria or hypochlorhydria can result in increased bacteria in the intestine. Therapy with histamine receptor antagonists and PPIs with the resultant decrease in gastric acidity has been shown to facilitate overgrowth.[4,13,14] Likewise, earlier surgical management for PUD, including antrectomy, vagotomy, and Billroth II, has the combined predisposing factors of decreased gastric acid output and altered intestinal motility.

Structural changes within the intestinal tract are also a cause of bacterial overgrowth. Patients with enteroenteric, gastrocolic, or gastrojejunocolic fistulae from Crohn's disease; ulcer disease; or even penetrating carcinomas are all predisposed to overgrowth and malabsorption. Additionally, retrograde seeding of the ileum with colonic flora has been demonstrated in patients after resection of the ileocecal valve.[4]

Table 16-1

ETIOLOGY OF BACTERIAL OVERGROWTH

- Intestinal stasis
  * Anatomic/postsurgical changes
  * Diverticula
  * Obstruction
  * Motility disorders
- Gastric acid disorders
  * Medication induced (PPIs and H_2RAs)
  * Peptic ulcer surgery
- Structural changes within the GI tract
  * Fistula
  * Ileocecal valve resection
- Immunodeficiency conditions
  * Common variable immunodeficiency
  * AIDS
  * Leukemia
  * T-cell deficiencies
- Other conditions
  * Chronic pancreatitis
  * Cirrhosis
  * End-stage renal disease
  * IBS

Several immunodeficiency conditions have been associated with bacterial overgrowth. Common variable immunodeficiency, the acquired immunodeficiency syndrome, chronic lymphocytic leukemia, and T-cell deficiencies are a few of the clinical entities in which bacterial overgrowth syndrome has been described.[15-17]

Although less well described and probably of multifactorial origin, bacterial overgrowth has been documented to occur in several other clinical conditions, including chronic pancreatitis,[18] cirrhosis,[19,20] and end-stage renal disease.[4,6,21] Recently, attention has focused on a possible association of small bowel bacterial overgrowth with irritable bowel syndrome.[21-26]

Pathogenesis

The pathogenesis of small bowel bacterial overgrowth can best be described as the result of the bacteria causing both impaired metabolism of intraluminal substances and mucosal injury. Fat malabsorption occurs with small bowel bacterial overgrowth as a result of the bacterial deconjugation of bile acids. Under normal conditions, fat absorption requires a critical concentration of conjugated bile acids to combine with dietary lipids to form mixed micelles that are then absorbed in the ileum. When there is bacterial overgrowth, the bile salts are deconjugated and form bile acids that are reabsorbed in the jejunum. As a result of this bile acid reabsorption there is decreased formation of mixed micelles and fat malabsorption occurs. Steatorrhea and malabsorption of the fat soluble vitamins (A, D, E, K) can occur.[4] If the fat malabsorption is clinically significant, signs and symptoms of night blindness, tetany, osteomalacia, neuropathy, and dermatitis can become apparent. As the bacteria synthesize vitamin K, a coagulopathy does not occur in small bowel bacterial overgrowth syndrome.[27]

Vitamin B_{12}/cobalamin deficiency is also associated with bacterial overgrowth. Vitamin B_{12} normally binds with gastric intrinsic factor and is absorbed in the ileum. With bacterial overgrowth, anaerobic bacteria will compete for the vitamin B_{12}.[4,28] As a part of the Schilling's test, vitamin B_{12} deficiency that does not correct with the addition of intrinsic factor but does so after antibiotic treatment is representative of small bowel bacterial overgrowth. Macrocytic and megaloblastic anemia and peripheral neuropathy are common clinical presentations in vitamin B_{12} deficiency.

Protein malabsorption may result from both intraluminal degradation of protein substrates by the bacteria, as well as from decreased uptake of amino acids secondary to mucosal injury.[29] There is also a protein-losing enteropathy associated with small bowel bacterial overgrowth in which mucosal injury leads to leakage of protein.[29] The resultant hypoproteinemia and hypoalbuminemia can become significant enough to lead to the development of peripheral edema.

Carbohydrate intolerance results from enterocyte injury with resultant decreased disaccharidase activity as well as from intraluminal degradation of the carbohydrates by the bacteria.[4] It is believed that the anaerobic bacteria produce glycosidases and proteases that effect hydrolases on the brush border of the enterocytes. Lactase activity has been reported to be one of the first enzymes to be effected, resulting in lactose intolerance and associated diarrhea.[27] Bacterial metabolism of carbohydrates results in an increased production of hydrogen and carbon dioxide which forms the basis for some of the diagnostic tests for small bowel bacterial overgrowth. This production of hydrogen and carbon dioxide, is also believed to be a factor in the development of the abdominal pain associated with this syndrome.[27] Lastly, the breakdown of carbohydrates by the intraluminal bacteria results in short chain organic acids that alter the chemistry of the intestinal fluid and lead to diarrhea.

Pathology

The histologic appearance of the small bowel in bacterial overgrowth does not differ significantly from that of the intestine with normal resident flora. However, in some cases there have been described evidence of villous atrophy and blunting, increased inflammatory cells in the lamina propria, as well as focal areas of erosion and ulceration. Biopsies are therefore primarily utilized to rule out other pathologic processes within the small intestine mucosa in particular celiac sprue.[9]

Clinical Presentation

The clinical manifestations of small bowel bacterial overgrowth are truly a direct consequence of the pathogenesis of the disorder (Table 16-2). As discussed above, patients present with fat, protein, and carbohydrate malabsorption. As such, diarrhea

Table 16-2

CLINICAL MANIFESTATIONS OF SMALL BOWEL BACTERIAL OVERGROWTH

Nutrient	Mechanism	Clinical Manifestation	Laboratory Findings
Fatty acids	Bacterial deconjugation of bile acids	Pale, voluminous stool without flatulence	Stool fat >6 g/day
Carbohydrates	Bacterial metabolism of carbohydrates Reduction of brush border disaccharides Decreased uptake of monosaccharides Proteases and glycosidases produced by aerobic bacteria destroy hydrolases on brush border	Watery diarrhea, flatulence, and milk intolerance	Increased breath hydrogen
Vitamin E	Refer to fat malabsorption	Peripheral neuropathy	Abnormal plasma or serum concentration of alpha tocopherol
Vitamin D	Refer to fat malabsorption	Paresthesia Tetany Pathological fractures Osteomalacia	Hypocalcemia Increased alkaline phosphatase Abnormal bone densitometry
Vitamin A	Refer to fat malabsorption	Follicular hyperkeratosis Night blindness	Decreased serum carotene
Vitamin B_{12}	Bacteria compete with host for vitamin B_{12} Breakdown of vitamin B_{12} to inactive metabolites	Anemia Subacute combined degeneration of spinal cord	

(continued)

Table 16-2

CLINICAL MANIFESTATIONS OF SMALL BOWEL BACTERIAL OVERGROWTH (CONTINUED)

Nutrient	Mechanism	Clinical Manifestation	Laboratory Findings
	Decreased peptide uptake	Peripheral neuropathy	Macrocytic anemia
	Impaired enterokinase activity		Abnormal Schilling's test
	Impaired activation of pancreatic proteases		Increased serum methyl-malonic acid
Proteins	Bacteria competing with the host for proteins	Edema	Hypoalbuminemia
		Muscle atrophy	Hypoproteinemia

Table 16-3

EVALUATION OF SMALL BOWEL

Laboratory Studies
- Serum: CBC with differential, prothrombin time (PT), partial thromboplastin time (PTT), albumin, total protein, calcium, magnesium, iron, folate, B$_{12}$ (if low, then proceed with the Schilling's test)
- Stool: Culture, ova and parasite, qualitative and quantitative fecal fat

Radiological Studies
- Small bowel series

Diagnostic Studies
- UGI endoscopy with small bowel biopsy and possible jejunal aspirate
- Breath tests: 14 C-D-xylose test, hydrogen test

and weight loss are often the most prominent and frequently occurring symptoms. Other common but nonspecific symptoms include abdominal pain, bloating, and dyspepsia. In more severe cases, vitamin and nutrient malabsorption may present with night blindness, tetany, osteomalacia, neuropathy, edema, and anemia.

Diagnosis

The diagnosis of small bowel bacterial overgrowth should be considered in any patient who presents with diarrhea, steatorrhea, weight loss, and other symptoms of malabsorption and is known to have a coexisting predisposition to this disorder. Often, however, it can become difficult to differentiate whether the symptoms are related to an exacerbation of the underlying disease or due to the development of bacterial overgrowth. As such, further evaluation should be undertaken (Table 16-3). Other causes of malabsorption and maldigestion included in the differential diagnosis of bacterial overgrowth such as celiac sprue, giardiasis, and pancreatic insufficiency must be ruled out.

After a thorough history and physical examination are completed, small bowel barium radiographs and basic laboratory evaluation should be performed. The barium radiographs are useful in detecting diverticula, strictures, fistulas, and postsurgical changes as well as providing evidence of dysmotility. Quantitative fecal fat measurement is used to document steatorrhea. Complete cell count and differential will demonstrate macrocytic anemia, and a sequential Schilling's test should then be performed in the presence of vitamin B$_{12}$ deficiency (Table 16-4).[4,6] If any of these tests demonstrate abnormalities, then further specific testing for small bowel bacterial overgrowth should be undertaken.

The gold standard for the diagnosis of bacterial overgrowth has been the findings of 10^5 colony-forming units per milliliter found on jejunal aspirate.[30,31] Obtaining an adequate sample for quantitative culture can be technically challenging. Utilizing a

Table 16-4

SCHILLING'S TEST

The Schilling's test is used in the evaluation of patients with low vitamin B_{12} levels.

The test measures 24-hour urinary excretion of radioactive Co-57.

Part I

The patient is given oral vitamin B_{12} (Co-57) followed by IV injection of non-radioactive vitamin B_{12}, which saturates liver storage, thus excess B_{12} is excreted in the urine. Urine is then collected for 24 hours, and the percentage of administered radioactivity is then measured.

Less than 7%:	Greater than 7%:
Intrinsic factor deficiency	Dietary deficiency
Intestinal malabsorption	

Part II

If the excretion is low, the patient is given oral Co-57 with intrinsic factor to differentiate between intrinsic factor deficiency and malabsorption. This test is done 5 to 7 days after the first part. Urine is again collected for 24 hours, and the percentage of administered radioactivity is then measured.

Less than 7%:	Greater than 7%
Intestinal malabsorption	Intrinsic factor deficiency

Part III

Patients with low excretion in parts I and II of the test are given tetracycline 250 mg QID for 10 days prior to repeating the test. Markedly improved excretion of radioactive Co-57 confirms intestinal malabsorption.

---

sterile suction catheter within an overtube that is passed through the biopsy channel during endoscopy of the small bowel is an effective means of obtaining an appropriate sample. Careful and appropriate handling of the aspirates is required because the samples need to be sent in the correct vials for both anaerobic and aerobic cultures. Even with careful collection technique, the culture may not yield appropriate results due to the possibilities of oral bacterial contamination, overgrowth occurring distal to the collection site, and the difficulty in performing anaerobic cultures.

Obtaining quantitative bacterial culture requires an invasive procedure, is expensive, and is not widely available. These factors have led to the development of alternative diagnostic testing for small bowel bacterial overgrowth. The 2 most frequently used tests are the xylose breath test and the hydrogen breath test.

Xylose is a pentose sugar that is catabolized by aerobic gram negative bacteria with resultant production of CO_2, which is then absorbed by the small bowel. After ingestion of 1 gram of carbon 14-labeled d-xylose, bacteria within the small bowel in bacterial overgrowth patients will catabolize the sugar to release the radioactive 14-CO_2. Within 60 minutes, elevated levels of the 14-CO_2 are detected in the breath. The sensitivity and specificity of this test has been documented to approach 90%.[32] The accuracy of the xylose test results have been questioned in cases of both delayed gastric emptying causing false negative results and in cases of rapid transit causing false positive ones. An additional limitation of this test is that use of the radioisotope is not recommended in children and in women of childbearing age.

The hydrogen breath test is based on the fact that human tissue does not produce hydrogen. After ingestion of a carbohydrate load of lactulose or glucose, there will be a rise in expired hydrogen due to the metabolism of the carbohydrate by the enteric bacteria. A positive test result demonstrates a double peak in the expired hydrogen levels, the first representing the metabolism by the bacteria overgrown within the small bowel and the second subsequently by the normal colonic flora. Although the hydrogen breath tests are simple tests and do not involve the use of radioactive isotopes, they are not without limitations. These tests have lower sensitivities (60% to 70%) and specificities (40% to 80%).[33] Patients undergoing this test need to refrain from eating bread, pasta, and fiber prior to the test because these foods can prolong hydrogen secretion. Cigarette smoking and vigorous exercise need to be avoided prior to the testing to avoid hyperventilation. Additionally, prior to testing, patients need to use an antiseptic mouthwash to eliminate any oral bacteria that could interfere with the test result. As in the xylose testing, false-positive results can occur in patients with rapid transit, while false negative results may occur due to the presence of flora unable to produce hydrogen.[34]

Treatment

The very first step in the management of the patient with small bowel bacterial overgrowth should consist of correction of fluid, electrolyte, and vitamin abnormalities. Vitamin D and calcium supplements, vitamin E, vitamin K, and cobalamin injections should be administered as indicated. Dietary modifications may also be useful. As mentioned earlier, lactase is one of the first enzymes to be affected by small intestinal mucosal injury. A lactose-free diet may therefore provide some relief from diarrheal symptoms. Additionally, because the bacteria readily ferment carbohydrates, substituting fats for carbohydrates may be of some benefit. The use of medium chain over long chain triglycerides probably has minimal value.

Once the diagnosis of bacterial overgrowth is made, initial treatment should then focus on correcting the underlying disorder. In cases due to intestinal stasis and structural abnormalities, this may involve both surgical and medical measures. Surgery may be indicated to treat strictures, adhesions, fistulae, and possibly revise prior surgical interventions. Stasis secondary to dysmotility may benefit from prokinetic agents. There have been limited studies investigating the use of these agents in small bowel bacterial overgrowth syndrome. Two reports of the beneficial use of octreotide and octreotide with erythromycin in patients with bacterial overgrowth have been cited in the literature.[35,36] In a small number of subjects, low dose octreotide given at bedtime was noted to stimulate phase 3 motor complexes. Subjects were noted to have decreased nausea, vomiting, and abdominal pain and noted to have cleared the bacterial overgrowth as evidenced by normalization of hydrogen breath testing. Cisapride had been demonstrated to be beneficial in decreasing transit time and clear-

Table 16-5

ANTIMICROBIAL AGENTS FOR THE TREATMENT OF SMALL BOWEL BACTERIAL OVERGROWTH

Antibiotic	Dosage (10-day course)
Amoxicillin – clavulanic acid	750 mg twice a day
Cephalexin + metronidazole	250 mg 4 times a day +
	250 mg 3 times a day
Trimethaprim – sulfamethoxazole	one double-strength tablet twice a day
Ciprofloxacin	500 mg twice a day
Norfloxacin	400 mg twice a day
Colistin + metronidazole	250,000 IU/kg/d +
	250 mg twice a day
Doxycycline	100 mg twice a day
Tetracycline	250 mg 4 times a day
Minocycline	100 mg twice a day
Chloramphenicol	250 mg 4 times a day
*Rifaximin	200 mg 3 times a day, 10 to 20 days

* currently being studied.

ing bacterial overgrowth in a small number of patients with cirrhosis and bacterial overgrowth.[37] However, because cisapride is no longer available, investigations with other prokinetic agents are warranted.

Unfortunately, the primary underlying disorder cannot be completely corrected in most cases of small bowel bacterial overgrowth. Management must therefore be directed at suppressing the bacteria with antibiotic treatment. Appropriate antibiotic treatment should have coverage against both aerobic and anaerobic bacteria. Tetracycline had previously been a first line agent in dosages of 250 mg 4 times daily. However, due to resistance patterns, up to 60% of patients with bacterial overgrowth are not responsive to tetracycline monotherapy. Broad spectrum coverage with amoxicillin-clavulanate has been shown to be successful in the empiric treatment of small bowel bacterial overgrowth.[38] Some of the other antibiotic regimens that have been utilized in bacterial overgrowth include cephalexin and metronidazole, trimethoprim-sulfamethoxazole and metronidazole, quinolone monotherapy, and chloramphenicol (Table 16-5). Recently, the use of rifaximin has demonstrated promise for treatment of small bowel bacterial overgrowth; however, further investigation is needed.

Treatment duration is variable and is clinically based. A single course of antibiotic therapy for 7 to 10 days may improve symptoms and patients may remain symptom free for several months. In patients with persistent or recurrent symptoms, prolonged therapy or a rotating schedule of antibiotic treatment is often required.

Lastly, as an alternative treatment modality for bacterial overgrowth, the use of probiotic therapy has also been investigated. Probiotic therapy is based on the belief that manipulating intestinal flora through live microbial supplements may influence enteric disease processes. Probiotic therapy has been documented in the management of *Clostridium difficile* and in IBD. In bacterial overgrowth, use of *Saccharomyces boulardii*, lactobacilli species, and bifidobacterium as adjuncts to antibiotic treatment as well as for primary therapy has been examined with variable results.[38,39]

References

1. Simon GL, Gorbach SL. The human intestinal microflora. *Dig Dis.* 1986;30(suppl19):147S.

2. Hanson LA, Dahlman-Hogund A, Karlsson M, et al. Normal microbial flora of the gut and the immune system. In: Hanson LA, Yolken RH, eds. *Probiotics Other Nutritional Factors, and Intestinal Microflora.* Philadelphia: Lippincott-Raven; 1999:217.

3. Adlerberth I. Establishment of a normal intestinal microflora in the newborn infant. In: Hanson LA, Yolken RH, eds. *Probiotics Other Nutritional Factors, and Intestinal Microflora.* Philadelphia: Lippincott-Raven; 1999:63.

4. Gregg CR, Toskes PP. Enteric bacterial flora and small bowel bacterial overgrowth syndrome. In: Feldman M, Friedman LS, Sleisinger MH, eds. *Sleisenger and Fordtran's Gastrointestinal and Liver Disease.* 7th ed. Philadelphia: Saunders; 2002:1783-1793.

5. Midvedt T. Microbial functional activities. In: Hanson LA, Yolken RH, eds. *Probiotics Other Nutritional Factors, and Intestinal Microflora.* Philadelphia: Lippincott-Raven; 1999:79.

6. Gregg C. Enteric bacterial flora and bacterial overgrowth syndrome. *Sem Gastrointest Dis.* 2002;13(4):200-209.

7. Hoeverstad T, Carlstedt-Duke B, Lingaas E, et al. Influence of oral intake of 7 different antibiotics upon fecal short chain fatty acid excretion in healthy subjects. *Scand J Gastroenterol.* 1986;21:997.

8. Riordan SM, McIver CJ, Wakefield D, et al. Small intestinal mucosal immunity and morphometry in luminal overgrowth of indigenous gut flora. *Am J Gastroenterol.* 2001;96:494.

9. Iivonen MK, Ahola TO, Matikainen MJ. Bacterial overgrowth, intestinal transit, and nutrition after total gastrectomy. Comparison of a jejunal pouch with roux-en-Y reconstruction in a prospective random study. *Scand J Gastroenterol.* 1998;33:63-70.

10. Levitt MD, Kuan M. The physiology of ileoanal pouch function. *Am J Surg.* 1998;176:384.

11. Kaye SA, Lim SG, Taylor M, et al. Small bowel bacterial overgrowth in systemic sclerosis: detection using direct and indirect methods and treatment outcome. *Br J Rheumatol.* 1995;34:265.

12. Pearson AJ, Brzechwa-Adjukiewicz A, Mc Carthy CF. Intestinal pseudo-obstruction with bacterial overgrowth in the small intestine. *Am J Dig Dis.* 1969;14:200.

13. Fried M, Slegrish H, Frei R, et al. Duodenal bacterial overgrowth during treatment with omeprazole in outpatients. *Gut.* 1996;35:23.

14. Shindo K, Machida M, Fukumura M, et al. Omeprazole induces altered bile acid metabolism. *Gut.* 1998;42:266.

15. Pignata C, Budillon G, Monaco G, et al. Jejunal bacterial overgrowth and intestinal permeability in children with immunodeficiency syndromes. *Gut.* 1990;31:879.

16. Smith GM, Chesner IM, Monaco G, et al. Small intestinal bacterial overgrowth in patients with chronic lymphocytic leukemia. *J Clin Pathol.* 1990;143:57.

17. Budhraja M, Levendoglu MD, Kocka F, et al. Duodenal mucosal T cell population and bacterial cultures in acquired immune deficiency syndrome. *Am J Gastroenterol.* 1987;82:427.

18. Lembeke B, Kraus B, Lankisch PG. Small intestinal function in chronic relapsing pancreatitis. *Hepatogastroenterology.* 1985;32:149.

19. Chang CS, Chen GH, Lien HC, et al. Small intestine dysmotility and bacterial overgrowth in cirrhotic patients with spontaneous bacterial peritonitis. *Hepatology.* 1998;28:1187.

20. Bauer TM, Steinbruckner B, Brinkmann FE, et al. Small intestinal bacterial overgrowth in patients with cirrhosis: prevalence and relation with spontaneous bacterial peritonitis. *Am J Gastroenterol.* 2001;96:2962.

21. Singh VS, Toskes PP. Small bowel bacterial overgrowth: presentation, diagnosis, and treatment. *Current Treatment Options in Gastroenterology.* 2004;7:19-28.

22. Pimental M, Chow EJ, Lin HC. Eradication of small intestinal bacterial overgrowth reduces symptoms of irritable bowel syndrome. *Am J Gastroenterol.* 2000;95:3503-3506.

23. Riordan SM, McIver CJ, Duncombe VM, et al. Small intestinal bacterial overgrowth and the irritable bowel syndrome. *Am J Gastroenterol.* 2001;96:2506-2508.

24. Pimental M, Kong Y, Park S. Breath testing to evaluate lactose intolerance in irritable bowel syndrome correlates with lactulose testing and may not reflect true lactose malabsorption. *Am J Gastroenterol.* 2003;98:2700-2704.

25. Pimental M, Chow EJ, Lin HC. Normalization of lactulose breath testing correlates with symptom improvement in irritable bowel syndrome: a double blind, randomized, placebo-controlled study. *Am J Gastroenterol.* 2003;98:412-418.

26. Lin HC. Small intestinal bacterial overgrowth. A framework for understanding irritable bowel syndrome. *JAMA.* 2004;292:852-857.

27. Li E. Bacterial overgrowth. In: Yamada T, ed. *Textbook of Gastroenterology.* 4th ed. Philadelphia: Lippincott, Williams and Wilkins; 2003:1717.

28. Welkos SA, Toskes PP, Baer H, et al. Importance of anaerobic bacteria in the cobalamin malabsorption of experimental rat blind loop syndrome. *Gastroenterology.* 1981;80:313.

29. King CE, Toskes PP. Protein losing enteropathy in the human and experimental rat blind loop syndrome. *Gastroenterology.* 1974;67:965.

30. Bouhnik Y, Alain S, Attar A, et al. Bacterial populations contaminating the upper gut in patients with small intestinal bacterial overgrowth syndrome. *Am J Gastroenterol.* 1999;94:1327-1331.

31. Stotzer P, Brandberg A, Kilander AF. Diagnosis of small intestinal bacterial overgrowth in clinical praxis: a comparison of the culture of small bowel aspirate, duodenal biopsies, and gastric aspirate. *Hepatogastroenterology.* 1998;45(22):1018-1022.

32. King CE, Toskes PP, Spivey JC, et al. Detection of small intestinal overgrowth by 14C-D-Xylosebreath test. *Gastroenterology.* 1979;77:75.

33. Corazzo GR, Menozzi MG, Strocchi A, et al. The diagnosis of small bowel bacterial overgrowth: reliability of jejunal culture and inadequacy of breath hydrogen testing. *Gastroenterology.* 1990;98:302.

34. Rhodes JM, Middleton P, Jewell DP. The lactulose hydrogen breath test as a diagnostic test for small-bowel bacterial overgrowth. *Scand J Gastroenterol.* 1979;14:333.

35. Soudah HC, Hasler WL, Owyang C. Effect of octreotide on intestinal motility and bacterial overgrowth in scleroderma. *N Engl J Med.* 1991;325:1461.

36. Verne GN, Eaker EY, Hardy E, et al. Effect of octreotide and erythromycin on idiopathic and scleroderma associated pseudoobstruction. *Dig Dis Sci.* 1995;40:1892.

37. Pardo A, Bartoli R, Lorenzo-Zuniga V, et al. Effect of cisapride on intestinal motility and bacterial overgrowth and bacterial translocation in cirrhosis. *Hepatology.* 2000;31:858.

38. Attar A, Flourie B, Rambaud JC, et al. Antibiotic efficacy in small intestinal bacterial overgrowth-related chronic diarrhea: a crossover, randomized trial. *Gastroenterology.* 1999;117:794.

39. Vanderhoof JA, Young RJ, Murray N, Kaufman SS. Treatment strategies for small bowel bacterial overgrowth in short bowel syndrome. *J Pediatr Gastroenterol Nutr.* 1998;28:155.

chapter 17

Irritable Bowel Syndrome

Rupa N. Shah, MD and Brenda J. Horwitz, MD

Background

IBS, a disorder in which bowel habits are altered in association with abdominal discomfort, is one of the most common functional GI disorders. Historically, IBS has been a disease that, once diagnosed, is difficult to treat, leaving the patient dissatisfied and the physician challenged. In the last several years, the advent of new pharmacologic therapies based on increased knowledge of the pathophysiology of IBS has expanded the therapeutic armamentarium available to the treating gastroenterologist. Current theories of the pathophysiology of IBS will be discussed as well as new and traditional therapies for this disorder.

The current definition of IBS is based on the Rome criteria (Table 17-1).[1] Although it is known that symptoms may change over time, it is useful to categorize patients with IBS into the following 3 symptom-based subgroups:

1. IBS associated with diarrhea.
2. IBS associated with constipation.
3. IBS alternating between diarrhea and constipation.[2]

Epidemiology and Societal Impact

IBS has a prevalence of 10% to 15% among adults in the United States and a similar prevalence worldwide.[3] The disease affects twice as many women as men in North America.[2] It is unclear whether this difference reflects a true predominance of the disorder among women or if it is due to the fact that women may be more likely to seek medical care. IBS is the most common diagnosis made by gastroenterologists in the United States,[4] accounting for 28% of their office visits, and it accounts for 12% of visits to primary care providers.[5] It is estimated, however, that only 15% to 25% of affected individuals seek medical care,[3,6,7] and studies suggest that those who seek care are more likely to have behavioral and psychiatric problems than those who do not seek medical care.[8] Although most cases present before age 45, elderly patients

Table 17-1

ROME CRITERIA FOR IRRITABLE BOWEL SYNDROME

Diagnostic Criteria

Abdominal discomfort or pain with 2 of the following 3 features for at least 12 weeks, not necessarily consecutive, during the past 12 months:

1. Relief with defecation.
2. Onset associated with a change in the frequency of stool.
3. Onset associated with a change in the form of stool.

Supportive Symptoms

- Abnormal stool form (hard or lumpy stools, loose or watery stools).
- Abnormal stool frequency (fewer than 3 bowel movements per week, more than 3 bowel movements per day).
- Sensation of abdominal fullness or bloating.
- Difficulty with stool passage (straining, urgency, feelings of incomplete evacuation).
- Passage of mucus during a bowel movement.

Adapted from Thompson WG, Longstreth GF, Drossman DA, et al. Functional bowel disorders and functional abdominal pain. *Gut.* 1999;45:II43-II47.

experience IBS symptoms up to 92% as often as young individuals.[3] Health care costs for IBS are high. Estimates suggest that the total direct cost of IBS-related medical services was between $1.7 and $10 billion in the United States during the year 2000.[9] Indirect costs of absenteeism and decreased productivity caused by IBS have been estimated at $20 billion per year.

Clinical Manifestations

IBS is a heterogeneous disorder with various presentations. Although patients with IBS may present with a wide variety and intensity of symptoms, abdominal discomfort and altered bowel habits are the primary characteristics. Affected individuals usually describe the pain as a crampy sensation in the lower abdomen ranging from mildly uncomfortable to debilitating pain.[10,11] Psychological stress and meal ingestion may exacerbate the pain, while defecation often provides relief. Patients with IBS report diarrhea, constipation, alternating bowel habits, or normal bowel habits alternating with either constipation and/or diarrhea. Diarrhea in patients with IBS is usually described as frequent loose bowel movements, small to moderate in volume, occurring postprandially during waking hours. In diarrhea-predominant IBS, bowel movements are often preceded by fecal urgency and followed by a sensation of incomplete evacuation. Patients with constipation may also experience a sensation of incomplete evacuation and report hard, pellet-like stools lasting from days to months. Other frequent symptoms include abdominal bloating and a feeling of increased gas production (belching/flatulence).

Patients with IBS may also experience heartburn, nausea, bloating, and early satiety more than twice as often as in the general population,[12] suggesting a significant overlap between IBS and functional dyspepsia. UGI symptoms occur more frequently in patients with constipation than in those with diarrhea-predominant IBS.[13]

Extraintestinal complaints are common and include pelvic pain, dyspareunia, dysmenorrhea, decreased libido, urinary frequency, nocturia, and a sensation of incomplete bladder evacuation (interstitial cystitis). There is a strong association between IBS and fibromyalgia.[14] Other symptoms include chronic fatigue, back pain and headaches.

Pathophysiology

Several interrelated factors have been implicated in the development of IBS, including altered GI motility, visceral hypersensitivity, dysregulation of neurotransmitters of the brain-gut axis, enteric infection, genetic predisposition, as well as psychosocial factors. Past studies have focused on small bowel and colonic motility with conflicting results despite intensive investigations. Although decreased fasting amplitude and cycle length of migrating motor complexes and increased frequency of clustered contractions have been shown in the small bowel of patients with IBS,[15] similar changes have been observed in some asymptomatic patients. Some studies have shown that in affected patients, pain is more frequently associated with abnormal motility of the small bowel and colon than in normal controls,[16,17] but other studies have not confirmed these findings.[18] Physical and psychological stress[19] as well as meal ingestion[20] may alter the contractility of the colon. In normal individuals, meal ingestion generates an increase in GI myoelectrical activity, known as the gastrocolonic response. In IBS patients, the gastrocolonic response to test meals causes prolonged restosigmoid motor activity in comparison to normal subjects[21] and may last up to 3 hours.[16] In the ileum and colon, patients with IBS show an augmented response to a variety of stimuli, including meals, distention, cholinergic stimulation, corticotropin-releasing hormone, cholecystokinin, neostigmine, and colonic perfusion of deoxycholic acid.[22,23] This response has not been shown to occur in the stomach or proximal small intestine. Although no consistent pattern of altered motility has been demonstrated as specific for IBS, accelerated small bowel transit is seen in patients with diarrhea, and delayed transit is seen in those with constipation.[24-26]

Studies on gas transit suggest possible explanations for the symptom of bloating in IBS patients. Although the total intestinal gas volume in patients with IBS has been shown to be normal,[27] a recent study showed abnormal gas retention associated with bloating and abdominal distention in IBS patients.[28]

Several studies have focused on the perception of abdominal sensation. Perception in the GI tract results from the stimulation of various chemoreceptors, mechanoreceptors, and nociceptors that transmit information via spinal afferent pathways to the brain. It is thought that IBS may result from sensitization of visceral afferent pathways such that normal physiologic events, which are not sensed by healthy individuals, are perceived as painful by patients with IBS. The hypersensitivity of visceral afferent nerves of the GI system may be a causative factor in the symptoms of IBS. This visceral hypersensitivity theory is supported by balloon-distention studies of the rectosigmoid[29] and the ileum,[30] which have shown that IBS patients experience pain and bloating at balloon volumes and pressures that are significantly lower than those that induce pain in control subjects. In addition, these patients are more likely than controls to notice intestinal contractions.[31] The underlying pathophysiology of IBS appears to involve a defect in visceral perception.

In addition to visceral hypersensitivity, CNS dysfunction has been implicated in the development of IBS. PET[32,33] and functional MRI[34,35] of the brain show different patterns of activation in the thalamus and anterior cingulate cortex (which mediates affective responses associated with pain) in response to balloon distention of the rectum in IBS patients compared to normal subjects. Subsequent studies have shown increased activity in other areas of the cortex and brainstem. Although these conflicting studies warrant further investigation, they implicate a defect in central processing of visceral pain sensation.

Recent studies have suggested that an imbalance in neurotransmitters of the enteric nervous system, including serotonin, calcitonin gene-related peptide, substance P, bradykinin, acetylcholine, vasoactive intestinal peptide, nitric oxide, and others, may be involved in the pathogenesis of this disorder.[36] Serotonin (5-hydroxytryptamine [5-HT]) plays a key role in the regulation of GI motility, secretion, and sensation. Five percent of serotonin is located within the CNS, whereas the remaining 95% lies within enterochromaffin cells, neurons, and mast cells of the GI system. Serotonin stimulates the enteric nervous system, resulting in intestinal secretion, peristalsis, nausea, bloating, and abdominal pain.[37] In a small pilot study, patients with diarrhea-predominant IBS were found to release more serotonin postprandially than healthy individuals.[38] Patients with constipation-predominant symptoms have increased numbers of serotonin-containing epithelial cells in the colon than do healthy individuals or diarrhea-predominant IBS patients.[39] The serotonin transporter protein (SERT), which terminates serotonergic neurotransmission by rapid re-uptake of 5-hydroxytryptamine (5-HT) back into the nerve terminal, has been the focus of current research studies. Preliminary evidence suggests that SERT (expressed on intestinal epithelial cells, serotonergic neurons, and platelet membranes) may be of lower density and binding affinity in diarrhea-predominant IBS patients, accounting for the reduced capacity of serotonin reuptake and severity of symptoms in these patients.[40] Another recent study supports the role of abnormalities related to SERT by showing decreases in the expression of SERT in patients with both diarrhea and constipation-predominant IBS.[41] This study also showed decreases in the expression of tryptophan hydroxylase, the rate-limiting enzyme in the biosynthesis of serotonin.

Another key player may be the N-methyl-D-aspartate (NMDA) receptor. This receptor, located on dorsal horn neurons of the spinal cord which are the recipients of afferent input from the GI tract, has also been implicated in the development of visceral hypersensitivity.[42] There appears to be a complex relationship between these neurotransmitters, bowel motility, visceral sensitivity, and the enteric and CNS.

Although psychiatric factors are not considered to be the major cause of IBS, there is abundant evidence that psychological disorders are more common in individuals with IBS who seek medical attention when compared to either the general population or to medical control patients such as those with IBD. The incidences of major depression, somatization disorder, generalized anxiety disorder, phobias, and panic disorder are higher in IBS patients than in healthy controls.[43] Psychological stress can alter motor function of the small bowel and colon, both in normal subjects as well as in patients with IBS. Stress triggers symptoms in many patients. A history of abuse during childhood (physical, sexual, or both) correlates with the severity of symptoms in patients with IBS.[44]

Alteration of the gut flora may be important in IBS. Patients with IBS may have a high prevalence of small intestinal bacterial overgrowth. In one study, 78% of IBS patients had bacterial overgrowth (as diagnosed indirectly by lactulose hydrogen breath test), and a small number of these patients reported improvement in Rome criteria symptoms following antibiotic treatment.[45] The results of this in similar studies warrant further investigation since lactulose breath tests may be falsely positive in conditions of rapid intestinal transit.

Recently, a role for infection in the genesis of IBS has been suggested. In a subset of cases, the development of IBS is related to antecedent GI infection. Several studies report persistent abnormal bowel function in 20% to 25% of patients for 6 or more months following bacterial gastroenteritis.[46,47] In patients with postgastroenteritis bowel dysfunction, the persistence of ongoing inflammation is suggested by increases in ileal and cecal mast cells, CD3 lymphocytes in the lamina propria, colonic enterochromaffin cells, and intraepithelial lymphocytes.[47] The cause of persistent or new altered bowel symptoms following an acute infection is unknown. Proposed theories include the association of persistent symptoms with more severe illness, reflecting the degree to which the pathogen invades the mucosa and changes in gut permeability due to increases in enteroendocrine cells.

Other factors that may contribute to existing symptoms of IBS may include malabsorption or intolerance to certain foods, elevated levels of short chain fatty acids in the stool, the development of bile acid malabsorption,[48] hormonal factors, and genetic factors. Hormonal factors may be responsible for the increased prevalence of IBS in women. Diarrhea, constipation, and abdominal discomfort increase just before and during menses.[49] Family members of patients with IBS often report altered bowel function, suggesting a genetic predisposition. Hereditary and environmental factors likely have a contributory role. In one study involving 6060 twin pairs, concordance for IBS was significantly greater in monozygotic (17.2%) than in dizygotic (8.4%) twins, supporting a role for genetic contribution to IBS.[50]

Diagnostic Approach

An appropriate diagnostic algorithm involves a cost-effective approach to identify symptoms consistent with IBS and the exclusion of other conditions having a similar clinical presentation (Table 17-2). The diagnosis of IBS begins with a thorough history, physical examination, and appropriate laboratory testing. A careful assessment of the patient's symptoms must be obtained, including a dietary history to identify factors and medications that may contribute to the symptoms of IBS such as sorbitol, lactose, caffeine, fatty foods, cruciferous vegetables, magnesium-containing products (which may cause diarrhea), calcium channel blockers, anticholinergics, and iron (which may cause constipation). Because a patient's definition of diarrhea and constipation may be different than the textbook definition, it is important to elicit a thorough history of the consistency, frequency, and volume of a patient's stools.

Patients aged <50 years should undergo the following laboratory studies: complete blood count, serum electrolytes, liver function tests, thyroid-stimulating hormone, guaiac stool testing, fecal leukocytes, ova, parasites, and *Giardia* antigen (in a patient with diarrhea).[5]

Table 17-2

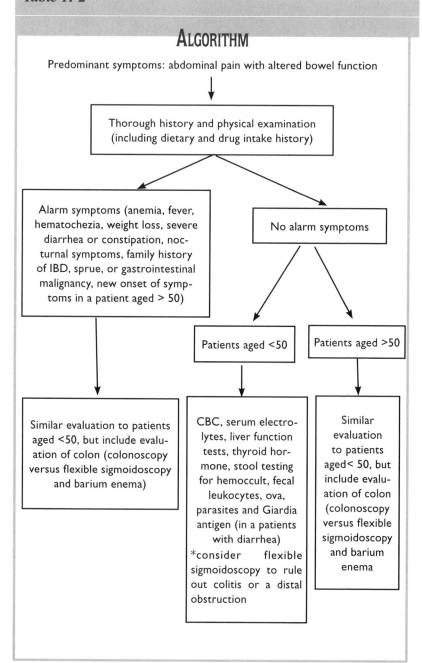

ALGORITHM

Predominant symptoms: abdominal pain with altered bowel function

Thorough history and physical examination
(including dietary and drug intake history)

Alarm symptoms (anemia, fever, hematochezia, weight loss, severe diarrhea or constipation, nocturnal symptoms, family history of IBD, sprue, or gastrointestinal malignancy, new onset of symptoms in a patient aged > 50)

No alarm symptoms

Patients aged <50

Patients aged >50

Similar evaluation to patients aged <50, but include evaluation of colon (colonoscopy versus flexible sigmoidoscopy and barium enema)

CBC, serum electrolytes, liver function tests, thyroid hormone, stool testing for hemoccult, fecal leukocytes, ova, parasites and Giardia antigen (in a patients with diarrhea)
*consider   flexible sigmoidoscopy to rule out colitis or a distal obstruction

Similar evaluation to patients aged< 50, but include evaluation of colon (colonoscopy versus flexible sigmoidoscopy and barium enema

A flexible sigmoidoscopy with biopsy may be considered to rule out colitis if diarrhea is present or a distal obstruction if constipation exists. In patients aged >50, a similar diagnostic evaluation should be performed with evaluation of the entire colon to rule out a colonic malignancy. This focused diagnostic approach excludes organic disease in over 95% of patients.[51,52] In the majority of cases, there are no abnormalities on physical examination or laboratory studies and findings suggestive of a structural disorder are not present.

If alarm symptoms are present (see Table 17-2), a more extensive investigation is indicated. Other disorders that may mimic IBS and should be excluded include lactase deficiency and other disorders of malabsorption, colon cancer, diverticulitis, IBD, mechanical obstruction of the small bowel or colon, enteric infection, ischemia, and gynecologic disorders such as dysmenorrhea or endometriosis.

Treatment

The comprehensive treatment of IBS involves patient education and reassurance, dietary modification, symptomatic treatment with medications, and/or psychologic intervention if indicated. Traditionally, practitioners have focused their efforts on treating the individual symptoms of IBS with multiple medications. As more information has become available providing insight into the pathophysiology of IBS, pharmacologic interventions have been developed to target more than one symptom of this disorder.

PATIENT EDUCATION

Once a diagnosis of IBS has been made, it is important to reassure and educate patients about the diagnosis. Patients should be encouraged to become active participants in the management of their symptoms. A trusting physician-patient relationship must be established in order to maximize the efficacy of treatment.

DIETARY MODIFICATION

A trial of dietary modification is a reasonable first choice in the treatment of IBS. Patients should be encouraged to keep a diary of food intake and symptoms allowing the identification and exclusion of symptom-causing foods.[53] Dietary modification may be useful since most IBS patients complain of symptom exacerbation after intake of certain food groups. Some patients may benefit from avoiding or limiting intake of caffeine, alcohol, fatty foods, gas-producing vegetables, and/or sorbitol-containing products such as sugarless gum and dietetic candy. In patients with diarrhea, a trial of a lactose-free diet should be instituted in the event of a concomitant lactase deficiency. Avoiding constipating foods and the addition of fiber either in the diet or in the form of supplements such as bran, polycarbophil, or a psyllium derivative equal to 20 to 30 grams per day may be helpful in treating patients with constipation. Fiber supplements have properties that should be beneficial in treating the altered bowel habits of IBS patients, including promoting water retention, helping to bulk the stool, and binding bile acids. Fiber is unlikely to provide relief in patients with symptoms of bloating and normal stool frequency as well as those with very slow colonic transit (>5 days between bowel movements).[54]

Table 17-3

MEDICATIONS FOR THE TREATMENT OF DIARRHEA/CONSTIPATION IN IRRITABLE BOWEL SYNDROME

Drug	Dose
Antidiarrheals	
Loperamide	4 mg/day orally up to 8 mg/day in single/divided doses
Diphenoxylate (2.5 mg) plus atropine sulfate (0.025 mg) (Lomotil [Pfizer Inc, Cambridge, Mass])	2 tabs orally QID
Cholestyramine resin	1 packet with fluid orally QD to BID
Antibiotics for bacterial overgrowth (rifaximin or ciprofloxacin and metronidazole)	Treat for 10 days
Probiotics (VSL #3)	1 packet with fluid QD to BID
Osmotic Laxatives	
Lactulose/sorbitol	10 mg/15 mL of syrup; 15-30 mL/day orally, titrate as needed
Polyethylene glycol solution	17 g dissolved in 240 mL (8 oz) of water orally daily
Milk of magnesia	15 to 30 mL/day orally as needed

MEDICATIONS

Medications for the treatment of IBS are chosen based on the patient's predominant symptoms. The treatment of diarrhea can be approached in a variety of ways (Table 17-3). Although not supported in randomized clinical trials, the use of low doses of fiber can occasionally help to reduce the frequency of bowel movements. Antidiarrheal agents include peripherally-acting opiate analogues such as loperamide and diphenoxylate. These agents stimulate receptors in the enteric nervous system, causing the inhibition of peristalsis and a decrease in fluid secretion. Loperamide decreases stool frequency and urgency and improves stool consistency.[55] It is the preferred agent because it lacks an anticholinergic component. Other agents used for IBS patients with diarrhea include bile acid binding resins and antibiotics. In refractory cases of uncontrolled diarrhea, cholestyramine may bind bile acids that may be responsible for increased colonic secretion and decreased colonic absorption of water.[56] Recent studies implicating an alteration of the intestinal bacterial flora as a pathogenic factor in the development of IBS have prompted investigations of therapy targeted toward reconstitution of the normal gut flora. In some cases, a short course of antibiotics may be tried in the hope of reducing refractory diarrhea by altering the intestinal bacterial flora.[45]

Probiotics are mixtures of bacteria and fungi thought to have efficacy in the treatment of some bowel disorders when an alteration of the normal gut flora appears to be a causative mechanism. There has been one randomized, placebo-controlled trial of the probiotic VSL #3 in diarrhea-predominant IBS. Although this study showed no change in gut transit time, global relief scores, abdominal pain, or bowel dysfunction, there was a significant reduction in bloating.[57] Other probiotic formulations have been evaluated as therapeutic agents in the treatment of IBS and may yield promising results.

For patients with IBS and constipation, the addition of supplemental fiber may help to normalize bowel movements and alleviate related symptoms such as tenesmus, dyschezia, and abdominal pain (see Table 17-3). There are numerous fiber supplements available over the counter; the decision regarding which one to choose depends primarily on the patient's preference (eg, liquid, capsule, or wafer). It is important to instruct the patient to consume adequate amounts of water with the fiber in order to avoid potential side effects.

Osmotic laxatives are often used in patients with constipation-predominant IBS who do not respond to therapy with fiber and can be used safely and indefinitely (see Table 17-3). Polyethylene glycol solutions have been shown to increase stool frequency and accelerate colonic transit in patients with slow transit constipation.[58] Other agents include lactulose, sorbitol, magnesium salts, and phosphate salts. Nonabsorbed carbohydrates such as sorbitol and lactulose may promote gas formation, which can cause discomfort. Long-term use of stimulant laxatives is not recommended because they have the theoretical potential to cause damage to enteric neurons and are associated with tachyphylaxis and dependency.

Antispasmodic medications are the most commonly prescribed drugs for IBS and are indicated in those patients in whom the predominant symptom is pain (Table 17-4). Antispasmodics may reduce abdominal pain via anticholinergic pathways or by direct relaxation of smooth muscle as with the use of nitrates and calcium channel blockers. The latter two therapies may cause unintentional hypotension and are, therefore, rarely prescribed for IBS. Anticholinergics act by the antagonism of muscarinic receptors innervated by the parasympathetic nervous system. In addition to the desired effect of relaxation of visceral smooth muscle, undesired effects such as sedation, salivary hyposecretion, and urinary retention can occur, limiting their use. Clinical trials of the anticholinergic medications in the United States have been suboptimal and are, therefore, difficult to evaluate. Although antispasmodic agents have been shown to reduce pain and decrease global symptoms,two recent meta-analyses show that they have no effect on symptoms of diarrhea and constipation.[59,60] Currently, 6 antispasmodic/anticholinergic agents are available for use in the United States: dicyclomine (Bentyl), hyoscyamine sulfate (Levsin [Schwarz Pharma, Inc, Milwaukee, Wis], NuLev [Schwarz Pharma, Inc, Milwaukee, Wis], IBS Stat), methscopolamine bromide (Pamine [Bradley Pharmaceuticals, Fairfield, NJ]), glycopyrrolate (Robinul), clidinium bromide chlordioxipoxide (Librax [F. Hoffmann-La Roche Ltd, Basel, Switzerland]), and belladonna with phenobarbital (Donnatal [PBM Pharmaceuticals, Gordonsville, NJ]).

The use of psychotropic medications has become popular in the treatment of functional bowel disorders, especially IBS (see Table 17-4). Both the tricyclic antide-

Table 17-4

MEDICATIONS FOR THE TREATMENT OF
PAIN IN IRRITABLE BOWEL SYNDROME

Drug	Dose
Anticholinergics/Antispasmodics	
Dicyclomine (Bentyl)	10 mg every 6 hours up to 40 mg every 6 hours if tolerated
Hyoscyamine (Levsin)	0.125 to 0.25 mg orally every 4 to 6 hours
(Levsin SL, Nulev)	0.125 to 0.25 mg sublingual every 4 to 6 hours
(Levinex, Levbid [Schwarz Pharma, Inc, Milwaukee, Wis])	0.375 to 0.750 mg orally every 12 hours
(IBS Stat)	1 to 2 sprays (1 to 2 mL) orally every 4 to 6 hours
Methscopolamine bromide (Pamine)	2.5 to 5 mg every 4 to 6 hours
Glycopyrrolate (Robinul)	1 mg orally TID
Clidinium bromide	
Chlordioxipoxide (Librax)	1 cap orally TID to QID
Belladonna with phenobarbital (Donnatal)	1 to 2 tabs/caps orally TID to QID Extended release: 1 tab orally every 8 to 12 hours
Tricyclic Compounds	
Nortriptyline (Pamelor)	10 to 75 mg/day
Desipramine (Norpramin)	10 to 75 mg/day
Selective Serotonin Reuptake Inhibitors	
Fluoxetine (Prozac)	20 to 80 mg/day
Paroxetine (Paxil)	20 to 50 mg/day

pressant medications (TCA) as well as the SSRIs can be utilized in IBS; however, the TCA medications have been more extensively evaluated for this purpose and may be more efficacious.

When choosing an antidepressant for therapy, the side effect profile should be utilized to the patient's advantage. In IBS patients with diarrhea, a TCA would be more appropriate given its side effect of constipation. Conversely, an SSRI should be chosen in IBS patients with constipation. When choosing a specific TCA, secondary amines should be used preferentially over tertiary amines because they have less overall side effects (nortriptyline [Pamelor {Mallinckrodt, Hazelwood, Mo}] instead of its

Table 17-5

5HT-RECEPTOR AGONISTS/ANTAGONISTS

Drug	Dose
IBS With Diarrhea	
Alosetron (Lotronex)	Starting dose 1 mg orally QD for 4 weeks increasing to 1 mg BID if tolerated/needed
IBS With Constipation	
Tegaserod (Zelnorm)	6 mg orally BID before meals

precursor amitriptyline [Elavil] or desipramine [Norpramin] instead of imipramine [Tofranil]). Low doses of the TCAs between 10 and 25 mg are used initially with the maximum benefit usually occurring at a dose of 50 mg each day. In addition, patients should be counseled that these medications are being used for pain modulation and not for the purpose of treating depression.

Little data are currently available about the SSRI antidepressant medications. However, preliminary studies have suggested possible efficacy with the use of paroxetine (Paxil [GlaxoSmithKlinie, Philadelphia, Pa]),[61] fluoxetine (Prozac [Eli Lilly and Company, Indianapolis, Ind]), and citalopam.[62] Standard antidepressant doses of these SSRI medications may be necessary. Preliminary evidence suggests that the use of naloxone, an opioid receptor antagonist, may be useful in the treatment of pain in IBS patients with constipation but larger scale studies are required before this recommendation can be made.[63] As will be discussed below, the 5HT-receptor agonists and antagonists can also be used in the proper circumstances for the treatment of pain.

The 5HT3-receptor antagonist alosetron (Lotronex [GlaxoSmithKline, Philadelphia, Pa]) has been shown to be effective in the treatment of women with IBS and diarrhea (Table 17-5). In clinical trials, alosetron was shown to improve stool frequency, stool consistency, and fecal urgency, as well as to significantly reduce abdominal pain.[64] Unfortunately, adverse reactions, such as severe constipation, ischemic colitis, and bowel perforation caused temporary withdrawal of alosetron from use; however, in June 2002, the FDA approved restricted marketing of alosetron for the treatment of women with severe, diarrhea-predominant IBS who have failed to respond to conventional IBS therapy. The starting dose is 1 mg QD for 4 weeks. If the patient experiences only partial relief after 4 weeks, the dose is increased to 1 mg BID. If there is no relief of symptoms after 4 weeks, the medication should be discontinued. Only physicians experienced in diagnosing and treating IBS patients are permitted to prescribe alosetron, and informed consent must be obtained from the patient prior to initiating therapy. Patients must be instructed to discontinue the medication and contact their physician if constipation or worsening abdominal pain occurs. Despite these restrictions, alosetron can be a very effective therapy in the appropriate patient.

Patients with IBS and constipation can be treated with the 5-HT4 agonist, tegaserod (Zelnorm [Novartis Pharmaceuticals USA, East Hanover, NJ]). Tegaserod is approved for the treatment of women with IBS whose primary bowel symptom is constipation. It is also approved in patients with chronic constipation. In clinical trials, tegaserod has been shown to accelerate colon and small intestine transit, increase the frequency of bowel movements, increase the softness of stools, decrease abdominal pain, reduce bloating, and improve patients' overall satisfaction with bowel habits.[65] Diarrhea and headache are the most common adverse events associated with the use of tegaserod (9% and 15%, respectively). Ischemic colitis has been reported in IBS patients taking tegaserod; however, the prevalence is lower than in IBS patients who are not taking tegaserod. ECG changes have not been seen with the use of tegaserod. The recommended dosage is 6 mg orally twice daily before breakfast and dinner (see Table 17-5). Renzapride, a 5HT4 receptor full agonist/5HT3 receptor antagonist, is currently under investigation for the treatment of IBS with constipation and has been shown to accelerate colon transit.[66]

Patients with IBS who actively seek care by a physician have a high incidence of psychological disorders, specifically depression and anxiety. A variety of psychological interventions have been utilized to treat the symptoms of IBS. Despite methodological flaws in most studies, there are some data to support the use of relaxation exercises, biofeedback, cognitive therapy, hypnotherapy, and psychotherapy.[67] The IBS-related symptoms most likely to respond to psychological intervention include abdominal pain and diarrhea. The factors influencing the choice between behavioral therapy include the availability of a skilled, interested therapist; patient preference; and cost.

Summary

IBS is a prevalent functional GI disorder of multifactorial pathogenesis, including abnormalities in GI motility, the enteric and CNS, as well as psychological function. Effective treatment of IBS includes an increased understanding of the pathophysiology of this disorder. It is a common disorder that accounts for a disproportionate share of health care costs. The advent of serotonin receptor agonists and antagonists allows treatment to be approached in a more global manner by addressing the multiple symptoms of IBS with a single therapeutic agent. A careful, concise diagnostic evaluation combined with the prompt institution of symptom-guided therapy can help improve the quality of life of patients who suffer from IBS.

References

1. Thompson WG, Longstreth GF, Drossman DA, et al. Functional bowel disorders and functional abdominal pain. *Gut.* 1999;45:1143-1147.
2. Brandt LJ, Bjorkman D, Fennerty MB, et al. Systematic review on the management of irritable bowel syndrome in North America. *Am J Gastroenterol.* 2002;97:S7-S26.
3. Drossman DA, Andruzzi E, Temple RD, et al. U.S. householder survey of functional gastrointestinal disorders: prevalence, sociodemography, and health impact. *Dig Dis Sci.* 1993;38:1569-1580.
4. Everhart JE, Renault PF. Irritable bowel syndrome in an office-based practice in the United States. *Gastroenterology.* 1991;100:998-1005.
5. Drossman DA, Whitehead WE, Camilleri M. Irritable bowel syndrome: a technical review for practice guideline development. *Gastroenterology.* 1997;112:2120-2137.

6. Jones R, Lydeard S. Irritable bowel syndrome in the general population. *BMJ.* 1992;304:87.

7. Heaton KW, O'Donnell LJ, Braddon FEM, et al. Symptoms of irritable bowel syndrome in a British urban community: consulters and nonconsulters. *Gastroenterology.* 1992;102:1962.

8. Drossman DA, Creed FH, Fava GA, et al. Psychosocial aspects of the functional gastrointestinal disorders. *Gastroenterol Int.* 1995;8:47-90.

9. Sandler RS, Everhart JE, Donwitz M, et al. The burden of selected digestive diseases in the United States. *Gastroenterology.* 2002;122:1500.

10. Lynn RB, Friedman LS. Irritable bowel syndrome. *N Engl J Med.* 1993;329:1940.

11. Swarbrick ET, Bat L, Hegarty JE, et al. Site of pain from the irritable bowel. *Lancet.* 1980;2:443.

12. Kennedy TM, Jones RH, Hungin AP, et al. Irritable bowel syndrome, gastroesophageal reflux, and bronchial hyper-responsiveness in the general population. *Gut.* 1998;43:770-774.

13. Schmulson M, Lee OY, Chang L, et al. Symptom differences in moderate to severe IBS patients based on predominant bowel habit. *Am J Gastroenterol.* 1999;94:2929-2935.

14. Sperber AD, Atzmon Y, Neumann L, et al. Fibromyalgia in the irritable bowel syndrome: studies of prevalence and clinical implications. *Am J Gastroenterol.* 1999; 94:3541-3546.

15. Kellow JE, Eckersley GM, Jones M. Enteric and central contributions to intestinal dysmotility in irritable bowel syndrome. *Dig Dis Sci.* 1992;37:168.

16. Rogers J, Henry MM, Misiewicz JJ. Increased segmental activity and intraluminal pressures in the sigmoid colon of patients with the irritable bowel syndrome. *Gut.* 1989;30:634-641.

17. Kellow JE, Phillips SF. Altered small bowel motility in irritable bowel syndrome is correlated with symptoms. *Gastroenterology.* 1987;92:1885-1893.

18. McKee DP, Quigley EM. Intestinal motility in irritable bowel syndrome: is IBS a motility disorder? 1. definition of IBS and colonic motility. *Dig Dis Sci.* 1993;38:1761-1772.

19. Almy TP. Experimental studies on the irritable colon. *Am J Med.* 1951;10:60-67.

20. Snape WJ Jr, Carlson GM, Matarazzo SA, et al. Evidence that abnormal myoelectrical activity produces colonic motor dysfunction in the irritable bowel syndrome. *Gastroenterology.* 1977;72:383-387.

21. Jepsen JM, Skoubo-Kristensen E, Elsborg L. Rectosigmoid motility response to sham feeding in irritable bowel syndrome: evidence of a cephalic phase. *Scand J Gastroenterol.* 1989;24:53.

22. Chey WY, Jin HO, Lee MH, et al. Colonic motility abnormality in patients with irritable bowel syndrome exhibiting abdominal pain and diarrhea. *Am J Gastroenterol.* 2001;96:1499-1506.

23. Fukudo S, Nomura T, Hongo M. Impact of corticotropin-releasing hormone on gastrointestinal motility and adenocorticotropic hormone in normal controls and patients with irritable bowel syndrome. *Gut.* 1998;42:845-849.

24. Cann PA, Read NW, Brown C, et al. Irritable bowel syndrome: relationship of disorders in the transit of a single solid meal to symptom patterns. *Gut.* 1983;24:405-411.

25. Lu CL, Chen CY, Chang FY, et al. Characteristics of small bowel motility in patients with irritable bowel syndrome and normal humans: an Oriental study. *Chinese Science.* 1998;95:165-169.

26. Vassallo MJ, Camilleri M, Phillips SF, et al. Colonic tone and motility in patients with irritable bowel syndrome. *Mayo Clinic Proc.* 1992;67:725-731.

27. Lasser RB, Bond JH, Levitt MD. The role of intestinal gas in functional abdominal pain. *N Engl J Med.* 1975;293:524-526.

28. Serra J, Azpiroz F, Malagelada JR. Impaired transit and tolerance of intestinal gas in the irritable bowel syndrome. *Gut.* 2001;48:14-19.

29. Whitehead WE, Engel BT, Schuster MM. Irritable bowel syndrome: physiological and psychological differences between diarrhea-predominant and constipation-predominant patterns. *Dig Dis Sci.* 1980;25:404-413.

30. Kellow JE, Phillips SF, Miller LJ, et al. Dysmotility of the small intestine in irritable bowel syndrome. *Gut.* 1988;29:1236-1243.

31. Kellow JE, Eckersley GM, Jones MP. Enhanced perception of physiological intestinal motility in the irritable bowel syndrome. *Gastroenterology.* 1991;101:1621.

32. Ringel Y, Drossman DA, Turkington TG, et al. Dysfunction of the motivational-affective pain system in patients with IBS: PET brain imaging in response to rectal balloon distention. *Gastroenterology.* 2000;118 (Suppl):A444.

33. Silverman DHS, Munakata JA, Ennes H, et al. Regional cerebral activity in normal and pathological perception of visceral pain. *Gastroenterology.* 1997;112:64-72.

34. Bonaz BL, Papillon E, Baciu M, et al. Central processing of rectal pain in IBS patients: an fMRI study. *Gastroenterology.* 2000;118(Suppl):A615.

35. Mertz H, Morgan V, Tanner G, et al. Regional cerebral activation in irritable bowel syndrome and control subjects with painful and nonpainful rectal distention. *Gastroenterology.* 2000;118:842-848.

36. Bueno L, Fioramonti J, Garcia-Villar R. Pathobiology of visceral pain: molecular mechanisms and therapeutic implications. III. Visceral afferent pathways: a source of new therapeutic targets for abdominal pain. *Am J Physiol Gastrointest Liver Physiol.* 2000;278:G670.

37. Gershon MD. Roles played by 5-hydroxytryptamine in the physiology of the bowel. *Aliment Pharmacol Ther.* 1999;13(Suppl 2):15-30.

38. Bearcroft CP, Perrett D, Farthing MJ. Postprandial plasma 5-hydroxytryptamine in diarrhea predominant irritable bowel syndrome: a pilot study. *Gut.* 1998;42:42-46.

39. Bose M, Nickols C, Feakins R, et al. 5-hydroxytryptamine and enteroendocrine cells in the irritable bowel syndrome. Abstract. *Gastroenterology.* 2000;118:2949.

40. Bellini M, Rappelli L, Blandizzi C, et al. Platelet serotonin transporter in patients with diarrhea-predominant irritable bowel syndrome both before and after treatment with alosetron. *Am J Gastroenterol.* 2003;98:2705-2711.

41. Coates MD, Mahoney CR, Linden DR, et al. Molecular defects in mucosal serotonin content and decreased serotonin reuptake transporter in ulcerative colitis and irritable bowel syndrome. *Gastroenterology.* 2004;126(7):1657-1664.

42. Willert RP, Woolf CJ, Hobson AR, et al. The development and maintenance of human visceral pain hypersensitivity is dependent on the N-methyl-D-aspartate receptor. *Gastroenterology.* 2004;126:683.

43. Creed F, Guthrie E. Psychological factors in the irritable bowel syndrome. *Gut.* 1987;28:1307-1318.

44. Drossman DA. Sexual and physical abuse and gastrointestinal illness. *Scand J Gastroenterol Suppl.* 1995;208:90-96.

45. Pimentel M, Chow EJ, Lin HC. Eradication of small intestinal bacterial overgrowth reduces symptoms of irritable bowel syndrome. *Am J Gastroenterol.* 2000;95:3503-3506.

46. Gwee KA, Graham JC, McKendrick MW, et al. Psychometric scores and persistence of irritable bowel after infectious diarrhea. *Lancet.* 1996;347:150-153.

47. Spiller RC, Jenkins D, Thornley JP, et al. Increased rectal mucosal enteroendocrine cells, T lymphocytes, and increased gut permeability following acute campylobacter enteritis and in post-dysenteric irritable bowel syndrome. *Gut.* 2000;47:804-811.

48. Niaz SK, Sandrasegaran K, Renny FH, et al. Postinfective diarrhea and bile acid malabsorption. *Journal of Royal College of Physicians Lond.* 1997;31:53.

49. Kane SV, Sable K, Hanauer SB. The menstrual cycle and its effect on inflammatory bowel disease and irritable bowel syndrome: a prevalence study. *Am J Gastroenterol.* 1998;93:1867-1872.

50. Levy RL, Jones KR, Whitehead WE, et al. Irritable bowel syndrome in twins: heredity and social learning both contribute to etiology. *Gastroenterology.* 2001;121:799.

51. Schmulson MW, Chang L. Diagnostic approach to the patient with irritable bowel syndrome. *Am J Med.* 1999;107:20 S.

52. Svendsen JH, Munck LK, Andersen JR. Irritable bowel syndrome—prognosis and diagnostic safety. A 5-year follow-up study. *Scand J Gastroenterol.* 1985;20:415.

53. Horwitz BJ, Fisher RS. The irritable bowel syndrome. *N Engl J Med.* 2001;344:1846-1850.

54. Mertz HR. Irritable bowel syndrome. *N Engl J Med.* 2003;349:2136-2146.

55. Cann PA, Read NW, Holdsworth CD, et al. Role of loperamide and placebo in management of irritable bowel syndrome (IBS). *Dig Dis Sci.* 1984;29:239-247.

56. Sciarretta G, Fagioli G, Furno A, et al. 75Se HCAT test in the detection of bile acid malabsorption in functional diarrhea and its correlation with small bowel transit. *Gut.* 1987;28:970-975.

57. Kim HJ, Camilleri M, McKinzie S, et al. A randomized-controlled trial of a probiotic, VSL #3, on gut transit and symptoms in diarrhea-predominant irritable bowel syndrome. *Aliment Pharmacol Ther.* 2003;17(7):895-904.

58. Cleveland MV, Flavin DP, Ruben RA, et al. New polyethylene glycol laxative for treatment of constipation in adults: a randomized, double-blind, placebo-controlled study. *South Med J.* 2001;94:478-481.

59. Poynard T, Regimbeau C, Benhamou Y. Meta-analysis of smooth muscle relaxants in the treatment of irritable bowel syndrome. *Aliment Pharmacol Ther.* 2001;15:355-361.

60. Jailwala J, Imperiale TF, Kroenke K. Pharmacologic treatment of the irritable bowel syndrome: a systematic review of randomized, controlled trials. *Ann Intern Med.* 2000;133:136-147.

61. Creed FH, Fernandes L, Guthne E, et al. The cost-effectiveness of psychotherapy and SSRI antidepressants for severe irritable bowel syndrome. *Gastroenterology.* 2001;120: A619.

62. Kurken SD, Burgers P, Tytgat GN, Boeckxstaens GE. Fluoxetine (prozac) for the treatment of irritable bowel syndrome: a randomized, controlled clinical trial. *Gastroenterology.* 2002;122:A551.

63. Hawkes ND, Rhodes J, Evans B. Naloxone treatment for irritable bowel syndrome—a pilot study. *Gastroenterology.* 2002;122:A552.

64. Camilleri M, Northcutt AR, Kong S, et al. Efficacy and safety of alosetron in women with irritable bowel syndrome: a randomized, placebo-controlled trial. *Lancet.* 2000;355:1035-1040.

65. Muller-Lissner SA, Fumigalli I, Bardhan KD, et al. Tegaserod, a 5-HT4 receptor partial agonist, relieves symptoms in irritable bowel syndrome patients with abdominal pain, bloating and constipation. *Aliment Pharmacol Ther.* 2001;15:1655-1666.

66. Camilleri M, McKinzie S, Fox J, et al. Effect of renzapride on transit in constipation-predominant irritable bowel syndrome. *Clin Gastroenterol Hepatol.* 2004;2:895-904.

67. Talley NJ, Owen BK, Boyce P, Patterson K. Psychological treatments for irritable bowel syndrome: a critique of controlled treatment trials. *Am J Gastroenterol.* 1996;91:277-286.

chapter 18

Evaluation and Management of Constipation

Benjamin Krevsky, MD, MPH

Constipation is a common, costly, and potentially dangerous condition that warrants careful consideration by clinicians. While epidemiologic studies vary greatly in the prevalence of constipation—from about 2% up to 30%—there is no doubt that many people are afflicted.[1-3] Accurate prevalence and incidence statistics are difficult to come by since a large number of patients self-treat themselves with dietary changes, over-the-counter medications, and food supplements. But one needs only to look at the size of the laxative aisle at a local drug or health food store to realize how many people are self-medicating and the cost of this problem. In addition, millions of people seek medical attention for constipation[2] and receive diagnostic workups and prescription medications, adding to the cost to society.

Beyond the direct cost to patients is the deterioration of quality of life attendant with constipation. Patients with functional GI disorders have higher than expected days lost from work and school. There is an increase in psychological disturbances.[4] Some patients become totally disabled.

Definition

To the patient, the definition of constipation is simple. Yet every patient's definition may be different. Self-reported symptoms may include stools that are too hard, too small, too infrequent, or too hard to expel. While some patients may have daily bowel movements, they clearly feel that they are constipated. It is the rare patient who reports constipation to the doctor, yet has none of these symptoms.

The traditional diagnostic criteria for constipation, and the one often used in clinical trials, is infrequent bowel movements. With the range of normal being about 3 bowel movements/week to 3 bowel movements/day, the definition was set at less than 3 spontaneous complete bowel movements/week. This is a difficult criterion to use clinically because many patients will not allow themselves to go that long without defecation. Others are clearly uncomfortable but are having more than 3 bowel movements/week.

A more practical approach to the definition of functional constipation is the use of the Rome II criteria.[5] The patient must have 2 of the following symptoms present for at least 12 weeks within the preceding year:

1. Straining >25% of the time.
2. Lumpy or hard stools >25% of defecations.
3. Sensation of incomplete evacuation >25% of defecations.
4. Sensation of anal blockage or obstruction >25% of defecations.
5. Manual maneuvers necessary to facilitate >25% of defecations.
6. Less than 3 spontaneous bowel movements/week.

It should be noticed that pain is not a component of the diagnostic criteria. In fact, the criteria for IBS should not be present to make the diagnosis of functional constipation.

Etiology of Constipation

There are many causes of constipation, including systemic, GI, and neurogenic diseases (Table 18-1).[1,2,6-10] Another large group of patients is constipated because of drugs that they are using. Finally, there are the small group of patients with misperception and the larger, often seriously ill group of patients with idiopathic constipation.

Commonly used drugs cause much of the constipation seen in clinical practice (Table 18-2). Although the classic group is the opioid analgesics such as codeine, oxycodone, and morphine,[11] many other classes of pharmaceutical agents can cause constipation. These include anticholinergics, antacids, iron supplements, neurally active agents, diuretics, antidiarrheals, and calcium supplements. Anticholinergics, like the opioids, cause constipation by slowing transit. Diuretics cause constipation by reducing the water available to hydrate the stool.

Systemic disorders associated with constipation include hypothyroidism, hyperparathyroidism, and diabetes, among others (see Table 18-1). It is important to recognize these potential causes in the evaluation of patients.

GI causes include obstruction of the GI tract, such as colon cancer obstructing the ascending colon or tuberculosis occluding the terminal ileum. Anorectal disorders, such as herpes, syphilis, and anal fissures, can cause constipation by causing so much pain that the patient is afraid to defecate.

Many neurological disorders can induce constipation and are generally divided between the central and peripheral categories. Among the most common problem of the peripheral type is the autonomic neuropathy seen in type I diabetics. Other peripheral causes include Hirschsprung's disease, Chagas' disease, and intestinal pseudo-obstruction. Central causes can include neurosyphilis, multiple sclerosis,[12,13] head trauma, and Parkinson's disease.

Occasionally, there is a patient who presents with a complaint of constipation but who is not constipated by any standard criteria. This is the "misperception" group. Usually, they are having fewer than one bowel movement per day and have been told that "normal" bowel function is to have a daily bowel movement. If they do not meet Rome II criteria and are otherwise comfortable, education and reassurance are the solution.

Patients with idiopathic constipation are among the most difficult to manage. Of course, this is a diagnosis of exclusion, with the other etiologies already ruled out. This

Table 18-1

MAJOR CAUSES OF CONSTIPATION

- Drugs (see Table 18-2)
- Systemic
  - * Hypothyroidism
  - * Hyperparathyroidism
  - * Diabetes mellitus
  - * Pregnancy
  - * Porphyria
  - * Systemic sclerosis
  - * Myotonic dystrophy
  - * Heavy metal poisoning
  - * Amyloidosis
  - * Uremia
  - * Immobility
- Gastrointestinal
  - * UGI
  - * Organic obstruction (intra- or extraluminal)
  - * Abnormal muscle function
  - * Rectal disorders
  - * Anal problems (eg, fissure)
- Psychogenic
- Neurogenic
  - * Peripheral
    - † Hirschsprung's disease
    - † Autonomic neuropathy
    - † Spinal cord damage
    - † Chagas' disease
    - † Intestinal pseudo-obstruction
  - * Central
    - † Trauma
    - † Syphilis
    - † Multiple sclerosis
    - † Parkinson's disease
- Misperception
- Idiopathic
  - * IBS
  - * Normal transit constipation
  - * Colonic inertia
  - * Functional rectosigmoid obstruction (outlet delay)

Table 18-2

DRUGS ASSOCIATED WITH CONSTIPATION

Class	Examples
Analgesics	
Opioids	Oxycodone
NSAIDs	Ibuprofen
Anticholinergics	
Antispasmotics	Belladonna
Antidepressants	Amitriptyline
Antipsychotics	Chlorpromazine
Antiparkinsonian drugs	Amantadine
Antihistamines	Diphenhydramine
Antacids/ulcer therapy (cation-containing)	
Aluminum-containing antacids	Aluminum hydroxide
Cytoprotective agents	Sucralfate
Iron supplements	Iron sulfate
Neurally active agents	
Vinca alkaloids	Vincristine
Calcium channel blockers	Verapamil
5HT3 antagonists	Alosetron
Anticonvulsants	Phenytoin
Diuretics	Hydrochlorothiazide
Antidiarrheal agents	Loperamide
Calcium supplements	Calcium carbonate

cause includes 4 subgroups:

1. IBS-constipation subtype.
2. Normal transit constipation.
3. Colonic inertia (also known as slow transit constipation).
4. Functional rectosigmoid obstruction (also known as outlet delay), which includes pelvic floor dyssynergia.

Patients with constipation who meet the Rome II criteria for IBS may have the IBS-constipation subtype or IBS-alternating subtype. These patients have significant abdominal pain and are managed according to Chapter 17 on IBS.

The small group of patients with idiopathic or functional constipation who have normal transit fall into this group. These meet the Rome II criteria, but testing of transit comes out within normal parameters. These patients may have a sensory or psychosocial disorder.

Table 18-3

PREVENTION OF CONSTIPATION

Method	*Example*
Activity	Avoid long periods of recumbancy
Diet	High fiber content
Habit	Try to defecate each morning after breakfast
Facilities	Bedside commodes for poorly ambulating patients
Early treatment	Don't wait for an impaction

Colonic inertia is defined by the delayed passage of markers through the entire colon, but in particular the proximal colon. This group is defined through the use of radiopaque markers[14] or through scintigraphic techniques.[15-17]

Patients with functional rectosigmoid obstruction (FRSO, also called dyssynergic defecation or obstipated defecation) have normal transit through most of the colon, but the markers are retained for an abnormal period of time in the rectosigmoid region. This delay may be due to an organic abnormality such as Hirschsprung's Disease, anal fissure, rectal cancer, and the like. In patients without an organic cause, the delay can be due to abnormal muscle function in the colon or pelvic floor dyssynergia. The latter is an abnormality of relaxation (or paradoxical contraction) of the pelvic floor musculature during defecation. This appears to be an acquired abnormality and may be more of a habit than an organic problem.

Prevention

The best way to treat constipation is to prevent it in the first place (Table 18-3). Encourage patients to increase their physical activity and be sure to have a diet high in fiber.[18,19] Many patients find that having a regular habit helps (eg, taking advantage of the gastrocolic reflex and going to the bathroom after breakfast). Many patients have difficulty getting to a bathroom down the hall and therefore train themselves to ignore the urge to defecate. Prevent this by putting a commode at the bedside. Finally, don't wait for an impaction. Inquire about bowel function during patient visits and start treatment early.

Evaluation

As with other disorders, it is always useful to start with a comprehensive history (Table 18-4). Exactly what are the symptoms that need to be addressed? Is the problem getting started or not getting an urge to defecate in the first place? Are the stools hard to pass? Is there pain associated with the constipation? Questions about the onset and chronicity will give clues as to the etiology. Often, the onset is associated with a life event that changes eating habits or activity level. Take a careful drug history because many agents are associated with constipation. Finally, a review of past medical history

Table 18-4

INITIAL EVALUATION

- History
  - * Chronicity
  - * Onset
  - * Drug use
  - * Systemic disorders
- Physical Examination
  - * Cutaneous sensations
  - * Anal tone and rectal movement
  - * ? fecal discharge
  - * Impaction
- Colonoscopy (or barium enema)
- Blood Tests
  - * Thyroid function
  - * Calcium
  - * Phosphorus
  - * Glucose
  - * CBC

and medication use may implicate a systemic disorder as the cause of the constipation.

Physical examination for constipation is limited. Palpate the abdomen for masses or tenderness. Sometimes impacted stool may feel like a mass. Check the deep tendon reflexes for hyporeflexia (hypothyroidism). The digital rectal exam can be very helpful. First, check for cutaneous sensation, its absence infers a neurological problem. Determine if anal tone is normal. Ask the patient to strain (try to defecate) with the finger in the anal canal. The finger should move posteriorly with straining as the puborectalis muscle relaxes. If the finger moves forward, pelvic floor dyssynergia should be suspected. If there is a large discharge of feces upon removal of the finger, Hirschsprung's disease may be the cause. Palpate for ulcers, fissures, stenoses, and masses. Finally, determine if an impaction is present, for this must be dealt with first before any further diagnostics or therapeutics can be initiated.

To rule out a mechanical obstruction of the colon, whether intrinsic (colon cancer, stricture, etc) or extrinsic (lymphoma, uterine mass, etc), the colon should be imaged. In most cases this means a colonoscopy, but in selected cases an air contrast barium enema will suffice. While many practitioners reserve colonoscopy for patients over 50, it should be remembered that cancer can occur at much younger ages. When other signs such as weight loss, anemia, Hemoccult (+) stool, or a mass are present, colonoscopy would be indicated in a much younger patient.

Table 18-5

ADDITIONAL STUDIES FOR THE EVALUATION OF CONSTIPATION

Test	Information Obtained
Anorectal manometry	Rectal sensation, internal anal relaxation
Colonic transit testing	Identifies normal and slow (regional) transit
Radiopaque markers	Inexpensive, qualitative
Colonic transit scintigraphy	Expensive, quantitative
Fecal defecography	Anatomical and functional abnormalities
Balloon expulsion test	Functional outlet obstruction
Rectal biopsy	Confirms Hirschsprung's disease
Anal endosonography	Identifies anatomical abnormalities
Colonic manometry	Motility evaluation (experimental)
Pelvic floor electromyography	Identifies pelvic floor dysfunction
Whole gut transit and/or UGI manometry	Colonic or entire gut malfunctioning
Rectal scintigraphy	Nuclear medicine version of defecography

A basic set of blood tests will help rule out the systemic disorders. These would include a CBC, thyroid panel, and chemistry panel, including glucose, phosphorous, and calcium. The CBC may indicate enteric blood loss, the thyroid panel hypothyroidism, the glucose diabetes, and the calcium/phosphorous hyperparathyroidism.

At this stage, assuming that a provisional diagnosis has been made and serious disorders such as colon cancer eliminated, a therapeutic trial of 20 to 30 g of fiber per day can begin. But if the trial is unsuccessful or the diagnosis seems elusive or inconclusive, further testing is indicated (Table 18-5). These tests take the form of motility tests, transit tests, and physiologic testing.

The first test obtained at this point is anal manometry.[20-22] This test can provide useful information on rectal sensation, anal pressure (tone), and presence of the rectoanal inhibitory reflex (Figure 18-1). A thin catheter with either ports for measuring pressure (low compliance pneumohydraulic system) or electronic pressure transducers is introduced into the rectum. A small balloon at the tip of the assembly simulates the arrival of fecal material into the rectum. After a "pull through" to measure resting tone of the internal and external anal sphincter, the pressure ports are repositioned to measure sphincter pressures. Then the rectal balloon is inflated stepwise to determine the rectal sensory threshold. Also measured are the presence and completeness of internal anal sphincter relaxation (Figure 18-2) and external sphincter contraction in response to balloon distention. Abnormalities can suggest pelvic floor dyssynergia, Hirschsprung's disease, etc.

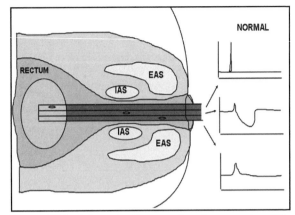

Figure 18-1. Schematic diagram of anal manometry. IAS= internal anal sphincter, EAS = external anal sphincter. A thin multi-lumen catheter is inserted into the anal canal, with a balloon at the tip, which is located in the rectum. Pressure ports are shown adjacent to the IAS and EAS. The normal response to balloon distension (simulating fecal arrival) is shown in the series of graphs on the right side of the figure. The top graph shows the increase in pressure with inflation of the balloon. The middle graph represents a typical IAS response (ie, an initial increase in pressure followed by a reflex relaxation) and then recovery. The bottom graph shows the EAS response to balloon distension. An increase in EAS pressure maintains continence when the IAS relaxes during fecal arrival.

Colonic transit testing is performed with radiopaque markers[14] or using scintigraphic techniques.[15,16,23,24] In the marker test, the patient swallows a capsule containing 24 small radiopaque plastic markers. Five days later, an abdominal x-ray is taken, the markers counted, and their location described. Modifications of the test include the sequential ingestion of markers on 3 consecutive days, the use of different shaped markers, and the use of multiple x-rays. All these modifications are aimed at improving the accuracy of the test. This is a simple, inexpensive test. It would seem to be the most useful in the case of a normal study, indicating that transit is normal. However, because the colon is highly variable in shape and the markers are not physiologic, the results are not highly reliable. The scintigraphic technique uses In-111-DTPA in water as a marker and its progression is followed though the colon over several days utilizing a gamma camera (Figure 18-3). The marker outlines the colon and is quantifiable. Using a simple formula (geometric center), the overall progression of the marker can be quantitated. This is used to differentiate colonic inertia from functional rectosigmoid obstruction (Figure 18-4). Variations on the test include the peroral intubation of the cecum (original method), ingestion of a dual labeled meal, and the use of a delayed release capsule. The advantage of the dual label meal is that gastric emptying for solids and liquids, small intestinal transit, and colonic transit can all be measured during the same test (see Figure 18-3).

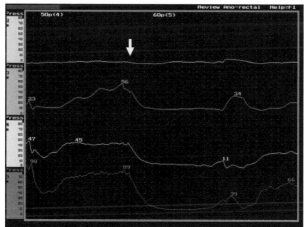

Figure 18-2. Actual tracing of a 4-channel recording during anal manometry in a normal individual. Channel numbers are on the left side, and actual pressures in mmHg are shown on the pressure tracings. Channel 2 is located in the rectum, with channels 3, 4, and 5 straddling the internal anal sphincter. When the rectal balloon is inflated (arrow), there is no response in the rectum, but a reflex relaxation of the internal anal sphincter occurs (rectoanal inhibitory reflex).

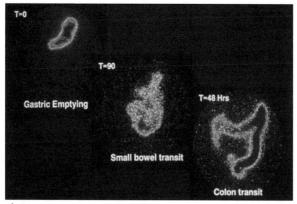

Figure 18-3. Scintigraphic images from a patient being evaluated with whole gut scintigraphy. After ingestion of the radiolabeled meal (T = 0) the stomach is outlined. Ninety minutes after ingestion (T = 90) most of the activity is in the small intestine. Forty-eight hours after ingestion, the activity is present in the colon, in this case primarily from the splenic flexure distally.

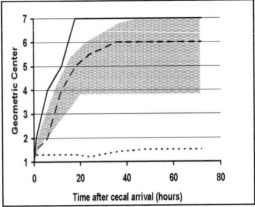

Figure 18-4. Quantitative analysis of several patients evaluated with colonic transit scintigraphy. The geometric center represents the center of activity of the radiolabel at any time point. This is calculated by first dividing the colon into 7 regions (1 = cecum and ascending colon, 2 = hepatic flexure, 3 = transverse colon, 4 = splenic flexure, 5 = descending colon, 6 = recto-sigmoid colon, and 7 = expelled feces). The geometric center is the sum of the fraction of activity in each region multiplied by the region number. The grey hatched area is the range of normal. The short dashed line shows the results in a patient with colonic inertia. The geometric center never gets higher than 1.5, indicating that the center of activity stayed in the cecum and ascending colon. The long dashed line shows the results in a patient with functional rectosigmoid obstruction. In this case, the progression was normal until the fecal material reached the recto-sigmoid. At that point, there was no progression for several days. The solid line shows the results in a surreptitious laxative abuser. The patient took laxatives immediately after ingestion of the labeled meal and defecated most of the label before 24 hours.

Defecography, while unpleasant for the patient, often yields valuable information about the defecation process.[22,25-27] After administration of a thick barium enema, the patient is asked to defecate while being monitored fluoroscopically. Anatomical abnormalities such as a rectocele or cystocele can be identified. Physiologic abnormalities such as inadequate pelvic floor descent can be visualized. The anorectal angle can be measured during straining and rest (Figure 18-5). If the angle does not widen or indeed narrows, pelvic floor dyssynergia is suggested. This test can also be performed with a simulated feces mixed with a radionuclide. Instead of fluoroscopy, a gamma camera is used to image the anorectal angle. This test is significantly more expensive than fecal defecography and does not yield as much anatomical information.

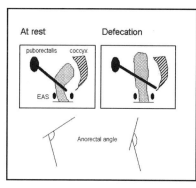

Figure 18-5. Schematic of defecation. At rest, the puborectalis muscle is contracted, creating a large angle represented by the intersecting axes of the anus and rectum. During defecation, the puborectalis muscle relaxes, resulting in an increase in the anorectal angle.

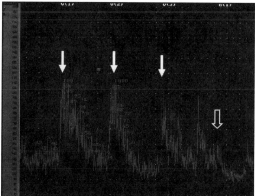

Figure 18-6. Tracing of a normal patient undergoing pelvic floor EMG. The tracing shows the EMG activity picked up by an anal electrode. The patient response to an instruction to squeeze (retain feces) is shown first (solid white arrow). An increase in EMG activity is shown. The response to an instruction to strain (defecate) is shown by the open arrow. There is a decrease in activity from the baseline.

Another test to evaluate the physiology of defecation is the balloon expulsion test.[21] This is a simple test that the patient either passes or fails. A small balloon is inflated with 50 mL of water and the patient is asked to expel it. If this is not accomplished in 1 minute, a pelvic floor abnormality is suggested, which may be confirmed with anorectal manometry or pelvic floor electromyography.

The rectal biopsy (full thickness) is used to confirm the presence of Hirschsprung's disease after a suggestive anorectal manometry.

Pelvic floor EMG measures the overall activity of the defecatory musculature.[28-30] A cylinder containing electrodes is placed into the anal canal. This apparatus is attached to an amplified physiologic recorder (polygraph), and the integrated activity is displayed on a monitor (Figure 18-6). An increase in activity should be seen when squeezing and a decrease in activity during straining (relaxation of the pelvic floor). An increase in EMG activity during bearing down (straining) is abnormal and suggests pelvic floor dyssynergia. The patient must be carefully instructed about procedures to avoid erroneous results. For example, the patient should "squeeze" by tightening the urethral sphincter and anus rather than by clenching the buttocks. In addition to diagnosing pelvic floor abnormalities, pelvic floor EMG may also be useful in the treatment of incontinence and pelvic floor dyssynergia by using biofeedback techniques.

Table 18-6

COMPLICATIONS OF CONSTIPATION

Systemic
- Laxative abuse
- Transient ischemic attacks
- Syncope
- Arrhythmias
- Myocardial infarction

Local
- Stercoral ulcer
- Proctitis
- Prolapse
- Hemorrhoids
- Infection
- Ischemia
- Perforation
- Incontinence
- Volvulus

Other tests less commonly utilized are anal endosonography and colonic manometry. Anal endosonography is most valuable in detecting anal sphincter abnormalities in patients with fecal incontinence. However, it has been used in constipation. Colonic manometry has been used to evaluate propulsive activity, but is difficult to perform and may not be very physiologic because of the necessary preparation and sedation often required to place the catheter. Further, interpretation of the results is problematic.

Complications of Constipation

Although unusual, constipation can result in severe and even fatal systemic complications (Table 18-6). Straining can provoke a Valsalva's response, inducing bradycardia or other arrhythmias. In the presence of underlying cardiovascular disease, these arrhythmias can provoke low flow states, resulting in transient ischemic attacks, syncope, or even myocardial infarction. Chronic laxative use or abuse can result in electrolyte imbalances or tolerance.

Local complications of constipation are distressing to the patient at the least but may result in chronic dysfunction and interfere with activities of daily living. Chronic stool retention in the rectum can cause a stercoral ulcer. If severe enough, this can go on to perforate or induce an abscess or fistula. Hemorrhoids are thought to be associated with constipation. A common sign of severe chronic constipation is fecal soiling. There may be an overflow of liquid fecal material around a large rectal impaction. The patient often presents complaining of incontinence or diarrhea when the problem is constipation. Other complications include proctitis, rectal prolapse, local ischemia, and volvulus.

Goals of Therapy

The primary goals of therapy in constipation are the elimination of the symptoms that caused the patient to present, normalization of bowel function, and the prevention of complications. Since each patient has a unique set of symptoms, it is important to address the concerns of the patient in directing therapy and ultimately deciding whether the treatment has been successful. A patient with stools that are hard to expel may not respond to the same treatment as a patient with infrequent defecation and bloating. Further, relieving the constipation may not relieve the pain in a patient with IBS-constipation subtype. Often, normalization of bowel function, whether ease of defecation, frequency of defecation, or stool hardness is the problem, will result in high patient satisfaction. All the symptoms may not be resolved, but the patient may feel the result is satisfactory. While not of immediate concern to the patient, the prevention of complications should always be considered by the physician. At the initial visit and during subsequent follow-ups, patient history and physical examination should be directed toward uncovering complications so that they can be addressed.

Approach to Therapy

Of course, prevention of constipation is the ideal method of treatment. This was discussed earlier in the chapter and centers on recognizing patients who are at risk for constipation and providing an environment that will prevent the onset of constipation. Physical activity, access to bathroom facilities, and diet all play an important role in preventing constipation and therefore its complications.

Once constipation has been diagnosed and the "red flags" of serious diseases such as cancer have been eliminated, therapy can commence (Table 18-7).

If a fecal impaction has been detected on physical examination, this must be addressed first. Digital disimpaction should be avoided. This practice has been associated with perforation, acute anal fissure formation, and even fatal arrhythmias. A series of enemas (eg, alternating tap water and mineral oil) is usually successful. When this fails, a milk and molasses enema (both osmotic and irritating) may be helpful. When enema therapy is unsuccessful, local anesthesia usually works. In females, a pudendal block in the lithotomy position will relax the anal canal and some of the pelvic floor muscles. Abdominal massage will usually "deliver" the impacted fecal material. In males, a local anal block will serve the same function.

In milder cases, improving exercise levels, fluid intake, and bathroom habits will often be successful. Moderate increases in exercise can improve colonic transit. If fluid intake is low, increasing it will help correct the problem. Bathroom facilities or a commode should be readily available. Patients should try to defecate after meals (eg, every day after breakfast) when the gastrocolic reflex is strongest.

Any cause of constipation that can be identified should be treated, if possible. Of course, any unnecessary drugs, whether prescription or over-the-counter, should be discontinued. Frequent problems are aluminum hydroxide antacids (Mg hydroxide

Table 18-7

TREATMENT MODALITIES FOR CONSTIPATION

- Clear impaction if present
- Exercise, habit
- Treat obvious causes
- Discontinue unnecessary drugs
- Laxatives (acute or chronic) and prokinetics
- Surgical intervention
- Other methods
  * Biofeedback
  * Combination therapy
  * Enemas
  * Mechanical devices

Table 18-8

AGENTS USED TO TREAT CONSTIPATION

Drug	*Example*
Bulk-forming agents	Psyllium
Emollient laxatives	Focusate
Lubricants	Mineral oil
Saline cathartics	Milk of magnesia
Stimulant cathartics	Bisacodyl
Hyperosmotic laxatives	Lactulose
Polyethylene glycol lavage	PEG-3350
Secretory agents	Misoprostol
Colchicine	Colchicine
Prokinetics	Tegaserod

can be substituted if renal failure is not present), iron tablets when iron deficiency anemia is not present, and opioid analgesic use.

The next step is the addition of laxatives and/or prokinetics (detailed below in the section on agents). There is a wide selection of agents available (Table 18-8), with differing mechanisms of action, cost, efficacy, dosing (Table 18-9), and side effect profiles. While it is standard therapy to start with prokinetics or osmotic agents, it may be necessary to utilize several agents simultaneously to reach a therapeutic goal.

Table 18-9

TYPICAL DOSES OF AGENTS USED IN THE TREATMENT OF CONSTIPATION

Drug	Dose
Psyllium	10 to 20 g/day in BID divided doses
Docusate	50 to 300 mg/day in TID divided doses
Mineral oil	15 to 45 cc daily
Milk of magnesia	30 to 60 cc daily at bedtime
Bisacodyl tablet	5 to 20 mg daily at bedtime
Lactulose	30 to 60 BID in divided doses
PEG-3350	17 g in 240 cc of water daily
Misoprostol	200 mcg TID
Colchicine	600 mcg TID
Tegaserod	6 mg BID

In addition to laxatives and prokinetic, there are other approaches to the treatment of constipation. Biofeedback may be helpful, especially in cases of pelvic floor dyssynergia. Enemas may be used as a "rescue" technique on occasion or for periodic (eg, weekly) therapy. Mechanical devices such as the Pulsed Irrigation Evacuation device (PIE* [PIE* Medical International, Duluth, Ga])[31] can be used for irrigation and cleansing. Usually a last resort, surgical intervention can be successful in alleviating constipation. This can range from the minimalist Malone antegrade continent enema (MACE)[32] procedure in which the appendix is anastomosed to the abdominal skin (appendicostomy) to afford access to an enema catheter, to the more radical total colectomy with ileostomy. There are also procedures in between these 2 extremes.

Agents Used to Treat Constipation

BULK-FORMING AGENTS

Mode of Action and Pharmacology

Fiber comes in many forms: soluble and insoluble, synthetic and natural, and tablet or powder. The differences are patient convenience and side effects. The most commonly used is psyllium. Like other fibers, psyllium absorbs water in the gut and swells to form an emollient gel. This enlarges the stool, softens it, and makes it easier to pass. Psyllium is the ground up husk of the psyllium plant seed and is available in pharmacies, health food stores, and under proprietary names such as Metamucil (Procter and Gamble, Cincinnati, Ohio). Psyllium is available as a powder to mix with water, a biscuit, and as granules in a capsule. Calcium polycarbophil is a synthetic fiber provided in tablet and chewable forms. Soy polysaccharide is a fiber added to tube-feeding formulas. Other fibers include methyl cellulose, guar, and bran.

Clinical Efficacy

Despite the generally accepted efficacy of these agents, reviewers in a systematic review[33] were less than impressed. Most of the above agents were listed as grade C recommendations, with psyllium as a grade B recommendation (moderate evidence in support of its use) without strong evidence for or against the use of these agents. It should be remembered that fiber, like many of the other older medications, has not been studied recently in carefully controlled double blinded studies, hence the low level of evidence strength in the studies.

Indication, Dosing, and Toxicity

These agents are often used as a first line treatment of constipation. Typical starting doses are 3 to 5 g/day, but most practitioners use higher dose recommendations (20 to 30 g/day). These doses are hard to achieve without toxicity or a problem with palatability. For example, the calcium polysaccharide tablets are only 0.5 g/tablet, requiring 40 tablets/day to achieve the 20 g dosing. Adding 3 teaspoons of psyllium to 8 oz of water quickly renders a mixture that is gritty, thick, and difficult to swallow. Common side effects are gassiness, bloating, and flatulence. This increases at higher doses and is more common in the natural fibers than in the synthetic ones. Fortunately, the gas problem usually subsides on its own after a week or two. Thus, warning patients to expect these problems and their resolution helps with compliance. Fiber is contraindicated in patients with a bowel obstruction.

EMOLLIENT LAXATIVES

Mode of Action and Pharmacology

Emollient laxatives such as docusate sodium are often used as over-the-counter remedies for constipation. It is conjectured that the docusate renders the stool softer and more slippery. Indeed, docusate liquid is slippery, although whether it has any effect at conventional doses is arguable. It is also thought to lower the surface tension of the stool, permitting better hydration. The 2 major emollients are docusate sodium and docusate calcium. They are available in several strengths.

Clinical Efficacy

These agents have been studied for years without much evidence that they work at all. Ramkumar and Rao list docusate as grade C and cannot recommend its use.[33] Other reviewers have not found any efficacy for this medication.[34]

Indication, Dosing, and Toxicity

Docusate sodium is often used by practitioners as a first line drug or prophylactic agent in hospitalized patients despite its apparent lack of efficacy. Typical starting doses are 50 mg TID, increasing to 300 mg TID. While generally safe and well tolerated, docusate sodium does provide a substantial sodium load and may be dangerous to those on sodium-restricted diets. Adverse reactions include bitter taste, throat irritation, nausea, and rash.

LUBRICANTS

Mode of Action and Pharmacology

Mineral oil is the prototypical lubricant. It is not absorbed by the GI tract and in essence, produces a steatorrhea. It is available in enema form or in bulk containers for oral use.

Clinical Efficacy

This is an effective medication for the treatment of constipation. The effect is often present at low doses, but higher volumes of the mineral oil may be needed to be effective.

Indication, Dosing, and Toxicity

Starting doses of mineral oil are 15 to 45 mL orally per day. This is usually given on an empty stomach. The enema is given as a single treatment, often after the failure of a standard tap water enema. This administration is thought to make the stool more slippery and ease defecation. Mineral oil is not without its problems, however. It interferes with the absorption of fat-soluble vitamins and drugs (hence the reason to avoid taking it with meals). Accidental aspiration can lead to fatal lipid pneumonia.

SALINE CATHARTICS

Mode of Action and Pharmacology

These agents are poorly absorbed electrolytes that act as hyperosmolar solutions, drawing water into the intestinal lumen until the stool is isosmolar with plasma. They may also act to release cholecystokinin (CCK), a gut hormone that stimulates antegrade motility. Examples of this type of agent include milk of magnesia, magnesium citrate, and sodium phosphate. The sodium phosphate formulation includes oral and enema forms. While milk of magnesia is typically administered at bedtime for overnight effect, magnesium citrate and sodium phosphate can have an effect within 1 hour.

Clinical Efficacy

There are not many trials of these agents in the recent literature, hence the grade C recommendation from Ramukar and Rao.[33] However, these agents are generally accepted to be efficacious.

Indication, Dosing, and Toxicity

These agents are indicated for the short-term treatment of constipation. A typical dose of milk of magnesia would be 30 to 60 mL at bedtime. Sodium phosphate can be used as an oral liquid 90 mL or as an enema (Fleet Enem [C.B. Fleet Company, Lynchburg, Va]). In the magnesium-containing formulations, magnesium absorption can lead to toxicity in patients with renal insufficiency. Likewise, phosphate overload can occur in renal failure. Sodium overload and resulting congestive heart failure can occur with the use of sodium phosphate solutions in susceptible patients.

STIMULANT CATHARTICS

Mode of Action and Pharmacology

This group of agents includes anthraquinones (senna, cascara, danthron), diphenylmethanes (bisacodyl and phenolphthalein), and castor oil. These drugs are available over-the-counter in many forms, including tablets, suppositories, and even "natural" teas. After activation by intestinal microorganisms, anthraquinones increase fluid and electrolyte secretion in the distal ileum and colon[35] and increase colonic peristalsis. They undergo hepatic metabolism but also enterohepatic circulation, explaining their sometimes prolonged effect. Diphenylmethanes are activated by endogenous esterases[36] and stimulate intestinal secretion and motility. Castor oil is hydrolyzed to ricinoleic acid by intestinal lipase. It inhibits water reabsorption, increases mucosal permeability, and stimulates motility via a mucosal enterochromaffin cell pathway.[36]

Clinical Efficacy

These agents have been available for quite some time, so placebo controlled trials are not available. There is no doubt, however, that they are effective in most patients for the short term.

Indication, Dosing, and Toxicity

These agents are indicated for the short-term treatment of constipation. Typical doses of cascara would be 325 mg, bisacodyl 5 to 20 mg, and castor oil 15 to 30 mL. These agents are typically administered at bedtime for overnight response. Anthraquinones are well known to increase the lipofuscin pigment in the colon, a condition called melanosis coli. This benign condition will reverse in most patients within 12 months of drug cessation. Tolerance to all these agents may occur. The most frequent side effect is cramping. These agents should be avoided for long-term use because of the potential for fluid and electrolyte imbalances. There is little evidence, though, that these drugs can cause "cathartic colon."[37]

HYPEROSMOTIC LAXATIVES

Mode of Action and Pharmacology

These agents, such as lactulose and sorbitol, are disaccharides that are resistant to intestinal disaccharidases. They reach the colon unmetabolized and unabsorbed, where they undergo fermentation by the intestinal flora. This results in the production of highly osmotic short chain fatty acids, drawing fluid and electrolytes into the colonic lumen. Sorbitol is available in a 70% solution that is equivalent to lactulose but at lower cost.

Clinical Efficacy

In Ramkumar and Rao's review,[33] lactulose received a grade B recommendation and sorbitol a grade C, although they are largely equivalent.

Indication, Dosing, and Toxicity

Osmotic agents such as lactulose are indicated for the acute or long-term treatment of constipation. Typical doses are 30 to 60 mL from 1 to 3 times a day. Common side effects include flatulence and bloating. These are understandable effects consistent with its fermentation in the colon.

POLYETHYLENE GLYCOL 3350

Mode of Action and Pharmacology

Polyethylene glycol 3350 (PEG) is available with (GoLYTELY [Braintree Laboratories, Inc, Braintree, Mass], NuLYTELY [Braintree Laboratories, Inc, Braintree, Mass], Colyte [Schwartz Pharma, Inc, Milwaukee, Wis]) or without (Glycolax [Schwartz Pharma, Inc, Milwaukee, Wis], Miralax [Braintree Laboratories, Inc, Braintree, Mass]) electrolyte additives. The form of PEG without electrolytes is indicated for the treatment of constipation, the form with electrolytes is used for gut purges before colonoscopy or surgery. The reason for the electrolytes in the purge formulation is to prevent large electrolyte changes because the volume is typically 4 L. Smaller volumes do not seem to be much of a problem. The PEG is not absorbed or metabolized in the gut and creates an isosmolar solution, thus keeping water in the lumen.

Clinical Efficacy

In either form, PEG is highly efficacious in the treatment of constipation. It received a grade A rating (good evidence in support of its use) by Ramkumar and Rao.[33]

Indication, Dosing, and Toxicity

PEG is indicated for the short-term treatment of constipation (<8 weeks), but seems to remain effective and safe with long-term use. Dosing is typically 17 g of PEG in 240 mL of water or other beverage daily. The 4-L lavage can be used for the acute treatment of constipation. The formulation containing electrolytes has a salty/bitter taste, with many patients finding it unpalatable. The formulation without electrolytes has no odor or taste. While equally efficacious to lactulose, it does not cause bloating and gassiness because its mode of action does not involve fermentation.

SECRETORY AGENTS

Lubiprostone

Mode of Action and Pharmacology

Lubiprostone is a new agent, approved by the FDA in January, 2006 for the treatment of chronic idiopathic constipation. A novel agent, it acts as a chloride channel activator, thereby stimulating the small intestinal mucosa to secrete more fluid. This in turn causes better hydration of the stool.

Clinical Efficacy

In two unpublished clinical trials, lubiprostone increased the frequency of bowel movements in as little as one week. The improvement continued for four weeks. In long term studies, the agent decreased constipation severity, bloating, and discomfort up to one year.

Indication, Dosing, and Toxicity

It is indicated for chronic idiopathic constipation. The dosing is 24 mcg bid. Contraindications are gastrointestinal obstruction and hypersensitivity to the agent. Side effects reported include nausea, diarrhea, abdominal pain and distension, headache and dizziness, among others.

Misoprostol

Mode of Action and Pharmacology

Misoprostol is a prostaglandin E1 analog indicated for the prevention of NSAID gastropathy. It was noted that many patients so treated developed diarrhea as a side effect. The mode of action is through increased intestinal secretion stimulated through a cAMP mediated pathway. The drug's mechanism of action is mucosal, and local concentration determines the extent of the effect. Thus, when given with food, gastric emptying is delayed and the agent is slowly delivered to the small intestine. When given while fasting, a higher concentration reaches the intestine and it has a greater effect.

Clinical Efficacy

There are few studies evaluating misoprostol as a treatment for constipation. Hence, its grade C rating.[33] However, the side effect of diarrhea is well established through clinical trials, so it is likely to be an effective agent.

Indication, Dosing, and Toxicity

Although not indicated for the treatment of constipation, misoprostol may be a useful adjunct when other agents are ineffective. Dosing is 200 µg before meals QID. This makes it an inconvenient dosing regimen for most patients.

COLCHICINE

Mode of Action and Pharmacology

Diarrhea is a well know side effect of colchicine when used for the treatment of gout. Although the exact mechanism is unknown, colchicine is thought to increase prostaglandin synthesis, thereby increasing intestinal secretion and perhaps increasing motility.

Clinical Efficacy

This medication has not been extensively studied for the treatment of constipation. One study, a double-blind, placebo controlled, crossover trial in 16 patients, found that colchicine significantly accelerated intestinal transit and increased the frequency of bowel movements.[38] However, due to a paucity of trials and patients tested, it is given a Grade C recommendation.[33]

Indication, Dosing, and Toxicity

The FDA has not approved colchicine for the treatment of constipation. Typical doses are 0.6 mg TID to start. Although generally well tolerated, colchicine is known to cause nausea, cramping, bone marrow suppression, neuropathy, and myopathy.

PROKINETICS

Mode of Action and Pharmacology

Prokinetics are agents that increase motility and specifically accelerate antegrade propulsion. Members of this class include metoclopramide, cisapride, and tegaserod. Metoclopramide does not seem to have an effect on the colon and is not used for constipation. Cisapride, a 5-HT4 serotonin agonist and 5-HT3 antagonist, accelerates colonic transit and may be useful for constipation, but has been removed from the US market. This leaves tegaserod, a 5-HT4 agonist. Tegaserod stimulates 5-HT4 receptors in the stomach, small intestine, and colon, thereby stimulating the peristaltic reflex. It also alters chloride secretion.

Clinical Efficacy

Several large, randomized, double blind controlled high quality trials have demonstrated the efficacy of tegaserod in the treatment of idiopathic constipation and IBS-constipation subtype.[39,40] Significant improvement was noted in the primary variable—number of complete spontaneous bowel movements/week. Based on these studies with level I evidence (best), tegaserod was given a grade A recommendation.[33]

Indication, Dosing, and Toxicity

Tegaserod is indicated for the short-term treatment of women with IBS, constipation subtype, and idiopathic constipation in both men and women. Typical starting dose is 6 mg BID. Side effects are uncommon, but include diarrhea, headache, and arthropathy.

Combination Therapy

It is important to note that a single agent may not suffice, especially in the refractory patient. Rather than pushing a single agent to toxic doses, several can be combined to effect laxation. Different physiologic mechanisms can be employed to obtain the desired effect. For example, fiber (psyllium) can be combined with an osmotic agent (lactulose) and a prokinetic (tegaserod) without going to high doses of any single agent.

Mechanical Approaches

Enemas may be useful in the acute treatment of constipation. They are inexpensive, easy to administer, rapid in action, and effective. Tap water enemas can be used in high volume (1 to 2 L) to relieve an impaction. Soap suds enemas should be avoided because of possible mucosal irritation. Enemas may contain laxatives more commonly used by mouth but also effective per rectum. These include mineral oil and sodium phosphate. Again, the sodium phosphate enema can be toxic in congestive heart failure and renal failure patients.

Another mechanical approach is the PIE* device from PIE* Medical International, Inc.[31] The PIE* device contains a reservoir of water and a computer controlled pump to irrigate the colon automatically after insertion of a catheter into the rectum. Fecal material is collected in a closed reservoir and easily discarded. The procedure usually takes less than an hour. It has been utilized in paraplegics and quadriplegics on a regular basis.

Biofeedback Training

Biofeedback for the improvement of constipation has received increasing acceptance in the past decade.[41,42] It is most useful in patients with pelvic floor dysfunction (dyssynergia). These patients contract their puborectalis muscle instead of relaxing it in the act of defecation. Through the use of 1 to 3(or more) biofeedback sessions, patients can be taught to correct this inappropriate muscle response. The relaxation of the pelvic floor muscles can be monitored through electromyographic or manometric pressure monitoring. Trained technologists are necessary to help the patients obtain the proper responses. There is some evidence that one-on-one coaching without biofeedback can also be successful.

Surgery

Surgery is usually the last resort for patients with refractory constipation. Before entertaining this option, it is mandatory to assess motility in the entire GI tract. Colectomy in patients with a generalized motility disorder (eg, chronic idiopathic intestinal pseudo-obstruction) is unlikely to be successful. Also, transit testing should demonstrate a colonic inertia pattern, not obstructed defecation.

The standard procedure is the total abdominal colectomy with ileorectal anastomoses.[43,44] This procedure is highly successful in selected patient groups.[45] However, this procedure should not be performed in patients with pelvic floor dysfunction unless the dyssynergia has been improved by biofeedback first. Further, this procedure is not likely to improve abdominal pain in these patients, although it does permit the use of opioid analgesics without the concern for their constipating effects. A more extreme surgical approach is total colectomy with ileostomy. This eliminates all colonic and defecatory problems in one procedure.

Another procedure is the Malone antegrade continent enema (MACE)[32,46,47] or laparoscopic antegrade continent enema (LACE).[48] In the MACE procedure, the tip of the appendix is anastomosed to the skin of the right lower quadrant, creating a small ostomy that is usually continent. A rubber or silicone catheter can then be inserted into the colon and the bowel irrigated with water or PEG solution, resulting in a prompt, controlled bowel movement (Figure 18-7).

Surgical resection of the aganglionic segment in Hirschsprung's disease is usually successful. Considerations include the length of the aganglionic segment, the age of the patient and experience of the surgeon.

References

1. Stewart RB, Moore MT, Marks RG, Hale WE. Correlates of constipation in an ambulatory elderly population. *Am J Gastroenterol.* 1992;87:859-864.

2. Sonnenberg A, Koch TR. Physician visits in the united states for constipation: 1958 to 1986. *Dig Dis Sci.* 1989;34:606-611.

3. Pare P, Ferrazzi S, Thompson WG, Irvine EJ, Rance L. An epidemiological survey of constipation in Canada: Definitions, rates, demographics, and predictors of health care seeking. *Am J Gastroenterol.* 2001;96:3130-3137.

4. Mason HJ, Serrano-Ikkos E, Kamm MA. Psychological morbidity in women with idiopathic constipation. *Am J Gastroenterol.* 2000;95:2852-2857.

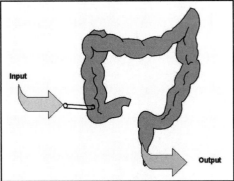

Figure 18-7. MACE procedure. In the classic procedure, the appendix is anastomosed to the skin of the right lower quadrant. This ostomy is then cannulated and fluid infused (input). The patient then has a prompt, yet controlled bowel movement (output).

Input

Output

5. Thompson WG, Longstreth GF, Drossman DA, Heaton KW, Irvine EJ, Muller-Lissner SA. Functional bowel disorders and functional abdominal pain. *Gut.* 1999;45:43-47.

6. Everhart JE, Go VL, Johannes RS, Fitzsimmons SC, Roth HP, White LR. A longitudinal survey of self-reported bowel habits in the united states. *Dig Dis Sci.* 1989;34:1153-1162.

7. Talley NJ, Fleming KC, Evans JM, et al. Constipation in an elderly community: a study of prevalence and potential risk factors. *Am J Gastroenterol.* 1996;91:19-25.

8. Campbell AJ, Busby WJ, Horwath CC. Factors associated with constipation in a community based sample of people aged 70 years and over. *J Epidemiol Community Health.* 1993;47:23-26.

9. Sandler RS, Jordan MC, Shelton BJ. Demographic and dietary determinants of constipation in the US population. *Am J Public Health.* 1990;80:185-189.

10. Whitehead WE, Drinkwater D, Cheskin LJ, Heller BR, Schuster MM. Constipation in the elderly living at home. definition, prevalence, and relationship to lifestyle and health status. *J Am Geriatr Soc.* 1989;37:423-429.

11. Maurer AH, Krevsky B, Knight LC, Brown K. Opioid and opioid-like drug effects on whole-gut transit measured by scintigraphy. *J Nucl Med.* 1996;37:818-822.

12. Hinds JP, Eidelman BH, Wald A. Prevalence of bowel dysfunction in multiple sclerosis. A population survey. *Gastroenterology.* 1990;98:1538-1542.

13. Hinds JP, Wald A. Colonic and anorectal dysfunction associated with multiple sclerosis. *Am J Gastroenterol.* 1989;84:587-595.

14. Metcalf AM, Phillips SF, Zinsmeister AR, MacCarty RL, Beart RW, Wolff BG. Simplified assessment of segmental colonic transit. *Gastroenterology.* 1987;92:40-47.

15. Krevsky B, Maurer AH, Fisher RS. Patterns of colonic transit in chronic idiopathic constipation. *Am J Gastroenterol.* 1989;84:127-132.

16. Maurer AH, Krevsky B. Whole-gut transit scintigraphy in the evaluation of small-bowel and colon transit disorders. *Semin Nucl Med.* 1995;25:326-338.

17. Bonapace ES, Maurer AH, Davidoff S, Krevsky B, Fisher RS, Parkman HP. Whole gut transit scintigraphy in the clinical evaluation of patients with upper and lower gastrointestinal symptoms. *Am J Gastroenterol.* 2000;95:2838-2847.

18. Tramonte SM, Brand MB, Mulrow CD, Amato MG, O'Keefe ME, Ramirez G. The treatment of chronic constipation in adults. A systematic review. *J Gen Intern Med.* 1997;12:15-24.

19. Tucker DM, Sandstead HH, Logan G Jr, et al. Dietary fiber and personality factors as determinants of stool output. *Gastroenterology.* 1981;81:879-883.
20. Rao SS, Azpiroz F, Diamant N, Enck P, Tougas G, Wald A. Minimum standards of anorectal manometry. *Neurogastroenterol Motil.* 2002;14:553-559.
21. Rao SS, Hatfield R, Soffer E, Rao S, Beaty J, Conklin JL. Manometric tests of anorectal function in healthy adults. *Am J Gastroenterol.* 1999;94:773-783.
22. Rao SS, Sun WM. Current techniques of assessing defecation dynamics. *Dig Dis.* 1997;15:64-77.
23. Bonapace ES, Maurer AH, Davidoff S, Krevsky B, Fisher RS, Parkman HP. Whole gut transit scintigraphy in the clinical evaluation of patients with upper and lower gastrointestinal symptoms. *Am J Gastroenterol.* 2000;95:2838-2847.
24. McLean RG, King DW, Talley NA, Tait AD, Freiman J. The utilization of colon transit scintigraphy in the diagnostic algorithm for patients with chronic constipation. *Dig Dis Sci.* 1999;44:41-47.
25. Karasick S, Ehrlich SM. Is constipation a disorder of defecation or impaired motility? Distinction based on defecography and colonic transit studies. *Am J Roentgenol.* 1996;166:63-66.
26. Jorge JM, Habr-Gama A, Wexner SD. Clinical applications and techniques of cinedefecography. *Am J Surg.* 2001;182:93-101.
27. Diamant NE, Kamm MA, Wald A, Whitehead WE. AGA technical review on anorectal testing techniques. *Gastroenterology.* 1999;116:735-760.
28. Podnar S, Vodusek DB. Standardization of anal sphincter electromyography: effect of chronic constipation. *Muscle Nerve.* 2000;23:1748-1751.
29. Fucini C, Ronchi O, Elbetti C. Electromyography of the pelvic floor musculature in the assessment of obstructed defecation symptoms. *Dis Colon Rectum.* 2001;44:1168-1175.
30. Xiong GY, Zhao ZQ. Clinical significance of functional constipation categorized by colonic transit time and pelvic floor electromyography. *Chin J Dig Dis.* 2004;5:156-159.
31. Constipation. Available at: www.piemed.com. Accessed 07/03, 2005.
32. Malone PS, Ransley PG, Kiely EM. Preliminary report: the antegrade continence enema. *Lancet.* 1990;336:1217-1218.
33. Ramkumar D, Rao SS. Efficacy and safety of traditional medical therapies for chronic constipation: Systematic review. *Am J Gastroenterol.* 2005;100:936-971.
34. Hurdon V, Viola R, Schroder C. How useful is docusate in patients at risk for constipation? A systematic review of the evidence in the chronically ill. *J Pain Symptom Manage.* 2000;19:130-136.
35. Yamada T, ed. *Textbook of Gastroenterology.* 4th ed. Philadelphia: Lippincott Williams & Wilkins; 2003.
36. Lembo A, Camilleri M. Chronic constipation. *N Engl J Med.* 2003;349:1360-1368.
37. Muller-Lissner SA, Kamm MA, Scarpignato C, Wald A. Myths and misconceptions about chronic constipation. *Am J Gastroenterol.* 2005;100:232-242.
38. Verne GN, Eaker EY, Davis RH, Sninsky CA. Colchicine is an effective treatment for patients with chronic constipation: an open-label trial. *Dig Dis Sci.* 1997;42:1959-1963.
39. Kamm MA, Muller-Lissner S, Talley NJ, et al. Tegaserod for the treatment of chronic constipation: a randomized, double-blind, placebo-controlled multinational study. *Am J Gastroenterol.* 2005;100:362-372.
40. Muller-Lissner S, Holtmann G, Rueegg P, Weidinger G, Loffler H. Tegaserod is

effective in the initial and retreatment of irritable bowel syndrome with constipation. *Aliment Pharmacol Ther.* 2005;21:11-20.

41. Bassotti G, Chistolini F, Sietchiping-Nzepa F, de Roberto G, Morelli A, Chiarioni G. Biofeedback for pelvic floor dysfunction in constipation. *BMJ.* 2004;328:393-396.

42. Rao SS, Welcher KD, Pelsang RE. Effects of biofeedback therapy on anorectal function in obstructive defecation. *Dig Dis Sci.* 1997;42:2197-2205.

43. Webster C, Dayton M. Results after colectomy for colonic inertia: a sixteen-year experience. *Am J Surg.* 2001;182:639-644.

44. Knowles CH, Scott M, Lunniss PJ. Outcome of colectomy for slow transit constipation. *Ann Surg.* 1999;230:627-638.

45. Redmond JM, Smith GW, Barofsky I, Ratych RE, Goldsborough DC, Schuster MM. Physiological tests to predict long-term outcome of total abdominal colectomy for intractable constipation. *Am J Gastroenterol.* 1995;90:748-753.

46. Herndon CD, Rink RC, Cain MP, et al. In situ Malone antegrade continence enema in 127 patients: a 6-year experience. *J Urol.* 2004;172:1689-1691.

47. Krogh K, Laurberg S. Malone antegrade continence enema for fecal incontinence and constipation in adults. *Br J Surg.* 1998;85:974-977.

48. Lees NP, Hodson P, Hill J, Pearson RC, MacLennan I. Long-term results of the antegrade continent enema procedure for constipation in adults. *Colorectal Dis.* 2004;6:362-368.

chapter 19

Fecal Incontinence

Arnold Wald, MD

Introduction

Of the many disorders of GI function in adults, fecal incontinence is among the most under-appreciated and poorly treated by practicing physicians, including those who specialize in GI diseases. It is under-appreciated because large numbers of embarrassed patients fail to report their problem to their physician and poorly treated because of lack of understanding of pathophysiology and inadequate training of physicians as to diagnostic testing and therapeutic options. Moreover, it is devastating to patients because of their diminished self-esteem and social isolation. In the elderly, the development of incontinence frequently leads to institutionalization. Yet, management of this disorder can be highly effective, often enabling sufferers of incontinence to return to emotional and physical well being.

This chapter reviews the relevant anatomy and function of the anorectum, the pathophysiology and major causes of fecal incontinence, and the evaluation and management of patients who present with this socially devastating disorder.

Epidemiology

Estimates of fecal incontinence vary depending on the population surveyed, differences in survey methods, and definitions used to identify incontinence. In general, incontinence increases with age in both men and women and affects almost 50% of elderly individuals who are institutionalized.[1] Most surveys document a significant impairment of quality of life with both adverse economic and social consequences. In many elderly individuals, fecal incontinence may be the factor that precipitates institutionalizing of an individual.

The cost of health care related to fecal incontinence, although not known precisely, is considerable because it encompasses loss of economic potential, diagnostic testing, treatment interventions and use of continence pads, skin care, and nursing care.[2]

Figure 19-1. Diagram of a sagittal view of the anal canal, rectum, and important components of the continence apparatus.

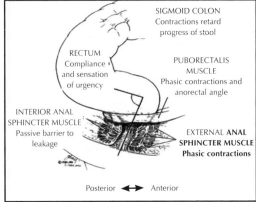

SIGMOID COLON
Contractions retard progress of stool

RECTUM
Compliance and sensation of urgency

PUBORECTALIS MUSCLE
Phasic contractions and anorectal angle

INTERIOR ANAL SPHINCTER MUSCLE
Passive barrier to leakage

EXTERNAL **ANAL SPHINCTER MUSCLE**
Phasic contractions

Posterior ◄─► Anterior

Pathophysiology and Anatomy

FUNCTIONAL ANATOMY AND ANORECTAL PHYSIOLOGY

The rectum serves as both a storage organ and as a conduit from the colon to the anal canal (Figure 19-1). The anal canal is defined proximally by the levator ani muscles, which form part of the pelvic floor, and includes the puborectalis muscle (PRM), which creates the anorectal angle. Two sphincters encircle the anal canal: the internal anal sphincter (IAS), which is a continuation of the circular smooth muscle of the rectum, and the external anal sphincter (EAS), which consists of striated muscles innervated by the pudendal nerves arising from S2, S3, and S4. Extrinsic innervation of the internal anal sphincter is by sympathetic and parasympathetic autonomic nerves.

Fecal incontinence relies heavily on the appropriate functioning of the puborectalis muscle, the internal anal sphincter, and external anal sphincter together with rectal storage capacity and anorectal sensation.

Continence during quiescent periods of bowel activity is largely a function of basal anal canal pressures, approximately 70% of which comes from the internal anal sphincter, together with compliance of the rectum and distal colon. When stool is delivered to the rectum, continence is maintained by contraction of both the puborectalis muscle and the external anal sphincter, the former by narrowing and elevating the anorectal angle and the latter by increasing anal canal resistance pressures. These are influenced by cognitive and behavioral factors and are also modulated by stool consistency and delivery to the rectum. Thus, derangements in one continence mechanism often can be compensated by others to maintain continence.

PATHOPHYSIOLOGY OF FECAL INCONTINENCE

The pathophysiology of fecal incontinence may be classified into a number of broad categories that occur alone or in combination (Table 19-1). These include overflow incontinence, impaired rectal and colonic storage functions, anal sphincter

Table 19-1

PATHOPHYSIOLOGY OF FECAL INCONTINENCE

1. Fecal impaction with overflow
2. Impaired rectal/colonic storage function
   A. Inflammation: IBD
   B. Surgery; proctectomy
   C. Fibrosis: radiation
3. Anal sphincter weakness
   A. Internal anal sphincter
      i. Trauma (sphincterotomy)
      ii. Neurological (diabetes)
      iii. Degenerative (scleroderma)
   B. External anal sphincter
      i. Trauma (vaginal delivery)
      ii. Neurological (pudendal neuropathy, spinal cord)
      iii. Degenerative (atrophy)
   C. Puborectalis
      i. Neurological (peripheral, CNS)
      ii. Trauma (high tear)
4. Rectal sensory impairment
   A. Neurological (ie, CNS)
   B. Muscle hypotonia (ie, megarectum)

and puborectalis weakness, and impaired rectal sensory mechanisms. In addition, alterations in stool consistency and delivery to the rectum are important cofactors in causing incontinence and also influence the management of patients with fecal incontinence.[3] For example, many patients with multiple sclerosis have weakness of the external anal sphincter and even rectal sensory impairment but remain continent when constipated, only to develop incontinence in the presence of diarrhea or too aggressive use of laxatives.

It is important to emphasize that the cause of fecal incontinence in any patient is often multifactorial. A careful history and a focused physical examination will often yield important clinical clues as to causation.[4] Also useful is to assess the severity of the problem and its impact on the patient and family members.[5] This information is often of value when designing appropriate treatment strategies.

Clinical Evaluation

HISTORY AND PHYSICAL EXAMINATION

Many patients present with a self-diagnosis of incontinence or are referred for evaluation by other physicians. Others may complain of diarrhea and do not volunteer that they have incontinence. Therefore, it is important that the physician asks about incontinence specifically and if acknowledged, attempts to characterize its frequency and characteristics. It is helpful to ask if a patient is incontinent for liquid and/or solid stools, whether there are major accidents or simply seepage of small amounts of liquid, if there is nighttime incontinence, and whether there is urge incontinence (ie, soiling despite all attempts to retain stool) or passive incontinence (ie, soiling occurs without awareness). The latter suggests possible loss of rectal sensory perception whereas the former may indicate altered delivery of stool to the rectum, impaired storage capacity, and/or anal sphincter weakness. These complaints are in contrast to minor seepage of mucus or liquid, which may indicate weakened resting anal pressures, especially if there are normal bowel habits. Although not entirely predictive of pathophysiology, such information may suggest possible clinical scenarios.

It may be helpful to grade the severity of fecal incontinence by using previously validated scoring systems such as the Cleveland Clinic or St Marks grading instruments.[6] Such systems are based on multiple parameters, ranging from absent to very severe. An example of such an instrument is shown (Table 19-2).

Comparisons of grading scores before and after treatment can also serve as an objective measure of response to treatments and are particularly important in treatment trials.

A directed physical examination often provides clues to pathophysiology. The salient elements of the examination include perineal inspection, digital rectal examination, and a focused neurologic assessment involving the lower extremities and back.

Examination of the perineum is best done with the patient in the left or right lateral position to obtain adequate exposure of the perineum and perianal area. Inspection assesses for perianal skin irritation and/or fecal soiling; mucosal or hemorrhoidal prolapse; gaping of the anus; atrophy of the gluteal muscles; and evidence of perianal scarring, inflammation, or drainage. If the patient is then asked to strain as if defecating, perineal descent of >3 cm suggests weakness of the pelvic floor, which may reflect neuromuscular disease. Although rectal prolapse may occur in the lateral position, it is best elicited with the patient squatting while using a mirror with a long handle to visualize the anal opening.

Assessment of perianal sensation should include determining the presence of the "anal wink," which is a reflex contraction of the external anal sphincter in response to gentle stroking of the perianal skin. This maneuver assesses both sensory and motor components of the nerves innervating this area, which arise from spinal cord roots S2, S3, and S4.

Lastly, a digital rectal examination should be performed. This may identify a fecal impaction, neoplasia, or rectal stricture but in experienced hands also assesses the pressures in the anal canal and the puborectalis muscle, as illustrated in Figure 19-2.

A more superficial digital examination should assess both resting anal canal tone and squeeze pressures as well as identifying any structural defects in the anal canal (see Figure 19-2A). The examining finger is then inserted deeper and oriented posteriorly

Table 19-2

INCONTINENCE INSTRUMENT

	Never	Rarely	Sometimes	Weekly	Daily
Incontinence for solid stool	0	1	2	3	4
Incontinence for liquid stool	0	1	2	3	4
Incontinence for gas	0	1	2	3	4
Alteration in lifestyle	0	1	2	3	4
				No	Yes
Need to wear a pad or plug				0	2
Taking constipating medicines				0	2
Lack of ability to defer defecation for 15 minutes				0	4

Never, no episodes in the past 4 weeks; rarely, 1 episode in the past 4 weeks; sometimes, >1 episode in the past 4 weeks but <1 a week; weekly, 1 or more episodes a week but <1 a day; daily, 1 or more episodes a day.

Add one score from each row; minimum score = 0 = perfect continence; maximum score = 24 = totally incontinent.

Reprinted from Vaizey CJ, Carapeti E, Cahill J, Kamm MA. Prospective comparative study of fecal incontinence grading systems. *Gut.* 1999;44:77-80 with permission from the BMJ Publishing Group.

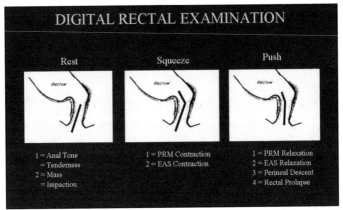

Figure 19-2. Illustration of the important components of the digital rectal examination in patients with fecal incontinence. At rest (A), tone of the anus indicates the integrity of the IAS whereas deeper insertion of the finger evaluates for fecal impaction, masses, and other structural abnormalities. Asking the patient to squeeze (B) allows assessment of EAS strength and fatigue; deeper insertion of the finger assesses the integrity of PRM contractions parameters. Asking the patient to bear down (C) allows assessment of PRM and EAS relaxation and perineal descent. Prolapse is best evaluated with the examining finger withdrawn and the patient in a squatting position.

to assess contractions of the puborectalis muscle (see Figure 19-2B). Digital examination can distinguish very weak muscles from normal ones but is not as accurate as manometry, which is considered the gold standard for measuring anal sphincter function.[3,4,7] Acquiring the experience of doing an appropriate digital rectal exam is very helpful for the front-line assessment of patients with fecal incontinence

DIAGNOSTIC STUDIES FOR FECAL INCONTINENCE

A wide array of diagnostic tests have been used to assess anorectal structure and function in selected patients with fecal incontinence.[4,7] These tests are most useful when the etiology of incontinence is uncertain after the initial evaluation, when the response to conservative management is suboptimal, and when making therapeutic decisions for which information obtained from testing may affect outcome. An example of the latter would be the finding of neuropathy in a patient with a structural defect of the anal sphincter in whom surgical repair is being considered because such a finding would lessen the chances of a good surgical outcome. The evidence to support such a diagnostic approach is often contentious, and the choice of testing is often influenced by physician beliefs and the availability of diagnostic studies.[8] Nevertheless, diagnostic studies often illuminate underlying pathophysiology and provide a greater understanding of causation, which in turn should lead to more rational decision making when choosing among treatment options. Diagnostic studies are listed in Table 19-3.

Table 19-3

DIAGNOSTIC TESTS FOR FECAL INCONTINENCE

Of Clinical Value
- Endoscopy of colon and rectum
- Anorectal manometry
- Anal ultrasound
- EMG of EAS and PRM

Of Uncertain Value
- Pudendal nerve terminal motor latency (PNTML)
- Barium proctography

Under Investigation and of Potential Value
- Pelvic MRI

Endoscopy

This test assesses the mucosa of the rectum and colon and is particularly valuable in patients who have diarrhea or a recent change in bowel habit. In the former situation, biopsies should be obtained even if the mucosa appears normal in order to exclude microscopic colitis. In patients older than age 50 or in whom a diagnosis of colon cancer is being considered, full colonoscopy should be performed.

Anorectal Manometry

This is the most helpful study to assess anal sphincter pressures, rectal sensation, and rectal compliance, all important components of continence.[7] The manometer consists of a catheter assembly that includes a balloon positioned in the rectum and water perfused or solid-state pressure transducers located in the anal canal. Essential parameters that should be measured include 1) resting pressure to assess IAS tone, which accounts for about 70% of basal pressures; 2) brief and sustained squeeze pressures to assess EAS strength and duration; and 3) thresholds for first sensation, constant urge to defecate, and maximum tolerable volume to assess sensory afferents and rectal storage capacity. Generally, characteristic abnormalities suggest pathophysiology and may direct therapeutic interventions (Table 19-4).

Anal Ultrasonography

Anal ultrasonography (EUS) is best performed using a rotating 7- or 10-MHz transducer, which provides a 360-degree view of the anal canal as it is slowly withdrawn from the rectum to the anal verge (Figure 19-3A). The IAS is identified as a dark homogeneous ring whereas the EAS has mixed echogenicity (Figure 19-3C). EUS reliably identifies anatomic defects or thinning of the IAS when done by experienced operators, whereas assessment of the EAS is less reliable, confounded by normal anatomic variations of the EAS, and more operator dependent.[9] EUS has largely replaced

Table 19-4

MANOMETRIC PATTERNS OF IDIOPATHIC FECAL INCONTINENCE

	IAS Weakness	EAS Trauma	Neurogenic Peripheral	Central
Resting P	/	NI	NI	NI
Squeeze P	NI	/	/	/
PRM	NI	NI	/	/
Sensation	NI	NI	NI	/
Compliance	NI	NI	NI	NI

NI = Normal
/ = Decreased in most or all

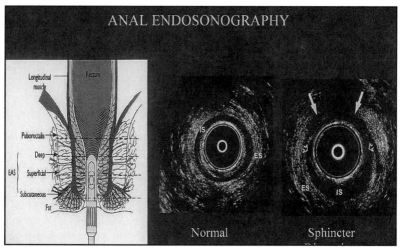

ANAL ENDOSONOGRAPHY

Longitudinal muscle · Rectum
Puborectalis
Deep
EAS — Superficial
Subcutaneous
Fat

IS · ES

Normal   Sphincter

Figure 19-3. Endoanal ultrasound images of the anal sphincters. (A) View of sonographic probe in the anal canal with important anatomic components of the IAS and EAS. (B) Sonographic images of the IAS (IS), which is hypoechoic, and EAS (ES), which is of mixed echogenicity (small arrow). (C) Anterior disruption of both the IAS and EAS (large arrows) in a patient with fecal incontinence following obstetric delivery.

needle EMG studies when mapping the integrity of the EAS and is most useful to exclude suspected structural causes of incontinence.

Electromyography

Needle EMG recordings of the EAS to identify structural defects have been replaced by EUS but remain useful to identify disturbances in innervation of the EAS and puborectalis muscle.[4] The source of such denervation injury can often be inferred by the pattern of muscle involvement but the importance of such a finding is that it substantially decreases the possibility that surgical correction of anal sphincter defects will be effective. EMG studies are highly operator dependent and require considerable experience in the interpretation of the study.

Pelvic Magnetic Resonance Imaging

This new and potentially important diagnostic test provides superior characterization of the EAS and puborectalis muscle compared to EUS.[9] It is the only imaging modality that can visualize both anal sphincter and pelvic floor anatomy as well as global pelvic floor motion in real-time without radiation exposure. The precise role of this new imaging study in clinical practice remains to be determined and is expensive.

Barium Proctography and PNTML

Although available in many centers, these tests are of uncertain utility and have serious shortcomings.[7] Barium proctography has been criticized because of poor inter-observer agreement on critical measurements, poor correlation of studies with symptoms and with other diagnostic studies, and a wide range of values in continent healthy control subjects. PNTML measurements lack sensitivity and specificity for the detection of EAS weakness caused by pudendal nerve damage. They often fail to predict outcome after surgical repairs of anal sphincter defects, and there is lack of reliable data concerning interoperator reproducibility. Finally, a normal PNTML does not exclude pudendal neuropathy because the presence of a few intact nerve fibers can produce a normal latency value. Neither of these tests can be recommended in the evaluation of fecal incontinence.[7]

Management of Fecal Incontinence

The treatment of patients with incontinence very much depends upon the clinical picture, focusing on correction of underlying disturbances of colorectal function that predispose the patient to incontinence. For the most part, patients with overflow incontinence or reduced storage capacity do not require more sophisticated testing, which is indicated for most incontinent patients with sensory and/or motor dysfunction (see Table 19-1). General interventions include skin and clothing protectors, measures that modulate bowel habits and delivery of stool to the rectum, modalities that are designed to correct sensory and/or motor abnormalities nonsurgically and surgically, and surgical and other invasive approaches.[3,4,10] Management can be tailored to patients who fall under subgroups of incontinence based on underlying pathophysiology.

OVERFLOW INCONTINENCE

A majority of patients in this category are children with encopresis and institutionalized elderly or psychotic patients. Such patients have fecal impaction, sometimes with megarectum or megacolon, and often have a history of constipation. The diagnosis should be suspected in the appropriate clinical setting and can be confirmed with a digital rectal examination. In some patients, impacted stool may be located beyond the reach of the examining finger; if stool retention is suspected, a plain abdominal x-ray will reveal excessive fecal loading.

In such patients, disimpaction followed by evacuation of the colon leads to rapid cessation of soiling. When impacted stool is hard, retention enemas containing warm water with mineral oil will help to soften the stool to allow easier passage. Once the obstructing bolus has been removed, osmotic laxatives such as PEG-electrolyte solution or magnesium salts should be given until the colon is emptied.[3,8] Most patients remain at increased risk for recurrent impactions and will require an ongoing bowel management program that involves regular attempts to defecate, sometimes with the assistance of laxatives. For children and ambulatory adults, daily ingestion of osmotic laxatives such as magnesium salts, polyethylene glycol-containing solutions, or nonabsorbable sugars such as sorbitol or lactulose can be titrated on a daily basis, with stimulant laxatives to be used if there is no defecation for 3 days. For bedridden patients, stimulant laxatives or enemas should be employed to periodically empty the colon. Dietary fiber restriction will help to minimize stool buildup in the colon. Short-term success rates of 60% to 80% have been reported in children, but high long-term recurrence rates require ongoing vigilance.

DECREASED COLONIC OR RECTAL STORAGE

In patients with incontinence associated with IBD, treatment is directed primarily toward healing the underlying inflammation to restore rectal and distal colonic storage capacity. If complete continence is not achieved or if there is an underlying condition that is not medically treatable (see Table 19-1), modifications of bowel habits by altering stool volume, consistency, and/or delivery are very effective approaches. Reduction of stool volume can be achieved by reducing dietary fiber combined with antidiarrheal agents; of the latter, loperamide is preferred because it has no CNS effects and may increase IAS tone to enhance continence.[11] Loperamide is best used pre-emptively (ie, before meals or when traveling outside the home where toilet facilities are not readily available). This provides confidence to the patient and often expands social and professional horizons. The pre-emptive use of loperamide is in contrast to the usual instructions to take antidiarrheal agents after each bowel movement, as with acute diarrheal illnesses. If the response to loperamide is sub-optimal, opioids that have CNS effects may be more effective. These agents include diphenoxylate, codeine, and deodorized tincture of opium, all of which should be monitored closely if used for long periods of time. In patients with diarrhea and IBS, medications with anticholinergic effects such as tricyclic agents[12] and smooth muscle relaxants may be highly effective, alone or with antidiarrheal agents. In women with IBS and diarrhea, the 5HT3 antagonist alosetron, currently available under a restricted program, may be useful.[3] For patients who develop occasional constipation with such a regimen, laxatives may be used periodically to prevent impaction and obstipation.

Minor Soiling (Isolated Internal Anal Sphincter Dysfunction)

This group of patients is easy to identify clinically on the basis of symptom patterns. Characteristically, they have minor spotting or soiling of liquid material in the presence of normal bowel habit. Examination may reveal diminished anal canal pressure with normal squeeze pressures reflecting IAS weakness in many but not all patients. Characteristically, they have no prolapse, protruding hemorrhoids, or other local causes of seepage.[8]

Treatment for minor soiling consists of a cotton plug to seal the anal orifice together with disposable underpads (panty liner) to prevent soiling of underwear.[13] The cotton plugs can be discarded when they become moist or before defecation after which they are replaced. This is an inexpensive approach that works well for many patients. Use of topical phenylephrine gel for isolated IAS dysfunction is attractive conceptually but has been a failure in clinical trials.[14]

Anal Sphincter and/or Sensory Impairment

Patients with major fecal incontinence generally exhibit one or a combination of rectal sensory and continence muscle abnormalities that are best documented by appropriate testing.[3] In addition to conservative treatment focused upon changes in stool consistency and delivery, a variety of treatments have been advocated and are available in centers specialized in colorectal disorders. In selected patients with verified structural defects of the EAS, surgical repairs have been recommended; for patients who are not candidates for surgery, there is pelvic floor training and biofeedback. Lastly, sacral nerve stimulation is a new and hopeful approach for patients who fail other forms of therapy and who have structurally intact anal sphincters.

Biofeedback

Both pelvic floor training and biofeedback, the latter based on the principles of operant conditioning first enunciated by Engel and colleagues,[15] have been reported to be effective in many patients with fecal incontinence associated with impaired functioning of the puborectalis muscle and the EAS. In contrast to pelvic floor retraining, which is directed exclusively at re-educating weakened or impaired muscles, biofeedback often includes techniques to alter rectal sensation and sphincter muscle responsiveness to intrarectal stimuli such as balloon distension. However, the biofeedback literature does not reflect a unified mechanistic approach.[16] Some investigators have emphasized enhancing the responsiveness of the EAS to rectal distensions, others have focused on increasing the force and duration of EAS contraction, and yet others have attempted to modify both. There appears to be a general consensus that improving thresholds of perceiving rectal sensation and synchronizing EAS contractions to rectal stimulation are important factors associated with improvement.[17] In contrast, increased striated muscle strength and endurance after biofeedback training have not been consistently shown.

There is widespread agreement that biofeedback is effective in approximately 75% of patients who fulfill entry criteria and has no adverse consequences.[17] Unfortunately, after almost 30 years following Engel's seminal report, the biofeedback literature has been plagued by methodological inadequacies, few long-term follow-up studies, and the absence of consistent and validated outcomes.[17] A recent Cochrane review concluded that there was insufficient evidence from trials of biofeedback and exercises for fecal incontinence to determine if such treatments are effective.[18] Moreover, there is no consensus as to which components of biofeedback are important, including the critical role of the patient-therapist relationship. To address these issues, a recent study examined critical components of the biofeedback process by randomizing 171 patients with fecal incontinence into four therapeutic groups.[19] In all groups, slightly more than 50% of patients reported clinical improvement on an intention-to-treat analysis. However, there were no differences among those patients who received only advice about strategies to reduce incontinence from nurse therapists, those who received both advice and verbal instructions about sphincter exercises, those who received advice together with a hospital-based biofeedback program, and those receiving both hospital and home EMG biofeedback. Moreover, improvement was maintained for at least 1 year, and anal sphincter pressure changes were similar in all groups. Determining those elements of biofeedback that are important to therapeutic efficacy is an area of needed study because biofeedback is both time consuming and provider intensive. At present, the evidence for using instrument-based training is insufficient but the value of dedicated and trained individuals to work with patients cannot be overstated.

Surgery

Surgical procedures for fecal incontinence may be classified as those that repair a damaged sphincter, those that create a neosphincter using nearby muscles or implantation of artificial material, and, as a last resort, diversion of the fecal stream.[20] A new technique based upon stimulation of the sacral nerves is under investigation.

Anal sphincteroplasty has been performed for many years and is based upon the straightforward premise of repairing an anatomically disrupted anal sphincter complex. The use of anal sonography to demonstrate disruptions of the anal sphincter has largely replaced the more invasive and painful EMG mapping of the external sphincter.[4,7,9] Although many studies have reported short-term improvement of fecal continence in up to 85% of patients, long-term follow-ups have been disappointing with failure rates of approximately 50% after 40 to 60 months.[20] In 3 recent representative series, full continence after sphincteroplasty was maintained in only 28% of patients after a mean follow-up of 40 months and in only 11% to 14% of patients followed for more than 69 months.[21-23] Suggested predictive factors for treatment failure include the presence of an IAS defect, prolongation of pudendal nerve terminal motor latencies, atrophy of the EAS as demonstrated by pelvic MRI, and the presence of IBS with diarrhea predominance.[8]

In the absence of demonstrable anal sphincter defects, the efficacy of surgical approaches designed to correct abnormalities of the pelvic floor such as anterior levatorplasty, postanal repair, and total pelvic floor repair is unproven. In one study, 8 of 12 patients after anterior levatorplasty and 7 of 12 after postanal repair failed to achieve continence compared to 4 of 12 after total pelvic floor repair.[8] Similarly, 6 of 11 patients after total pelvic floor repair and 6 of 9 after postanal repair showed no change of incontinence.[8] A Cochrane review concluded that there was insufficient evidence to determine if clinically important differences between various alternative procedures exist to guide clinical practice.[24] These procedures cannot be recommended for patients with neurogenic incontinence and in the absence of structural defects.

Other Surgical Approaches

Replacement of a damaged or nonfunctioning anal sphincter complex has been reported using nearby muscles (dynamic graciloplasty) or an artificial implanted sphincter.[20] Recent reviews of both procedures suggest that improved continence occurs in more than 50% of patients on intention-to-treat analyses but this is tempered by significant morbidity, including infections, device malfunction, and—in the case of the artificial sphincter—a high percentage of explantation of the device. Such procedures are best done for the therapeutically desperate by surgical teams with considerable experience.

For those with severe refractory incontinence, a diverting colostomy may provide dramatic improvement although no formal assessment of quality of life has been published.[10]

Sacral Nerve Stimulation

Sacral spinal nerve stimulation is a new therapeutic approach for patients with fecal incontinence that is associated with structurally intact anal sphincters. This technique arose as an extension of the successful use of this modality for urinary voiding and continence disorders together with the realization that stimulating electrodes implanted into pelvic floor muscles are prone to infection, migration, and fibrous tissue reactions.[25]

The procedure involves the following 3 phases:

1. Location of sacral spinal nerves by percutaneous probing with a needle electrode to identify the nerve root that maximally stimulates anal sphincter contraction.

2. Temporary placement of an electrode to chronically stimulate the nerve root identified as the most efficient during acute testing.

3. Permanent implantation of a neurostimulator for chronic therapeutic stimulation.

In patients who successfully complete the first 2 phases, clinical improvement of fecal incontinence has been confirmed in both short- and long-term studies,[26] especially in patients who have fecal incontinence at the first urge to defecate ("urge incontinence"). Clinical parameters include substantial decrease in episodes of liquid and solid stool incontinence and significant improvement of quality of life parameters as assessed by validated quality of life questionnaires for periods ranging from 6 months to more than 5 years. Objective physiologic changes have included increases in both resting and squeeze pressures, increased squeeze durations, decreased thresholds of rectal sensation, and increased time of retention of a saline load. It has been hypothesized that there may be possible transformation of type II fast twitch muscles to slow twitch type I fibers, which are more resistant to fatigue although there is little evidence to support this. A multicenter study in the United States is currently in progress.

Conclusions

Fecal incontinence is a socially devastating disorder with multiple and often complex etiologies. Appropriate management begins with a detailed history and physical examination that either reveal the probable cause or require additional diagnostic studies to elucidate pathophysiology. A large array of therapeutic options are available, many with little evidence to support efficacy, but together they allow most patients to be managed effectively. Figure 19-4 details a suggested algorithm for the evaluation and management of patients who present with fecal incontinence.

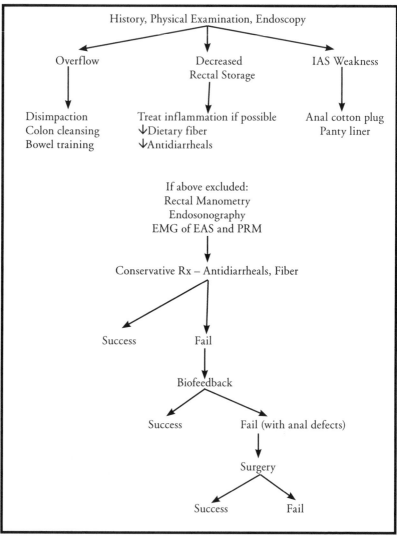

Figure 19-4. Suggested algorithm for the evaluation and management of the patient with fecal incontinence.

Acknowledgement: The author wishes to thank Helen Gibson for her expert assistance in preparing the manuscript.

References

1. Nelson RL. Epidemiology of fecal incontinence. *Gastroenterology.* 2004;126:S3-S7.
2. Miner PB Jr. Economic and personal impact of fecal and urinary incontinence. *Gastroenterology.* 2004;126:S8-S13.
3. Rao SSC. Diagnosis and management of fecal incontinence. *Am J Gastroenterol.* 2004;99:1585-1604.
4. Bharucha AE. Fecal incontinence. *Gastroenterology.* 2003;124:1672-1685.
5. Rockwood TH. Incontinence severity and QOL scales for fecal incontinence. *Gastroenterology.* 2004;126:S106-S113.
6. Vaizey CJ, Carapeti E, Cahill J, Kamm MA. Prospective comparative study of fecal incontinence grading systems. *Gut.* 1999;44:77-80.
7. Diamant NE, Kamm MA, Wald A, Whitehead WE. AGA technical review on anorectal testing techniques. *Gastroenterology.* 1999;116:732-760.
8. Cheung O, Wald A. Review article: management of pelvic floor disorders. *Aliment Pharmacol Ther.* 2004;19:481-495.
9. Bartram C. Radiologic evaluation of anorectal disorders. *Gastroenterol Clin N Am.* 2001;30:55-75.
10. Whitehead WE, Wald A, Norton NJ. Treatment options for fecal incontinence. *Dis Colon Rectum.* 2001;44:131-144.
11. Sun WM, Read NW, Verlinden M. Effects of loperamide oxide on gastrointestinal transit time and anorectal function in patients with chronic diarrhea and fecal incontinence. *Scand J Gastroenterol.* 1997;32:34-38.
12. Santoro GA, Ertan BZ, Pryde A, Bartolo DC. Open study of low-dose Amitriptyline in the treatment of patients with idiopathic fecal incontinence. *Dis Colon Rectum.* 2000;43:1676-1682.
13. Mortensen N, Humphreys MS. The anal continence plug: a disposable device for patients with anorectal incontinence. *Lancet.* 1991;338:295-297.
14. Carapeti EA, Kamm MA, Phillips RKS. Randomized controlled trial of topical phenylephrine in the treatment of fecal incontinence. *Br J Surg.* 2000;87(1):38-42.
15. Engel BT, Nikoomanesh P, Schuster MM. Operant conditioning of rectosphincteric responses in the treatment of fecal incontinence. *N Engl J Med.* 1974;290:646-649.
16. Wald A. Biofeedback for fecal incontinence. *Gastroenterology.* 2003;125:1533-1535.
17. Norton C, Kamm MA. Anal sphincter biofeedback and pelvic floor exercises for fecal incontinence in adults—a systematic review. *Aliment Pharmacol Ther.* 2001;15(8):1147-1154.
18. Norton C, Hosker G, Brazzelli M. Effectiveness of biofeedback and/or sphincter exercises for the treatment of fecal incontinence in adults. Cochrane Electronic Library. 2003;Volume 1.
19. Norton C, Chelvanayregam S, Wilson-Barnett J, Redfern S, Kamm MA. Randomized controlled trial of biofeedback for fecal incontinence. *Gastroenterology.* 2003;125:1320-1329.
20. Madoff RD. Surgical treatment options for fecal incontinence. *Gastroenterology.* 2004;126:S48-S54.
21. Karoui S, Leroi AM, Koning E, et al. Results of sphincteroplasty in 86 patients with anal incontinence. *Dis Colon Rectum.* 2000;43(6):813-820.

22. Malouf AJ, Chambers MG, Kamm MA. Clinical and economic evaluation of surgical treatments for fecal incontinence. *Br J Surg.* 2001;88(8):1029-1036.

23. Halverson AL, Hull TL, Long-term outcome of overlapping anal sphincter repair. *Dis Colon Rectum.* 2002;45(3):3451-3458.

24. Bachoo P, Brazzelli M, Grant A. Surgery for fecal incontinence in adults. Cochrane Electronic Library. 2000;(2):CD001757.

25. Pettit P, Thompson JR, Chen AH. Sacral neuromodulation: new applications in the treatment of female pelvic floor dysfunction. *Curr Opin Obstet Gynecol.* 2002;14(5):521-525.

26. Matzel KE, Stadelmaier U, Hohenfellner M, Hohenberger W. Chronic sacral spinal nerve stimulation for fecal incontinence: Long-term results with foramen and cuff electrodes. *Dis Colon Rectum.* 2001;44(1):59-66.

Intestinal Gas

Harvey Licht, MD

Many people have symptoms that they attribute to intestinal gas. These include complaints of bloating, distention, excessive belching, and the passage of flatus. A small proportion of this group will seek medical attention for these complaints, and these symptoms may also be prominent in people with IBS. Some people have significant distress from gaseousness, and it has an adverse impact on the patient's daily activities.

The Physiology of Intestinal Gas

An understanding of the normal physiology of intestinal gas will allow the physician to educate and to reassure the patient and to attempt to alleviate the symptoms. Studies suggest that the volume of gas in the GI tract is approximately 200 mL and is the same in people with or without symptoms of "excessive gas." Approximately 50 mL of gas is in the stomach with very little in the small intestine and the remainder in the colon. Symptoms attributed to excessive gas may be a function of abnormal perception of the gas rather than an absolute increase in volume. Although the amount of gas within the GI tract is relatively stable at approximately 200 mL, the volume expelled may vary greatly from approximately 200 mL to 1500 mL per day depending on the diet and the amount of nondigestible food products that reach the colon. Much of the gas that is expelled as flatus is produced by bacterial fermentation of these food products. The average number of passages of flatus appears to vary from 12 to 20 per day for normal subjects.

The sources of GI gas include swallowed air, gas formed in the intestine from the malabsorption of food products, and gas that diffuses into the gut from the blood. The major components of GI gas include oxygen and nitrogen from swallowed air and gases that are produced by intestinal bacteria, including carbon dioxide, hydrogen, and methane (Figure 20-1). These gases are all free of odor. The unpleasant odor of flatus is predominantly from small quantities of sulfur-containing gases, such as hydrogen sulfide, that are produced by colonic bacteria from food products contain-

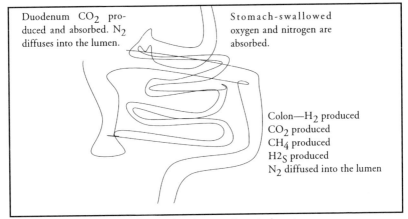

Figure 20-1. Distribution of gas within the gastrointestinal tract.

ing sulfur. Foods high in sulfur include egg yolks, onions, garlic, cabbage, broccoli, Brussels sprouts, and nuts. Short chain fatty acids from nondigestible carbohydrates such as bran and other trace compounds present in flatus such as skatoles and ammonia may also contribute to the odor. Skatoles are trace compounds found in beets, and ammonia is derived from protein breakdown. A diet high in nondigestible carbohydrates can help bacteria to incorporate ammonia as they grow and replicate and can reduce the amount of ammonia excreted in flatus. Gases produced by colonic bacteria are either excreted in flatus or may be absorbed into the blood and are then exhaled via the lungs. This may result in halitosis.

Although oxygen and nitrogen are swallowed, their concentrations vary through the GI tract depending on diffusion into or out of the lumen. This is determined by the differences in the partial pressures of the gases between the lumen and the blood. Concentrations of oxygen and nitrogen are high in the stomach from swallowed air. Therefore, oxygen diffuses out of the lumen of the stomach and upper intestine and undergoes net absorption into the blood and is found in low quantities entering into the colon. This is also true for nitrogen, which also diffuses out of the stomach into the blood. However, because the partial pressure of nitrogen is low in the colon, it diffuses from the blood into the colonic lumen and is the predominant gas expelled in flatus. Nitrogen may account for 50% to 80% of the gas in flatus.

The other gases found within the lumen of the GI tract are produced in it. Carbon dioxide is formed in the duodenum by the reaction of hydrochloric acid secreted by the stomach with bicarbonate secreted by the duodenal mucosa, pancreas, and hepatobiliary system. The resulting carbon dioxide undergoes diffusion from the duodenum into the circulation. Each milliequivalent of hydrochloric acid that is neutralized by bicarbonate creates 25 cc of carbon dioxide. Approximately 40 to 50 meq of gastric acid is secreted with each meal, and the acid that is not neutralized by food is available to react with duodenal bicarbonate and potentially may lead to the production of up to 1000 cc of carbon dioxide. Carbon dioxide is also produced in the proximal small intestine as a byproduct of the digestion of triglycerides to free fatty acids. These acids are also neutralized by bicarbonate, resulting in the production of carbon dioxide. Such large volumes of carbon dioxide raise the partial pressure within the lumen and lead to the diffusion of carbon dioxide into the blood stream. Very little of the carbon dioxide that is produced in the small intestine passes into the colon. The carbon dioxide that is passed in flatus is predominantly from the bacterial fermentation of undigested carbohydrates and is produced in the colon. With the presentation of increased amounts of carbohydrate to the colonic bacteria, more carbon dioxide will be formed. This occurs when foods containing nondigestible carbohydrates are eaten in large quantities. Examples include beans or foods in the cabbage family. The ingestion of lactose- or fructose-containing foods in patients who are deficient in the enzymes needed to digest these carbohydrates will also increase the load of carbohydrate delivered to the colon.

Hydrogen is also produced in the colon by bacterial fermentation of non-digested carbohydrates or proteins. The ingestion of beans exemplifies this. Beans contain the nondigestible oligosaccharides raffinos and stachyose. These are fermented by colonic bacteria and produce hydrogen. This can also occur in the small intestine in the presence of bacterial overgrowth syndromes. The hydrogen that is produced can be absorbed by diffusion into the blood and circulate to the lungs where it is expired. The exhaled gas may be collected and measured, and this is the basis of the hydrogen breath test that is used to assess bacterial overgrowth or carbohydrate malabsorption. Hydrogen that remains in the lumen of the colon can be expelled in flatus unchanged; however, it can also be utilized by bacteria to produce methane (CH_4) or hydrogen sulfide (H_2S). This results in a reduction of the total amount of expelled gas. The production of methane results from the reaction $4 H_2 + CO_2 \rightarrow CH_4 + 2 H_2O$. Thus, 5 molecules of gas are utilized to produce one molecule of methane. The production of methane is variable from person to person and is partially determined by the concentration of methane-producing bacteria within the colon as well as other environmental factors. Approximately one third of people produce significant amounts of methane. Much of the hydrogen and methane that is produced in the colon diffuses into the circulation because of the high intraluminal partial pressures compared to the blood. The amount of these gases expelled in flatus is a function of the quantity produced within the gut in balance with the amount that diffuses from the lumen into the blood.

Gas Disorders

ERUCTATION

Eructation or belching is generally a consequence of the normal swallowing mechanism. With each swallow of food or liquids, there is a small volume of air that is trapped and swallowed. The air accumulates in the stomach and then may pass back into the esophagus when there is relaxation of the LES. This may represent the teleological explanation for the transient relaxation of the LES. The esophagus enters the stomach in the right upper aspect of the stomach. Gastric air is expelled into the esophagus more readily in the upright position because the gas bubble interfaces with the anatomic position of the LES in this position. In contrast, when the patient is recumbent, gastric contents and fluid collect over the area of the LES. This position predisposes to acid reflux into the esophagus and allows air to pass to the antrum and into the small intestine. Lying on the left side also allows air to rise to the area of the

LES and reduces nocturnal acid reflux; although perhaps predisposing to the likelihood of belching if one eats soon before lying down. Air passing from the stomach into the esophagus causes distention of the esophagus that can result in secondary peristalsis that propels the air back into the stomach. However, esophageal distention can also result in relaxation of the UES, and air then erupts (more correctly, eructs) as a belch. Thus, eructation is an involuntary and normal physiologic mechanism to release swallowed air from the stomach.

Belching commonly occurs from swallowing excessive amounts of air during meals. The patient is usually unaware of this. Anxiety, eating quickly, and gulping food or liquids can contribute to increased amounts of swallowed air. Because air is swallowed with saliva, actions that increase salivation may also result in increased swallowed air. Such activities include gum chewing, smoking, and sucking on hard candies. Excessive air is often swallowed with hot liquids in an attempt to cool it. Drinking hot liquids or carbonated liquids also increases the amount of gas in the stomach. The amount of swallowed air may also be increased in patients with sinus congestion or difficulty breathing who are forced to mouth breathe. In addition to swallowing more air, frequent belching can also be the result of relaxation of the LES, which then allows more air to pass back into the esophagus. This occurs after eating certain foods such as fats, chocolate, and mints (carminatives) and may be associated with GER. Perhaps insight into belching can be garnered from ancient Roman eating habits; the word eructate derives from the Latin word *eructare*, which is similar to the Latin word *rugire*, meaning to roar.

Thus, involuntary belching, which is the most common type, typically occurs following a meal. However, some patients have chronic, repetitive belching that can occur throughout the day. This is a result of air that is voluntarily swallowed but does not enter the stomach. The air remains in the esophagus, which becomes distended. This results in relaxation of the UES, which releases the swallowed air and produces the belch. This pattern may become a habit, although the patient is often not aware of the association of swallowing air and belching. This may be seen with anxiety or may accompany UGI diseases such as reflux if the patient achieves relief of symptoms with belching.

Belching rarely requires evaluation unless there are accompanying warning symptoms suggesting the presence of GI diseases such as abdominal pain, heartburn, vomiting, or weight loss. Treatment is directed toward counseling the patient regarding eating habits and making the patient aware of aerophagia (Table 20-1). There is no evidence that treatment with simethicone is efficacious, although this is frequently tried. The patient should be questioned regarding the use of baking soda (ie, sodium bicarbonate), which could lead to the production of large volumes of carbon dioxide in the stomach because it neutralizes hydrochloric acid.

FLATULENCE

The volume of flatus passed per rectum varies between individuals ranging from several hundred mL to 1500 mL per day. The number of passages also varies with an average of 10 to 20 times per day. Patients may complain of the passage of increased amounts of gas or of an increased frequency of passing flatus. However, some studies suggest that most patients with such complaints pass volumes of flatus that fall within the accepted range of normal values. The other major complaint of patients regard-

Table 20-1

TREATMENT OF COMPLAINTS OF BELCHING

- Avoid drinking hot liquids.
- Avoid drinking carbonated liquids (eg, soda, seltzer).
- Do not chew gum or smoke.
- Do not suck on hard candy.
- Eat slowly.
- Avoid chocolate, mints, and fatty foods (if associated with reflux).
- Counsel and reassure patient regarding aerophagia.

Table 20-2

TREATMENT OF COMPLAINTS OF MALODOROUS FLATUS

- Trial restricting sulfur-containing foods (eg, egg yolk, onions, garlic, nuts, cabbage, Brussels sprouts).
- Trial restricting skatoles (eg, beets).
- Suggest high carbohydrate diet in proportion to meat to reduce ammonia.

ing flatus is that of malodor. As previously noted, flatus is composed of nitrogen and lesser amounts of oxygen that pass into the colon from diffusion from blood. The other components of flatus include hydrogen, carbon dioxide, and methane, which are produced by bacterial fermentation of non-digested carbohydrates in the colon. These gases all have no odor. As mentioned previously, the gases responsible for the odor of flatus are predominantly derived from the bacterial action on sulfate, which is present in foods such as garlic, onions, cabbage, broccoli, and nuts. Sulfate is also used as an additive to bread and beer. The gases formed, hydrogen sulfide and methanethiol as well as others, are found in trace quantities but are the major contributing agents causing flatus to be malodorous. A study has demonstrated that zinc acetate reacts with these compounds and reduces odor, although activated charcoal may be more effective (Table 20-2).[1]

Excessive volumes of flatus most commonly occur due to bacterial fermentation of an increased substrate of non-digested carbohydrates entering the colon. Examples of oligosaccharides that are not well digested include raffinose and stachyose, which are found in beans, broccoli, cabbage, Brussels sprouts, and asparagus. High-fiber diets with large amounts of bran and other whole grains also contain poorly digestible carbohydrates that are presented to the colon and are fermented by colonic bacteria. This results in increased production of hydrogen, carbon dioxide, and (in some people) methane.

Table 20-3

TREATMENT OF COMPLAINTS OF FLATUS

- Avoid poorly digestible carbohydrates (eg, beans, broccoli, cabbage, Brussels sprouts, bran).
- Trial of lactose-free diet.
- Trial restricting fructose-containing foods (eg, fruits [dates, oranges, cherries, apples, pears, honey] and fructose additives in processed food).

In addition to eating a diet high in nondigestible carbohydrates, another mechanism that results in an increased carbohydrate load to the colon is malabsorption of carbohydrate. This may occur in various diseases of the small intestine such as celiac sprue but may also be seen with deficiency of brush border enzymes of the small intestine. Examples of the latter include the maldigestion of fructose and lactose. Fructose is used as a sweetener in soda, fruit juices, and candy and also is naturally present in fruits such as apples, peaches, pears, and oranges. Its absorption in the small intestine is via carriers using facilitative diffusion and is limited. Therefore, when ingested in amounts greater than can be absorbed by this system, the unabsorbed fructose enters the colon and undergoes bacterial fermentation to gases and short chain fatty acids. This may be associated with cramps, gaseousness, or diarrhea, and the development of these symptoms correlates with the quantity of fructose ingested.[2] A diagnostic and therapeutic option would be a trial of a fructose-restricted diet. This diet should stress avoidance of fruits and fructose as an additive in processed foods. High-fructose corn syrup is commonly used as a sweetener in processed foods and usually does not need to be restricted. It is a mixture of glucose and fructose. The ingestion of glucose increases the absorption of fructose and thereby reduces the amount delivered to the colon. This reduces the substrate available for bacterial fermentation to gas and explains the ability of most patients who are fructose intolerant to use this sweetener. However, sorbitol, which is used as a sweetener in some diet foods, reduces the absorption of fructose, and foods containing this combination should be avoided by the fructose intolerant patient (Table 20-3).

Malabsorption of lactose may also result in increased gas production in the colon and be associated with cramps, gaseousness, and diarrhea. Lactose is the major carbohydrate of milk and dairy products and is digested by the brush border enzyme lactase. Lactase deficiency is a common finding in people around the world. After young children are weaned, there typically is a reduction in intestinal lactase levels. A minority of people have an autosomal dominant gene that maintains elevated enzyme levels into adulthood. The persistence of elevated levels of lactase is most commonly seen in people of northern European descent. Most other people develop the enzyme deficiency as they age. Seventy-five percent of the world population is lactase deficient, and depending on the amount of enzyme that persists, symptoms may develop when dairy products are eaten. Affected people will complain of symptoms of gaseousness, cramps, and diarrhea when large amounts of lactose-containing foods are consumed.

Table 20-4

LACTOSE CONTENT OF DAIRY PRODUCTS

	Units	Lactose (g)
Milk	1 cup	10 to 12
Buttermilk	1 cup	10
Cottage cheese	1 cup	6 to 8
Hard cheese	1 oz	0.5
Yogurt	1 cup	11 to 15
Ice cream	1 cup	10
Butter	2 pats	0.1

Lactose content varies with different dairy products (Table 20-4). The ingestion of 1 quart of milk, which contains 50 g of lactose, will cause symptoms in most lactase-deficient individuals. Milk and ice cream have the greatest amount of lactose. Although yogurt is fermented and should be expected to have minimal lactose, commercial yogurt has milk or cream added during processing after fermentation and therefore contains significant amounts of lactose. Some people with lactase deficiency will be able to tolerate hard cheeses because of the lower amounts of lactose found in hard cheeses. Lactose is concentrated in whey, which is separated from hard cheeses during processing. Soft cheeses have milk or cream added and will therefore have higher amounts of lactose (see Table 20-4).

Some people wrongly attribute symptoms to lactose intolerance. A study of people who thought themselves to be severely lactose intolerant were tested with hydrogen breath tests, and only two thirds were documented to have lactose intolerance. Thus, one third had symptoms that were clearly from another cause. The total group was studied and given one glass of milk with or without lactase pretreatment daily for 1 week and then crossed over to the other arm of the trial. None of the people developed significant symptoms during either test period. By history, each person in the study had attributed GI symptoms to the ingestion of smaller amounts of milk than was taken during the study. This suggests that history alone may not be an adequate way to establish that symptoms are secondary to lactose intolerance. This study demonstrated that some people with presumed lactose intolerance can tolerate small quantities of dairy products, and the symptoms that they attributed to lactose containing foods may be secondary to another cause.[3]

The colon is the organ in which most gas is produced by bacterial fermentation; however, bacterial fermentation can also occur within the small intestine in patients with bacterial overgrowth. In health, the bacterial counts in the small intestine are low and orders of magnitude less than those in the colon. This is the result of 2 factors. First, acid in the stomach retards growth and replication of bacteria that are swallowed and thus reduces the bacterial counts entering the duodenum. Secondly, motility of the small intestine, which is regulated by the migrating motor complex, leads to peristalsis that sweeps the contents out of the small intestine during fasting and night time and in this way reduces the time for bacterial growth and colonization that otherwise would occur. Diseases that result in stasis of small intestinal contents may result in proliferation of bacteria in the small intestine. This can occur with anatomic abnormalities of the small intestine such as strictures or diverticula. Stasis can also be the result of diminished peristaltic activity, which can be associated with scleroderma or diabetes. Ingested carbohydrates and proteins within the small intestine that have not yet been absorbed are then exposed to high bacterial counts, and fermentation to gases occurs and may result in distention of the intestine accompanied by symptoms of bloating or cramps. These gases may then diffuse into the circulation or be passed into the colon. Bacterial overgrowth should be suspected in patients with these symptoms who also have the associated symptoms or findings of malabsorption or vitamin B_{12} deficiency. Diagnosis can be established by hydrogen breath test, by a 3-part Schilling test, or by quantitative cultures of small intestine bacterial flora. Treatment is with antibiotics.

BLOATING AND DISTENTION

Bloating and distention are frequent complaints for which people seek medical attention and also are common complaints of patients with IBS. These may be very difficult symptoms to treat. Although often considered to be caused by excessive gas, this has not been supported by clinical studies. A study using CT scan of the abdomen to evaluate for objective evidence of distention has documented an increase in the abdominal profile of patients complaining of distention, although there was no increase in the amount of intraluminal gas and no change in the lumbar lordosis or position of the diaphragm to explain the perception of distention.[4] Another study found no correlation of the amount of gas seen on abdominal x-ray with symptoms of distention in patients with IBS.[5] This suggests that the perception of distention is not related to the amount of gas within the intestine.

To elucidate the cause of these symptoms, one study[6] compared patients with IBS with healthy controls and infused a gas mixture into the jejunum and calculated the retention of gas in the intestine in these 2 groups. Patients with IBS retained more gas. There was no difference if a rectal tube was placed, thus indicating that gas retention was not attributable to tightening of the anal sphincter. Gas infusion in the group with IBS reproduced the symptoms of distention and bloating, although the measured girth was only minimally increased. Another study[7] infused gas into the small intestine or into the rectum and found that, with jejunal gas infusion, most of the gas was present in the small intestine and cecum, whereas, with rectal gas infusion, most of the gas was in the left colon. Lipid was then infused into the jejunum in an attempt to reproduce the postprandial state and this decreased tone in the rectum but increased tone within the duodenum, thus changing the compliance characteristics of the intestinal muscle. With the infusion of gas after lipid infusion, it was noted that more gas was accommodated more comfortably in the left colon with fewer symptoms than when the gas was infused into the jejunum.

This suggests that with similar amounts of gas retention, gas pooling in the small intestine was associated with more symptoms of bloating, cramps, and distention and appeared to be related to the increased muscle tone of the intestine. These 2 studies offer insight into the cause of the symptoms of distention and bloating in IBS patients.

It has been postulated that because of increased tone of the small intestinal muscula-ture and because of delayed transit, there may be segments within the intestine where gas pools and is associated with a hypersensitive perception by the patient. Symptoms do not appear to be related to increased amounts of gas within the bowel.

Other studies agree with this postulate. In one study,[8] healthy people were given lactulose, psyllium, or methylcellulose. There was a sensation of increased bloating with each diet; however, there was no increase in the amount of gas formed with the addition of either psyllium or methylcellulose. Gas production and the passage of flatus was only increased after lactulose. Another study[9] evaluated the correla-tion between gas production and bloating in 3 groups of patients. A group with IBS was compared with a group with lactose intolerance and a control healthy group. Hydrogen breath tests and symptoms of cramps and bloating were assessed after a diet. Symptoms were greater in the patients with IBS, although hydrogen breath tests were similar in all groups. Thus, these studies indicate that symptoms of bloating and distention are not dependent on and do not correlate with gas production. A study[10] was also done to alter the colonic flora in an attempt to affect gas production. A group of patients with IBS and symptoms of gaseousness, bloating, and cramps were given either *Lactobacillus plantarum* for 4 weeks or placebo and kept a diary of symptoms. The treated group had a decrease in flatulence but there was no effect on symptoms of cramping or bloating.

It is common for patients with IBS to have complaints of bloating and distention. Symptoms tend to increase as the day progresses with worsening of symptoms follow-ing meals. Although patients and physicians attribute these symptoms to excessive gas formation after eating, these studies suggest that the symptoms of bloating and disten-tion are not associated with excessive gas within the lumen of the GI tract. Instead, recent studies suggest that these symptoms are caused by a defect in propulsion of intestinal contents and an increased tone within the intestine that is accompanied by hypersensitivity and abnormal perception within the gut wall.[5,6] This requires further study but suggests that treatment directed at reducing gas formation with restrictive diets may not have a significant effect on symptoms of bloating and distention.

When beginning treatment, a dietary diary should be kept to determine if particu-lar foods correlate with the development of symptoms. With these data, it is possible to more appropriately suggest a restrictive diet. A patient's memory without a diary correlating symptoms with diet is often misleading and inaccurate (Table 20-5). Low-dose antidepressants have also been tried to reduce symptoms of bloating and cramps in patients with IBS. Drugs that affect GI muscle tone and motility and hyper-sensitivity may prove more beneficial. Drugs that modulate serotonin receptors and opioid receptors can affect these parameters, and more study is needed to determine if pharmaceutical agents in these classes will have an important role in the treatment of such complaints.

References

1. Suarez FL, Springfield J, Levitt MD. Identification of gases responsible for the odor of human flatus and evaluation of a device purported to reduce this odor. *Gut.* 1998;43:100-104.
2. Choi YK, Johlin FC Jr, Summers RW, Jackson M, Rao SSC. Fructose intolerance: an under-recognized problem. *Am J Gastroenterol.* 2003;98:1348-1353.

Table 20-5

TREATMENT OF COMPLAINTS OF BLOATING

- Create dietary diary to correlate with symptoms.
- Trial of restrictive diet based on diary results.
- Trial of low-dose antidepressant.

3. Suarez FL, Savaiano DA, Levitt MD. A comparison of symptoms after the consumption of milk or lactose-hydrolyzed milk by people with self-reported severe lactose intolerance. *N Engl J Med.* 1995;333:1-4.
4. Maxton DG, Martin DF, Whorwell PJ, Godfrey M. Abdominal distension in female patients with IBS: exploration of possible mechanisms. *Gut.* 1991;32:662-664.
5. Koide A, Yamaguchi T, Odaka T, et al. Quantitative analysis of bowel gas using plain abdominal radiograph in patients with IBS. *Am J Gastroenterol.* 2000;95:1735-1741.
6. Serra J, Azpiroz F, Malagelada J-R. Impaired transit and tolerance of intestinal gas in the IBS. *Gut.* 2001;48:14-19.
7. Harder H, Serra J, Azpiroz F, Passos MC, Aguade S, Malagelada JR. Intestinal gas distribution determines abdominal symptoms. *Gut.* 2003;52:1708-1713.
8. Levitt MD, Furne J, Olsson S. The relation of passage of gas and abdominal bloating to colonic gas production. *Ann Intern Med.* 1996;124:422-424.
9. Haderstorfer B, Psycholgin D, Whitehead WE, Schuster MM. Intestinal gas production from bacterial fermentation of undigested carbohydrate in IBS. *Am J Gastroenterol.* 1989;84:375-378.
10. Nobaek S, Johansson ML, Molin G, Ahrne S, Jeppsson B. Alteration of intestinal microflora is associated with reduction in abdominal bloating and pain in patients with IBS. *Am J Gastroenterol.* 2000;95:1231-1238.

Index

WAIT
...*There's More!*

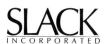

DATE DUE

GAYLORD   #3523PI   Printed in USA